Lectures on Perception

Lectures on Perception: An Ecological Perspective addresses the generic principles by which each and every kind of life form—from single celled organisms (e.g., difflugia) to multi-celled organisms (e.g., primates)—perceives the circumstances of their living so that they can behave adaptively. It focuses on the fundamental ability that relates each and every organism to its surroundings—namely, the ability to perceive things in the sense of how to get about among them and what to do, or not to do, with them.

The book's core thesis breaks from the conventional interpretation of perception as a form of abduction based on innate hypotheses and acquired knowledge, and from the historical scientific focus on the perceptual abilities of animals, most especially those abilities ascribed to humankind. Specifically, it advances the thesis of perception as a matter of laws and principles at nature's ecological scale, and gives equal theoretical consideration to the perceptual achievements of all of the classically defined "kingdoms" of organisms—Archaea, Bacteria, Protoctista, Fungi, Plantae, and Animalia.

Michael T. Turvey is Board of Trustees' Distinguished Professor of Experimental Psychology at the University of Connecticut and a Senior Scientist at Haskins Laboratories in Connecticut. He is the recipient of Guggenheim and Catell Fellowships, the American Psychological Association Early Career Award, Fellow of Society of Experimental Psychologists (SEP), Bernstein 2009 Prize in Motor Control, SEP Lifetime Achievement Award, Association for Psychological Science Lifetime Mentor Award, and two honorary doctorates.

Lectures on Perception

An Ecological Perspective

Michael T. Turvey

Routledge
Taylor & Francis Group
NEW YORK AND LONDON

First published 2019
by Routledge
605 Third Avenue, New York, NY 10017
4 Park Square, Milton Park, Abingdon, Oxon OX14 4RN

Routledge is an imprint of the Taylor & Francis Group, an informa business

Library of Congress Cataloging-in-Publication Data
A catalog record for this title has been requested

ISBN: 978-1-138-33525-7 (hbk)
ISBN: 978-1-138-33526-4 (pbk)
ISBN: 978-0-429-44387-9 (ebk)

Typeset in Goudy
by Florence Production Ltd, Stoodleigh, Devon, UK

To the graduate students who suffered through the course that is the foundation of this book. And to the cats—including Ralph, Daisy-Danny, FloJo, Coco, and the many nameless visitors who made their way to my office window—whose countless feats of perception–action provide daily confirmation of an ecological perspective.

Contents

Preface

A primary inspiration for the intellectual themes expressed in this book is owing to James J. Gibson, themes he established in *The Senses Considered as Perceptual Systems* (1966) and *The Ecological Approach to Visual Perception* (1979). The lure is the wide variety of scientific and philosophical challenges faced in detailing an account of perception that is, at its core, not peculiar to humans but generalizable to all organisms. The behavioral challenges posed by cluttered surroundings provide an exemplary case. Any organism from any one of the Six Kingdoms—Animalia to be sure but also Plantae, Fungi, Protoctista, Archaea, and Bacteria, too—confronts impediments to its motion or growth that require adaptive behavior. The behavior will be uniquely characteristic of the organism and its scale: Behavior by a member of the Kingdom Fungi, for example, would be measured in tens of meters; behavior by a member of the Kingdom Archaea would be measured in tiny fractions of a millimeter.

The investigation of perception has a long but, in some sense, narrow history: a focus predominantly on perception by one species—namely, *Homo sapiens*; predominantly perception by one modality—namely, vision; and predominantly perception as an intellectual, logical process—namely, inference. The last of these, in particular, motivates the interpretation of *perception as indirect*. The ecological perspective taken by this book, in contrast, gives consideration to all Six Kingdoms. And the primary proposal is that perceiving of self and surroundings by all organisms in all Kingdoms is unmediated. Said differently, *perception is direct*. Direct perception is a matter of the laws that configure nature at the ecological scale. If such were not the case—that is, if perception were inferential, then organism as perceiver would necessarily have to embody certain antecedents. In particular, if epistemic mediators—whatever their proposed incarnation—are to be taken seriously, then the organism must embody a theory of its niche and habitat as well as a theory of how its niche and habitat structure energy distributions. Nothing less will suffice as a basis for discerning the meaning of patterned energy distributions registered by the multiplicity of kinds of perception–action systems across the Six Kingdoms. For any epistemic mediator advanced as an answer to the *mechanism question* of "How does it work?" one must advance an accompanying answer to the *origin question* of "How did it arise?" But eschewing epistemic mediation, as in the case presented in the current volume, means that answers to "How does it work?" must be in terms of law and answers to "How did it arise?" must be in terms of the physics of self-organization.

A few words on logistics: This book is largely based on a graduate course on perception given by the author at the University of Connecticut (hence the use of "Lecture" to label the chapters), a course that evolved in content over 40 years. This origin also underlies the extensive use of illustrations. In addition to aiding general understanding, their purpose is twofold. They are designed to assist those who choose to build their own presentations from the book. Additionally, many are intended to encourage students to craft, where possible, cartoon-like visual depictions of concepts as regular accompaniments to their note taking (not everything has to be anatomically correct). The sequence of concepts here has been chosen to facilitate pedagogy. Coming to terms with perception as direct (unmediated, lawful) as opposed to perception as indirect (mediated, inferential) requires a deep appreciation for the issues and conceptions that constitute the ground for theorizing about perception, both in its historical and contemporary forms. The roles of Part 1 (Lectures 1–15: *Foundational Concepts*) and Part 2 (Lectures 16–19: *Computational–Representational Perspective*) are to provide the aforementioned appreciation of perception's indirect form. The role of Part 3 (Lectures 20–26: *Ecological Perspective*) is to reveal why perception must be direct and in what manner it can be so.

I should also point out that many concepts addressed here make generic points and have implications for a variety of domains in science and philosophy. During the last 10 years or so, passages of particular timeliness have been incorporated in various chapters and articles that I've directed at specific issues. The interested reader can see extensions of coordination dynamics, impredicativity, the perception–action divide, awareness by single-celled organisms, and quantum issues in those chapters and articles (Turvey, 2004a, b, 2013, 2015; Chemero & Turvey, 2007). These elaborations serve to demonstrate once again that perception weaves through not only the history of science and philosophy but their future as well.

References

Chemero, A., & Turvey, M. T. (2007). Complexity, hypersets, and the ecological approach to perception-action. *Biological Theory*, *2*, 23–36.

Gibson, J. J. (1966). *The senses considered as perceptual systems*. Boston, MA: Houghton Mifflin.

Gibson, J. J. (1986). *The ecological approach to visual perception*. Mawah, NJ: Erlbaum (original work published 1979).

Turvey, M. T. (2004a). Impredicativity, dynamics and the perception-action divide. In V. K. Jirsa & J. A. S. Kelso (Eds.), *Coordination dynamics: Issues and trends* (pp. 1–20). Berlin: Springer Verlag.

Turvey, M. T. (2004b). Space (and its perception): The first and final frontier. *Ecological Psychology*, *16*, 25–29.

Turvey, M. T. (2013). Ecological perspective on perception-action: What kind of science does it entail? In W. Prinz, M. Beisert, & A. Herwig (Eds.), *Action science: Foundations of an emerging discipline* (pp. 139–170). Cambridge, MA: MIT Press.

Turvey, M. T. (2015). Quantum-like issues at nature's ecological scale (the scale of organisms and their environments). *Mind & Matter*, *13*, 7–44.

Acknowledgments

The Center for the Ecological Study of Perception and Action (CESPA) has provided a unique social–intellectual environment in which ideas and people can thrive. I am grateful to the University of Connecticut for establishing the Center in 1987. I am indebted to several colleagues and dear friends: Claire Michaels, one of my earliest Ph.D.s (my first woman, as she is fond of saying), whose humor and general acumen keep me on my toes (even if I don't always get the joke); Robert Shaw, who helped to build and sustain the Center and whose intellectual engagement is an inspiration; Claudia Carello, whose 27-year tenure as Center Director established what has been referred to as the "CESPA Way"; J. Dixon, the current Director, who is overseeing a period of exciting intellectual growth; and to the countless visitors who have enhanced the richness of CESPA through their insights, challenges, and new perspectives (not to mention their kimchi, Pão de Queijo, and Douwe Egbert).

The National Science Foundation provided funding for *Haptic Perceptual Instruments* for 25 years (particularly evident in Lectures 8, 9, and 25). The thermodynamic perspective that is apparent throughout the book (explicitly in Lecture 20) led to eventual support from DARPA (*Physical Intelligence* subcontract HRL 000708-DS) and the National Science Foundation (under INSPIRE Track 1 grant BCS-1344725, *Development of Perception–Action in Non-Living, Dissipative Systems* awarded to J. Dixon).

I am especially indebted to my wonderful wife, Claudia, who did an embarrassing amount of work to bring this book across the finish line. As my dear old Mum used to say, "There's nothing she can't do!" No one has benefited from her astonishing range of capabilities more than I.

Part 1

Foundational Concepts

Lecture 1
What Kinds of Systems Do We Study?

In abstract terms, a beginning student of perception (and by implication, action) has embarked on the study of *epistemic, intentional systems*. The focus is in respect to the function of perception more than its content. Perception's universal function is to coordinate the individual organism (specifically, its activity) with its surroundings. The content of perception, the specific varieties of an organism's awareness of body and environment (see Gibson, 1979/1986), will vary with the organism-niche specifics. In this initial lecture, we begin with the concept of system, proceed to the qualifier intentional, and end with the qualifier epistemic.

1.1 System

The word *system*, like many of the important words in the study of perception and action, is vague. It refers to a loose concept, one that is readily intuited but not easily codified. This is not a damaging criticism. Science is infested with loose concepts that play constructive and creative roles (Elkana, 1970; Löwy, 1992). Denying them, or awaiting their strict codification before use, would hamper progress. That said, the needed deployment of loose concepts must be coordinate with the nurturing of respect for precise well-formulated concepts.

Given the potential for vagueness in defining *system* (e.g., Berlinski, 1976; Marchal, 1975), it might be more fruitful to begin with the opposite notion. What can be meant by *non-system?* A set of isolated pieces that don't interact, or interact so weakly that their influences upon each other are negligible, seems to fit the bill. Even better, perhaps, is the notion of a collection of related pieces where the relations have no implications for the properties or behaviors of the pieces. Certainly lacking in the image of a non-system is the sense of shared influences or mutual dependencies; intuitively, a non-system exhibits no coherence or functional unity. Also lacking is the sense of a boundary, a separation of the pieces into "ground" (pieces that surround) and "figure" (pieces that are surrounded).

Heaps and aggregates are sometimes promoted as intuitive examples of non-systems (Bunge, 1977; Grobstein, 1973). In a heap or aggregate, the properties of any one component when it is excluded from the aggregate is the same as when it is included in the aggregate. A rock in a rock pile is related to the other rocks in terms of distance, weight, and shape, but these relations make no difference to the individual rock. Remove it from the pile and it possesses the same properties that it had in the pile. Minimally, one would think, a system is distinguished from a non-system by the fact that, in a system, the relation "makes some difference to its relata (Bunge, 1979, p. 6)." It helps to distinguish between what might be called *bonding* and *non-bonding* relations (Mahner & Bunge, 1997). A relation between two things x and y is bonding if and only if the states of y alter when the relation to x holds. The examples above of relations of distance, size and weight are non-bonding. A non-bonding relation such as the distance between x and y does not itself bring about a change in the state of y but it may allow that x can act upon y.

A problem with the use of heaps and aggregates as non-systems is that straightforward heaps (in the form of sand piles and rice piles, for example) and common biological aggregates (a collection of amoeba, for example) can, under certain conditions, exhibit self-organized coherent behavior (Bak, 1996; Garfinkel, 1987). Apparently, *non-system* is not a permanent designation. In recognition of this fact, the terms *facultative* and *obligate* have been suggested to distinguish, respectively, between (a) systems that assemble from and disassemble to non-systems and (b) systems that persist as systems once assembled (Grobstein, 1973; Juarrero, 1999).

Although our willingness to ponder the curious notion of non-system has proven fruitful, the enterprise fails to convey fully what *system* must mean because, for non-system, boundary is vacuous. A system, unlike a non-system, has a distinguishable "inside" and "outside." A wall (or boundary, or interface, or dynamical process) separates and shields the inner from the outer components (Krieger, 1992). Of particular significance is how to interpret the outside. Is a system individuated by its inner components alone or by the inner and outer components together? The latter of the two alternatives is the answer given by Figure 1.1.[1]

In Figure 1.1, we arrive at a definition or model of a system s by considering (i) the inner degrees of freedom (DF) that compose it, $C(s)$ (ii) the outer DF with which it interacts, $E(s)$ and (iii) the relations, both bonding and non-bonding, among inner DF and between inner and outer DF constituting its structure, $S(s)$. This model comprising *composition*, *environment* and *structure*, a CES model, is a *minimal* starting point for understanding any system of interest at any level of interest (Mahner & Bunge, 1997). The environment $E(s)$ within the CES model is always relative to a given system s. As such, an environment is not defined without a system (there are no empty environments), there are as many environments as there are systems (excluding the universe as a whole), and an environment of a system is not an entity, not itself a system.[2] Because environment is not an entity, it cannot be that $E(s)$ as a whole acts upon or interacts with s; rather, members of $E(s)$ act upon or interact with members of $C(s)$.

Figure 1.1 permits an overview of scientific predilections. Inquiry restricted to $C(s)$ defines reductionism. Inquiry restricted to $E(s)$ defines environmentalism. Inquiry restricted to $S(s)$ defines structuralism. Inquiry that gives due consideration to all members of the triple $\langle C(s), E(s), S(s)\rangle$ defines systemism (Bunge, 1979). Less dryly, we can contrast the latter with holism, the view that every thing is connected to every other thing, and atomism, the view that every thing operates in isolation from every other thing. For systemism, every thing is connected with *some* other thing or things (Mahner & Bunge, 1997).

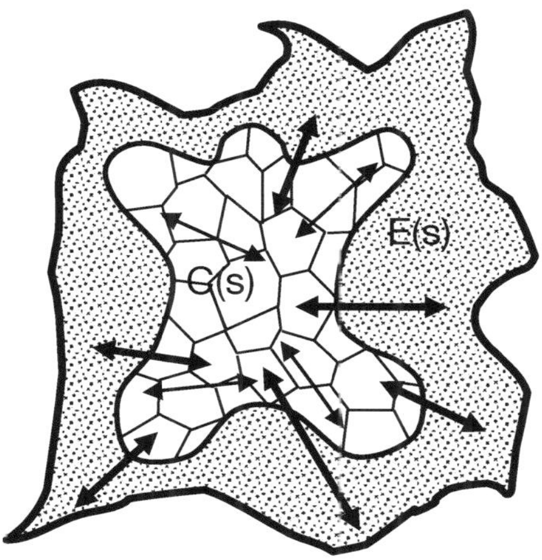

Figure 1.1 The minimal model of any arbitrary material system is: $m(s) = \langle C(s), E(s), S(s)\rangle$. $C(s)$ is the collection of all the parts of s, its composition. $E(s)$ is the collection of all those things other than s that can influence s or be influenced by s, the composition of s's environment. The thin arrows are the relations among the parts of s, its internal structure $S_{int}(s)$. The thick arrows are the relations among s's components and environmental things, its external structure $S_{ext}(s)$. The union of the internal and external structure is $S(s)$.

(From Figure 25, Bunge, 1979, adapted with permission from Dover Publications.)

1.1.1 *Partial Systems*

Taking nature apart to find systems is a necessary scientific strategy. It's how we make nature manageable. It is, nonetheless, a strategy fraught with difficulty. There is always the risk of slipping by the system that is actually exhibiting the phenomena of interest. There are two unwelcome consequences of over-decomposing (Turvey & Shaw, 1979). First, the phenomena may appear indeterminate, lacking reference to any underlying law, when in fact, at their proper and coarser grain size of analysis, the phenomena are deterministic and lawful (Humphrey, 1933). Second, erroneous content or function may be ascribed to the partial system (Ashby, 1963; Casti, 1989). Where a selected system is at the wrong grain size of analysis for the phenomena of interest, that system must be endowed with properties that are conjectured to have the ability to generate the phenomena.

With respect to the first consequence, imagine that the phenomena of interest are (a) the short-period diurnal and semidiurnal tides and (b) the long period tides whose rhythms range from 14 days to 19 years. If attributed to the Earth–Water system, these short- and long-period oscillations in sea level would look capricious. Alternatively, they might invite the hypothesis that there are two different systems in operation on different time scales. In contrast, if these temporal tidal events are recognized as the phenomena of a larger system, the Sun–Moon–Earth–Water system to be exact, then they will be seen as lawful. The latter, more inclusive system embodies the laws of which the tides are necessary consequences. Those laws are not embodied by the Earth–Water system (Figure 1.2).

With respect to the second consequence, we can take an example from Ashby (1963). This example makes the general point that if the total system (from the perspective of the phenomena of interest) is unobservable, then the partial system that can be observed may assume "remarkable, even miraculous properties" (Ashby, 1963, p. 114). The paradigmatic case is the magician's trick. It looks miraculous because not all of the significant variables are observable.

Consider a system composed of two interconnected devices A and B and the input I that influences both of them (Figure 1.3). Thus, A's inputs are both B and I. The device A shows some characteristic behavior R only when B is at state z and I is at state y. It is the case that B is in state z only subsequent

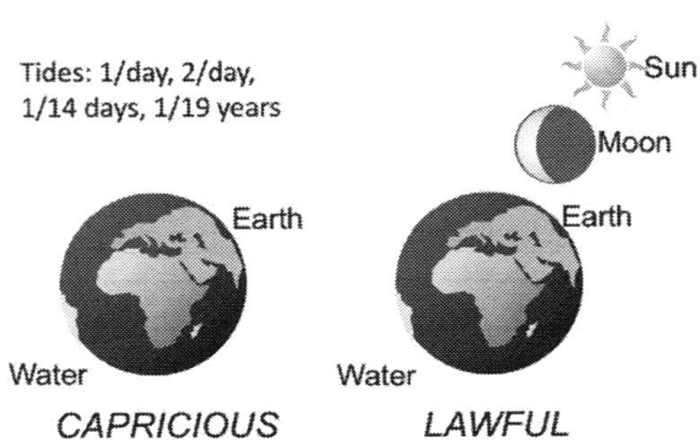

Figure 1.2 Partial system (*left*) and total system (*right*) in the explanation of tides.

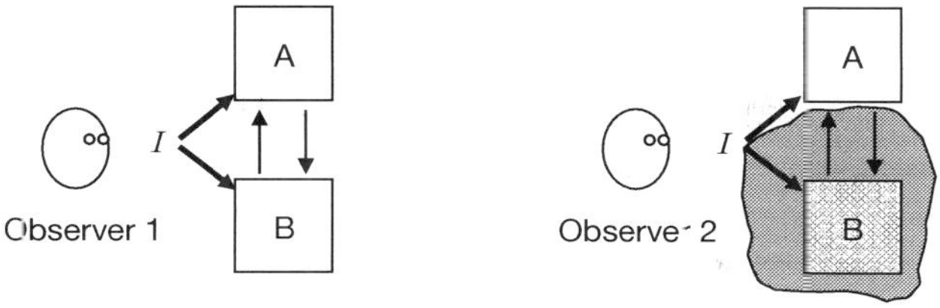

Figure 1.3 Two observers try to explain the behavior *R* of a system. Observer 1 sees the total system *A* + *B* + *I*; Observer 2 sees only the partial system *A* + *I*. Observer 1 explains *R* through the present states of the system; Observer 2 has to appeal to past states, to memory, to explain *R*. See text for details.

to I taking the value x. There are two observers. Observer 1 sees the total system and is able to conclude that R occurs whenever the total system shows a state with B at z and I at y. Observer 2 cannot see B (or does not take it into account). Consequently, knowing the states of A and I is insufficient to predict reliably the occurrence of R. After all, I is sometimes y and sometimes some other state. Nevertheless, Observer 2, by paying attention to earlier states of I can make reliable predictions about R. If I passes successively through states x and y, then R will occur and not otherwise. It follows, therefore, that Observer 2 can make reliable predictions by using successive values of I that are in fact observable.

Suppose the two observers now get into an argument about the "system." Observer 1 will claim that R is fully accounted for by the *present* state of the system. Observer 2 will claim that R can only be accounted for by considering the *past* states of the system—that is, only when memory is assumed. The point is, however, that the two observers are arguing about different systems. Observer 1 is discussing A + B + I, Observer 2 is discussing A + I. Observer 2 is ascribing memory to the system as a substitute for failure to observe (or to take into account) B.

The point is, perhaps, obvious, but it can escape notice. The possession of some property by a system is not wholly an objective property of the system. It depends on whether the observer is able to observe the events in question in all the significant variables. For cases similar to that of Figure 1.3, the fewer the observable variables, the more likely is it that past events will have to be credited with playing a part in the system's behavior (Ashby, 1963). The commonplace appeal to memory as explanation of an organism's behavior or to memory loss as an account of a human failing could be misplaced.[3]

1.1.2 Mereology

Mereology is the technical term for the examination of part-whole relations. It is an enterprise aimed at "the rules for constructing coherent discourses involving reference to parts and wholes" (Harré & Llored, 2013, p. 127). For our purposes, the enterprise has identified two major mereological fallacies, one semantic and one ontological (Harré & Llored, 2011, 2013). The mereological semantic fallacy is that of ascribing to a subsystem a predicate that gets its meaning from its use as an attribute of the system (cf. note 3). Bennett and Hacker (2003) have argued that the practice of Cognitive Neuroscience as a discipline is particularly prone to this fallacy. The discipline is founded upon the premise that psychological predicates—those that refer to the capabilities of a person, such as perceiving, planning, remembering—can be individually ascribed to particular subsystems instantiated in specific areas of the person's brain. On the foregoing premise, it only seems that a whole system (a person) perceives, plans, and remembers. In actuality, it is individual subsystems (parts of the person) that perceive, plan, and remember.

It will be important for future lectures to appreciate that one *could*, in practice, commit the mereological semantic fallacy in regard to nonliving things.[4] Consider an old-fashioned pendulum clock.[5] It has multiple parts: a pallet fork, an escape wheel, a center wheel, a main wheel (together with several other wheels), a weight, a pendulum, clock hands, a minute wheel, an hour wheel and a connector wheel. As examples, one could predicate "time keeping" of the pallet fork and escape wheel (the clock's energy control), or predicate "hour measuring" of the hour wheel. Both predications would be fallacious. Time keeping and hour measuring are achievements of the whole clock.

The mereological ontological fallacy is inferring that the products of an analytical procedure applied to a system are the subsystems of the system on which the procedure was performed. Here is a homely example. The parts of a bicycle made manifest when the bicycle is dismantled with spanner and screwdriver are ontologically right. They were the original constituents—the original subsystems. The parts of a bicycle made manifest when the bicycle is dismantled with an acetylene torch are ontologically wrong. They were not the original constituents—not the original subsystems. It would be a mereological ontological fallacy to claim that they were.[6] The fallacy is transparent in the homely bicycle example but likely to be opaque in the elaborate practices of science. At the very least we can appreciate what the fallacy warns: Any particular methodology can yield outcomes suggestive of parts that do not in fact compose the original material entity.

1.2 Intentional

The qualifier *intentional* does not correspond with the common use of the word "intentional" to mean "deliberate." It is a technical term of philosophers. Qualifying *system* by *intentional* means that the system's states have the quality of *aboutness*—that is, they have the power or capacity to refer to or be about other states of affairs (Searle, 1983). Perceptions are about objects and events, and actions are about goals. An organism cannot perceive without perceiving something, and an organism cannot act without its acting referring to something. These things that perceiving and acting are about should not be confused with the crass physical objects that compose an organism's material surroundings. By this, one means that the things in question are not describable in the ordinary (organism-neutral, observer-independent) terms of classical physics. Accordingly, they need to be distinguished by a special name. For the time being, we can call them by the name often used by philosophers: They are *intentional objects*.

The notions of *intentional* and *intentionality*, and the various ideas surrounding them, come to us primarily from the 19th-century psychologist–philosopher Franz Brentano (1874/1973). For him, mental states but not physical states are "directed upon an object" (Dennett, 1969). This distinction derives from the observation that intentional objects need not exist. Consider the intentional state of wanting something. It does not follow from the fact of my wanting a balcony outside my office door that there exists a balcony outside my office door that I want. In contrast, consider the physical action of standing on something. It *does* follow from the fact of my standing on the balcony outside my office door that there exists a balcony outside my office door on which I stand. The thing wanted does not have quite the same status as the thing stood upon.

Now consider the intentional state of perceiving. It does not follow from the fact that I perceive myself to be walking backwards over the ground that there is a state of affairs "I am walking backwards over the ground" that I am currently perceiving.[7] Compare this with the physical action of walking backwards. It *does* follow from the fact that I am walking backwards over the ground that there is a state of affairs "I am walking backwards over the ground" that is currently being realized.

Hopefully, you can gather from these cursory remarks why Brentano felt that purely physical systems could not be intentional.[8] How could the states of purely physical systems ever be about nonexistent things? How could reliable laws of physical interaction hold if nonexistent states were part and parcel of the ordinary behavior of physical systems?

There is a practical side to the qualifier *intentional*. It implies that one can do a pretty good job of explaining and predicting the behaviors of these systems by ascribing to them beliefs, desires, goals, and so on (Dennett, 1971, 1989). The *intentional stance*, as a strategy for interpreting systems, contrasts with the so-called physical and design stances. Adopting the physical stance, one attempts to explain and predict through the intensive application of physical laws and principles. In the design stance, one might liken a system to a particular artifact, a system built for some purpose, and base explanation and prediction upon the regularities of that artifact. A fact of homeostasis, such as a constant body temperature, invites comparison with the thermostat. From that comparison, certain expectations about the system's thermoregulatory behavior can be framed. A more general example of the design stance is the strategy that would typify an ideal neurobiology: explanation and prediction based on a blueprint of the nervous system and the ability to trace the causal chain (Lecture 3) of relevant neural interactions.

1.3 Epistemic

The qualifier *epistemic* simply brings into emphasis one particular intentional property: *knowing about*. What is perhaps most tantalizing about the systems of interest to the student of perception and action is the very obvious fact that they are knowledgeable. Each such system is knowledgeable, in a very practical sense, about itself and its surroundings. An ant of the minor worker caste relates to its nest in 27 different knowledgeable ways (Wilson, 1976). Despite its humble status, the worker ant is a sophisticated and challenging epistemic, intentional system.

The term *epistemic* partners the term *epistemology*. The latter is the label for the branch of philosophy concerned with hypotheses about what knowledge is and how knowledge is possible. Among the most central and most enduring questions of epistemology are whether perceptual knowing about, or non-perceptual knowing about, or either kind of knowing about, can be trusted. Although the study of such matters has been a long-term philosophical endeavor, it has, relatively speaking, only recently become a serious scientific endeavor. A crude assessment of the 19th and 20th centuries is that their major scientific achievements were a formal and rigorous understanding of the previously intuitive ideas, respectively, of "energy" and "information" (at least as the latter idea bears on issues of communication). It is not unreasonable to hope that the 21st century is going to provide a similar comprehension of the intuitive idea of "knowing about" as a property that some material systems possess with respect to themselves and other material systems.

In good time, we will review arguments that substantial progress has already been made toward this latter goal. We will consider the possibility that the desired understanding can be founded on the exact idea of computation, an idea clarified last century as an integral component of science's formal grasp of information. From this perspective, "knowing about" is a species of computation over discrete symbol strings that are presumed to stand for, to represent, the knowledge in question. We will also consider the possibility that the desired understanding will follow from an enriched comprehension of neural networks. How does "knowing about" emerge in the parallel communication of continuously graded signals among very many, computationally simple, processing elements? The neural network perspective regards "knowing about" as a species of dynamics—specifically, of the time evolution of neural-like states. In either perspective, meeting the challenge of "knowing about" is equated with developing and understanding mechanisms that simulate cognitive phenomena (e.g., memory, language, perception, learning) and collecting them into a single unified theory (e.g., Newell, 1990).

As the lectures unfold, we will address a very different possibility (Turvey & Shaw, 1995)—namely, that understanding epistemic, intentional systems and, thereby, knowing about, will demand "a dramatic, and far from obvious, overhaul of our fundamental orientations, physically and philosophically, toward living things, their surroundings and the relations that hold between them" (p. 145).

Minimally, the overhaul requires the transformation of physics into the science of complex systems. The concept of *complex* is notoriously loose. At this juncture, it can be remarked glibly that complex does not refer to complication but to the possession of an essential semantic component. For the past two centuries, the various sciences of living things have sought to interpret their subject matter by the extension of laws inferred by physicists from the study of simple systems and mechanisms. Rosen (1985, 1987, 1991, 2000) regards that historical enterprise as a matter of putting the cart before the horse (Harold, 2001). The simple systems studied by physics, such as gases and planetary orbits, are the special cases. Complex systems—for example, the multiple living things that exhibit perception and action—represent the general case. The conventional doctrine would have us believe that the material systems that express perception and action are too special an aspect of nature to yield universal generalizations. Rosen (1987, 1991) argues that the doctrine should be turned on its head—that is: *material systems of the kind that express perception and action are more general in respect to the principles that underlie them than the material systems traditionally addressed by physics*. The disquisition of epistemic, intentional systems can be expected to disclose nature's most general principles (Turvey, 1990; Turvey & Shaw, 1995). George Gaylord Simpson (1964) said it best (especially if one permits substitution of "psychology" for "biology"):

> [L]iving things have been affected for . . . billions of years by historical processes . . . The results of those processes are systems different in kind from any nonliving systems and almost incomparably more complicated. They are not for that reason necessarily any less material or less physical in nature. The point is that *all* known material processes and explanatory principles apply to organisms, while only a limited number of them apply to nonliving systems . . . Biology, then, is the science that stands at the center of all science . . . where all the principles of all the sciences are embodied . . .
>
> (pp. 106–107)

Notes

1 The 19th-century Russian scholar Ivan Sechenov (1960, p. 501) was unambiguous on this issue: "Any organism is inconceivable without an external environment for its existence; hence, a scientific definition of organism should include also the environment by which it is influenced. Since the organism cannot exist without

the external environment, all the talk about what is more important for life—the environment or the organism itself—is absolutely senseless."

2 In respect to the latter point, there will be cases where a concept of environment as a self-existing entity will be needed. For this purpose, a different term is recommended (Lewontin, 1983; Mahner & Bunge, 1997). It could be *habitat*.

3 Reinforcing this point, Ashby (1952, p. 41) commented: "It should be noted that from now on 'the system' means not the nervous system but the whole complex of the organism and its environment. Thus, if it should be shown that 'the system' has some property, it must not be assumed that this property is attributed to the nervous system: it belongs to the whole; and detailed examination may be necessary to ascertain the contributions of the separate parts."

4 The reader may note that the references cited on mereology are mainly from the field of chemistry.

5 See Lecture 13, Figure 13.2.

6 There are implications that an adequate theory of mereology will have to recognize cases in which parts, when combined, are no longer the same parts they were prior to combination (Earley, 2005).

7 Experimenters can create a room with a stationary floor but movable walls and ceiling. If a person in the room is walking forward at a certain pace, and if the walls and ceiling are moving away from the person at a greater pace, the person may perceive that he or she is walking backwards (Lishman & Lee, 1973), a phenomenon addressed in Lecture 23.

8 It should be underscored that the distinction here has nothing to do with consciousness. Intentionality and consciousness are not equated (Searle, 1983). Many conscious states are not intentional and many intentional states are not conscious. Examples are, respectively, a momentary feeling of elation and a certain belief that you have but which you have not, up to this point in time, considered (Searle, 1983).

References

Ashby, R. A. (1952). *Design for a brain*. London: Chapman & Hall.

Ashby, R. A. (1963). *An introduction to cybernetics*. New York: Wiley.

Bak, P. (1996). *How nature works*. New York: Springer Verlag.

Bennett, M. R., & Hacker, P. M. S. (2003). *Philosophical foundations of neuroscience*. Oxford, UK: Blackwell.

Berlinski, D. (1976). *On systems analysis*. Cambridge, MA: MIT Press.

Brentano, F. (1973). *Psychology from an empirical standpoint*. London: Routledge & Kegan Paul (original work published 1874).

Bunge, M. (1977). *Ontology I: The furniture of the world*. Dordrecht, Netherlands: D. Reidel.

Bunge, M. (1979). *Ontology II: A world of systems*. Dordrecht, Netherlands: D. Reidel.

Casti, J. L. (1989). *Alternate realities: Mathematical models of nature and man*. New York: Wiley.

Dennett, D. (1969). *Content and consciousness*. London: Routledge & Kegan Paul.

Dennett, D. (1971). Intentional systems. *Journal of Philosophy*, 68, 87–106.

Dennett, D. (1989). *The intentional stance*. Cambridge, MA: MIT Press.

Earley, J. E. (2005). Why there is no salt in the sea. *Foundations of Chemistry*, 7, 85–102.

Elkana, Y. (1970). Helmholtz's 'kraft': An illustration of a concept in flux. *History of Studies in the Physical Sciences, 2*, 263–298.

Garfinkel, A. (1987). The slime mold Dictyostelium as a model of self-organization in social systems. In F. E. Yates (Ed.), *Self-organizing systems: The emergence of order* (pp. 181–212). New York: Plenum Press.

Gibson, J. J. (1986). *The ecological approach to visual perception*. Mahwah, NJ: Erlbaum (original work published 1979).

Grobstein, C. (1973). Hierarchical order and neogenesis. In H. H. Pattee (Ed.), *Hierarchical theory: The challenge of complex systems* (pp. 29–48). New York: Braziller.

Harold, F. M. (2001). *The way of the cell: Molecules, organisms and the order of life*. Oxford, UK: Oxford University Press.

Harré, R., & Llored, J-P. (2011). Mereologies as the grammars of chemical discourses. *Foundations of Chemistry, 13*, 63–76.

Harré, R., & Llored, J-P. (2013). Molecules and mereology. *Foundations of Chemistry, 15*, 127–144.

Humphrey, G. (1933). *The nature of learning*. New York: Harcourt Brace.

Juarrero, A. (1999). *Dynamics in action*. Cambridge, MA: MIT Press.

Krieger, M. H. (1992). *Doing physics: How physicists take hold of the world*. Bloomington: Indiana University Press.

Lewontin, R. C. (1983). Gene, organism and environment. In D. S. Bendall (Ed.), *Evolution from molecules to man* (pp. 273–285). Cambridge, UK: Cambridge University Press.

Lishman, J. R., & Lee, D. N. (1973). The autonomy of visual kinaesthesis. *Perception, 2*, 287–294.

Löwy, I. (1992). The strength of loose concepts—boundary concepts, federative experimental strategies and disciplinary growth: The case of immunology. *History of Science, 30*, 371–396.

Mahner, M., & Bunge, M. (1997). *Foundations of biophilosophy*. New York: Springer.

Marchal, J. (1975). On the concept of a system. *Philosophy of Science, 77*, 45–72.

Newell, A. (1990). *Unified theories of cognition*. Cambridge, MA: Harvard University Press.

Rosen, R. (1985). Organisms as causal systems which are not mechanisms: An essay into the nature of complexity. In R. Rosen (Ed.), *Theoretical biology and complexity* (pp. 165–204). San Diego, CA: Academic Press.

Rosen, R. (1987). Some epistemological issues in physics and biology. In B. J. Hilley & F. D. Platt (Eds.), *Quantum implications: Essays in honor of David Bohm* (pp. 315–327). New York: Routledge & Kegan Paul.

Rosen, R. (1991). *Life itself*. New York: Columbia University Press.

Rosen, R. (2000). *Essays on life itself*. New York: Columbia University Press.

Searle, J. (1983). *Intentionality*. Cambridge, UK: Cambridge University Press.

Sechenov, I. (1960). *Selected physiological and psychological writings*. Moscow: Foreign Languages Publishing House.

Simpson, G. G. (1964). *This view of life*. New York: Harcourt, Brace & World.

Turvey, M. T. (1990). The challenge of a physical account of action: A personal view. In H. T. A. Whiting, O. Meijer, & P. van Wieringen (Eds.) *A natural-physical approach to movement control* (pp. 57–93). Amsterdam, Netherlands: Free University Press.

Turvey, M. T., & Shaw, R. E. (1979). The primacy of perceiving: An ecological reformulation of perception for understanding memory. In L.-G. Nilssen (Ed.), *Perspectives on memory research: In honor of Uppsala University's 500th anniversary* (pp. 167–222). Hillsdale, NJ: Erlbaum.

Turvey, M. T., & Shaw, R. E. (1995). Toward an ecological physics and a physical psychology. In R. Solso & D. Massaro (Eds.), *The science of the mind: 2001 and beyond* (pp. 144–169). Oxford, UK: Oxford University Press.

Wilson, E. O. (1976). Behavioral discretization and the number of castes in an ant species. *Behavioral Ecology and Sociobiology*, *1*, 141–154.

Lecture 2

Organism–Environment Dualism

For the human species, the world comes to be known largely through sight. "Knowing about" is very much a matter of vision. It is for this reason, perhaps, that from the time of Plato, sight has been both the primary example of knowing and the source of its leading metaphors (Zajonc, 1993).

A cornerstone of most attempts to address how one knows the world by sight has been the metaphysical position of *dualism*. The most famous dualism is that which posits two distinct types of substances—mental and material—characterized by two mutually exclusive sets of properties. This combined *substance dualism* and *property dualism* (Kim, 1998) is justifiably attributed to Descartes (see Lecture 6). Although there were many prior advocates (e.g., Plato), none developed the idea of the mind as a distinct substance with unique non-material properties as thoroughly as did Descartes. For the most part, contemporary science and philosophy has rejected Descartes' idea of two substances: the only existing things are material things (Bunge, 1977; Kim, 1998). Modern thinking, however, has not been able to let go of Descartes' idea that there are two kinds of properties. Reasonable grounds can be identified for the claim that mind may be fundamentally material but its physical properties are not reducible to the physical properties that define non-mental matter (Kim, 1998). Cleaving close to Descartes, a complete account of knowing the world by sight seems to require two mutually exclusive languages that might be termed "mentalese" and "physicalese" (Fodor, 1975) or intentional and extensional (Dennett, 1969, 1971; Lecture 6).

Although the classical opposition of mind and body has drawn most attention, it is not the sole example of polar opposites impressing themselves upon the theory of how one knows the world by sight. Others of note are symbol–matter, subject–object, appearance–reality, private–public, semantics–syntax and perception–action.[1] Each of these dualisms, however, can be regarded as subordinate to an overarching dualism—that of organism and environment (Järvilehto, 1998a, 1998b; Michaels & Carello, 1981; Shaw & Turvey, 1981, 1999; Turvey & Shaw, 1979, 1995, 1999). Arguably, this dualism is more pervasive and influential than the aforementioned dualisms, though less obvious and less heralded. It can be readily appreciated in respect to the issue of adaptation in evolutionary theory.

2.1 The Notion of Adaptation

The notion that organisms adapt, either through evolution or learning, implies that there is something to which they are being adapted or fitted. A useful metaphor is that of grinding a key to fit a lock (Lewontin, 1982). The lock is a circumstance that exists prior to and independently of the key. The lock can be seen as a challenge to which the key is a response or, synonymously, as a problem to which the key is a solution. Similarly, the notion of adaptation begins with an environment defined without reference to the organism, as a well-defined state of affairs to which the organism becomes adapted. More particularly, the starting point is a world partitioned into pre-existent ecological niches with evolution producing progressively better fits of organisms to those niches. In Lewontin's (1982) words: "Environment begins as alienated from the organism, which must then bring itself into conformity with the given world" (p. 159).

The adaptive view of evolution can be given a compact portrayal as a pair of differential equations (Lewontin, 1983). The first equation describes the change in organisms, O, as a function of organism and environment, *E*: $\dot{O} = f(O, E)$. The second equation describes the autonomous change of the environment: $\dot{E} = g(E)$. One immediate benefit of this portrayal is the elucidation of the presumed causal structure of adaptation. As expressed by the first equation, organisms are the effects of autonomous causes originating internally (O interpreted as inheritable factors) and externally (*E*). Thinking of extant organisms as optimal solutions to their environments raises the question of what might motivate further evolution. Befitting the causal direction identified by the preceding differential equations is an answer known, picturesquely, as the *Red Queen hypothesis* (Van Valen, 1973). Roughly, organisms are like the Red Queen in Lewis Carroll's *Through a Looking Glass*. They are always running simply to keep up with an environment that is constantly undergoing change. By this hypothesis, the rate of evolution is governed by $\dot{E}$ implying that understanding the evolution of living things is tantamount to understanding the laws of environmental change, $g(E)$.

2.2 Newton's Dualism of States and Dynamical Laws

The prominence of organism–environment dualism in the sciences of living things and their capabilities is for good reason: it is compatible with the primary epistemological preconception of Newton's mechanics—the dualism of system and environment or, more precisely, the dualism of states and dynamical laws. Rosen (1991) is forthright in his assessment:

> It is this dualism between states and dynamical laws that, more than anything else, has determined the character of contemporary science. (p. 95)

The assessment should be read as including the sciences that address perception and action. Theorizing about perception and action in the past three centuries has been largely modeled on Newton's mechanics.

Despite his famed remark *hypothesis non fingo* ("I frame no hypothesis"), Newton did make hypotheses. In particular, he hypothesized that once the system for investigation has been identified, so has the system's environment (Rosen, 1988, 1991). Given a single particle as system,[2] its environment is everything else in the universe. Appreciating the logical independence of system and environment begins with the observation that *states* or *phases* can be assigned to the system but not to the environment. This distinction means that the environment and the system cannot be causal in the same sense. A few preliminary concepts are required to illuminate this fundamental dualism.

Central to Newton's mechanics are the concepts of state and recursion. A particle's state is characterized by its position x at time t, that is, $x(t)$, and by its motion at time t as given by the successive time derivatives of $x(t)$: $\dot{x}(t)$, $\ddot{x}(t)$, $\dddot{x}(t)$, and so on, ad infinitum. Recursion, roughly, is the conversion of a present state to a future state or the entailment of the future by the present. A recursively defined function f is one in which successive values are obtained by applying a fixed operation or mapping T to its preceding value. An example is $f(n) = T^n(r)$, where r is an initial arbitrary value and n is the number of times (the nth instance) the operation has been applied.

For Newton's mechanics, the essence of the concept of state is its recursive[3] character (Rosen, 1991; see also Arnold, 1990): A particle's state in the future must be entailed[4] from the particle's state now. The instant-to-instant change in a state variable composes a chronicle or time series with as many chronicles as there are state variables. Together, the chronicled variables defining a particle's evolving state form a recursive set $\{x^{(k)}(t)\}$. This is Taylor's theorem that a function can, under certain conditions, be represented as a power series in the neighborhood of a point where it can be differentiated infinitely. The various order derivatives evaluated at that point are the coefficients of the series.

The potentially very large number of quantities defining the state of a single particle (remember the ad infinitum from above?) prohibits the same state description for the particle's environment Clearly, if the environment is all other particles, giving a parallel description of the *state* of the environment is unthinkable. Newton's resolution of this dilemma was to express environment by its effects on the particle—more precisely, by the particle's change of state. Newton embodied the concept of a system's environment in the concept of the force F acting on the particle or system of mass m. From the second law, $F(x, \dot{x}) = m\ddot{x}$, three things follow. First, the particle's state is reduced from infinity to two variables $(x, \dot{x})$ often referred to as the *phase* of the particle. Second, the environment's effects are proportional to the particle's acceleration $\ddot{x}$. Third, the environment's effects are functions of the particle's state defined by position and velocity, that is, the phase $(x, \dot{x})$. And fourth, the environment's effects on the particle are modulated by the parameter m.

To summarize to this point, and to use Rosen's (1988, 1991) terms, the environment is encoded into force and system is encoded into a formalism in which the only entailment is a recursion rule such that, given the phase at t_0,

$$(x_0, \dot{x}_0) \rightarrow (x_0 + \dot{x}_0 dt, \dot{x}_0 + F dt) \tag{2.1}$$

This encoding of system, in the context of system–environment dualism, is of great significance: *It reduces the notion of causality to a sequence of state transitions*. Bohm (1969) refers to it as an "automorphism[5] of motion": There is a limited field of possible phases and each change corresponds to a transition from one phase to another in this limited field. A particle's motion in Newtonian mechanics is simply a process of going from one position and velocity to another position and velocity.

We can sharpen the logical independence between Newton's system and Newton's environment via Aristotle's mutually exclusive (and collectively exhaustive) causal categories. These causes are provided as answers to the question "why?" For example, "Why is this artifact like it is?" The answer is: (a) because of the artifact's material composition (*material cause*); (b) because of the physical work performed and energy spent to make it as it is (*efficient cause*); (c) because of the plan or design that was followed to make it as it is (*formal cause*), and (d) because the agent wanted it to be like it is (*final cause*). In terms of the Aristotelian categories, system is material cause and environment is efficient cause. As anticipated, system and environment are not causal in the same sense. Looking at the state transition identified above, the present state is what it is because of the system's initial state $(x_0, \dot{x}_0)$—the material cause—and because of the environment's dynamical law $F(x, \dot{x}) = m\ddot{x}$—the efficient cause. It should be added, also, that in this context, m is the formal cause modulating the system–environment relation. The larger lesson to be learned from applying Aristotle's causal categories is that it makes precise the paradigm of system description inherited from Newton: causal categories should be reflected in logically independent aspects of system description (Rosen, 1987).[6]

2.3 Consequences of Organism–Environment Dualism

We can now return to the organism-environment dualism presupposed by the notion of adaptation. Its linkage to Newton's dualism is fairly plain. The environment is clearly the source of forces impressed upon the organism (Figure 2.1). More subtly, the environment must also be the origin of the initial conditions, but through processes other than those encoded in the formalism for force. Everything of real significance is in the environment for

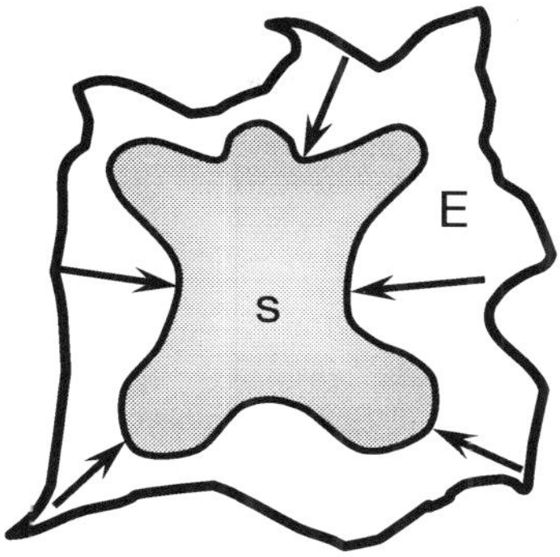

Figure 2.1 Newton's dualism. The environment (*E*) is the efficient cause (a source of forces) acting upon system (*s*), a material cause. Externality is an essential mark of efficient causation: an external influence producing changes in *s*.

(From Figure 25, Bunge, 1979, adapted with permission from Dover Publications.)

Newton, but there is no description of the environment apart from its effect on system (Rosen, 1988). This same paradox inflicts the notion of adaptation (Lewontin, 1978). The necessity of defining environments—more specifically, niches without organisms—supposes a finite number of preferred combinations of factors that compose niches to be distinguished from an infinite number of combinations that do not compose niches. Lacking, however, is the law that would select the possible niches and, further, be responsible for the changes that occur in them. Just as Newton's environment is known only through its effect on system, the environments or niches of adaptation theory are known only through their organisms.

The implicit assumption that organism and environment are two logically independent components has had profound consequences for understanding how organisms know their environments by sight. The most obvious consequence is that it sharply demarcates the organism that does the visual "knowing" from the environment that is visually "known" (to adopt terms from James, 1909/1975 and Dewey & Bentley, 1949).

The division of scientific labor parallels this demarcation (Mace, 1974). Historically, the students of *what* vision has to work with—the qualities of the illuminated environment and the nature of light—have been geometers and physicists. In contrast, the students of *how* vision performs its work to yield "knowing about" have been philosophers, psychologists, physiologists, etc. On the presumption that the division of labor is proper, those who would seek to explain the workings of visual perception accept as their starting point the results of those who would seek to determine the stimuli for visual perception. Any dissonance between the achievements of vision and the physical–geometric conditions of vision can then be accepted as fact and, thus, grist for the theory mill. The conclusion frequently drawn from the fact that the physical–geometric conditions for color vision do not account for the psychology of color vision is that colored objects do not exist (e.g., Sekuler & Blake, 1994): "[O]bjects themselves have no color; nor is the light reflected from those objects colored. Instead, color is a psychological phenomenon, an entirely subjective experience" (p. 182).

Organism–environment dualism gives license, as the preceding quotation perhaps implies, to the promotion of a particular kind of theorizing about perception. Its hallmark strategy is that of situating internal subjective states (for want of a better phrase) between the conditions of the environment and the organism's perceptual experience. These in-between states are the intentional objects that we encountered in Lecture 1. Their function is to mediate the all-important epistemic contact between the organism and its environment. In other words, the proximal cause for perceptual experience is not the environment as such, but one of the links in a hypothesized chain of cause-and-effect that connects the organism as perceiver to its environment (Russell, 1927). We might call these proximal causes *epistemic mediators* (Shaw & Bransford, 1977; Turvey, 1977).

According to a theory of this kind that incorporates epistemic mediators, one only knows the world by sight in a roundabout way, usually by inference. The organism doesn't know about the current environment as such. More precisely, it knows about the epistemic mediator that is, somehow, standing in for the environment. An appealing metaphor is that of *organism as sleuth.* Much like a detective assiduously putting together the events at the scene of a crime, the organism's perception of its environment must be constructed: "from fleeting fragmentary scraps of data signaled by the senses and drawn from the brain's memory banks—themselves constructions of snippets of the past" (Gregory, 1972, p. 707).

To pursue the metaphor, the organism (sleuth) knows about the environment as reconstructed by its own efforts (the reconstructed crime), rather than about the environment as such (the actual crime). It should be emphasized how befitting is organism-as-sleuth to the notion of adaptation in evolutionary theory and, by implication, organism-environment dualism. Both quotations just given encrypt the history of perceptual psychology. As we shall see in subsequent lectures, decoding them will take us from the early Greek mathematicians and philosophers to the international computer-oriented perceptual scientist of the 21st century. There is much for the beginning student of perception and action to learn from this history.

2.4 Epistemic, Intentional Systems may not be Approachable from the Doctrine of Organism–Environment Dualism

The assumed dualism of organism and environment sanctifies two prominent explanations of knowing about (cf. Järvilehto, 1998a, b). One is in terms of the causal powers of an organism's mind or brain. It is a style of explanation that focuses only on $C(s)$ ignoring $E(s)$ and $S(s)$. The other is in terms of the causal interaction between an organism and its environment treated as rigidly separable things. Here, explanation ignores $S(s)$ and interprets $E(s)$ as a self-existing (independent-of-s) entity that can induce changes in $C(s)$. Because these forms of explanation are so ingrained historically, it is valuable to examine some very psychological phenomena that highlight the importance of adopting the minimal model depicted in Figure 1.1 (or something much like it) in order to achieve understanding.

2.4.1 Reinforcement

A classical concern of the experimental investigation of learning—namely, the nature and mechanism of reinforcement—highlights the possibility that major aspects of knowing about may not be approachable from the doctrine of organism-environment dualism (Turvey & Shaw, 1999).

It is self-evident that a behavior can be facilitated, improved and rendered more likely to occur by particular consequences historically referred to as *reinforcements*. Efforts to achieve a viable theory of the self-evident fact of reinforcement have been thwarted, however, by the difficulties of identifying reinforcers and the mechanism by which they work. The questions to be answered are: "What determines whether something can function as a reinforcer or, synonymously, how can reinforcers be predicted?" and "How does a reinforcer produce its effects—that is, how does it bring about an increase in the probability of a behavior?"

In earlier conceptions, reinforcers were identified with a special class of stimuli. These special stimuli were viewed as categorically distinct from the behaviors that they reinforced and their effect was interpreted as one of strengthening the instrumental response. The preceding ideas were repudiated by the observation that reinforcers were oftentimes behaviors rather than stimuli of a particular kind (Premack, 1965). Response R_n can act as a reinforcer of response R_m but not because of anything intrinsic to R_n. Rather, it is the probability with which R_n occurs relative to R_m. Premack's differential probability principle says that the reinforcing response R_n is simply a response that is more likely to occur than the instrumental response R_m (Domjan, 1998). If conditions rendered R_n less probable than R_m, then the roles would be reversed; R_m would be the reinforcer for R_n. Reinforcers do not exist in any absolute, context-independent sense.

Research inspired by Premack's principle has led to an even more radical understanding. Far from being absolute, reinforcers are created online by the contingencies of instrumental learning. Any behavior that functions as a reinforcer is a restricted behavior. It is restricted in the sense that the opportunity to engage in the reinforcing behavior is contingent upon engaging in the instrumental behavior. A low-probability behavior, so restricted, will act as an effective reinforcer of a high-probability behavior. It is not the relative response probabilities that matter, as Premack had presumed, but rather the degree to which the instrumental response–reinforcer contingency disrupts behavioral stability. Apparently, the success of the contingency in increasing the instrumental response rests on its forcing the organism away from a preferred or optimal distribution of activities and on the organism's inclination to so behave as to maintain that distribution (e.g., Allison, 1989; Domjan, 1998; Timberlake, 1980). In sum, reinforcers are predictable and the resultant increases in behavior are understandable in the light of a broad principle of behavioral regulation.

2.4.2 CES Spectroscopy

Given the preceding observations, it is evident that the theory of reinforcement will demand much of science. The notion of a preferred distribution of behaviors invokes principles of a particular physical theory of complexity referred to as *homeokinetic physics* (e.g., Iberall & Soodak, 1987; Soodak & Iberall, 1978). The identification of these principles in relation to behavioral regulation begins with the observation that an organism is marginally unstable within its environment (when at rest, it cannot stay at rest; when active, it cannot stay active). This inherent instability is a patterning of a limited (but reasonably large) number of behavioral modes (Iberall & McCulloch, 1969). The patterning is in the form of cycling among the modes–a pattern of recurrences. There is nothing fixed about the patterning except that all modes are visited a requisite average number of times (e.g., eat 2–4 times a day, groom about every 10 minutes). An organism "threads" its way among the modes ergodically,[7] meaning that there is global stability of behavior in the statistical mechanical sense (Bloch, Cardon, Iberall, et al., 1971). For adaptive success, however, the organism must, in addition, thread its way *comfortably*. The pattern of behavioral recurrences should fit, rather than oppose or be indifferent to, the environmental recurrences. That is, the behavioral recurrences should be entrainable and preferably in small numbers. Humans eat, void, sleep just a few times a day. Such recurrences can fit the circadian cycle comfortably.

Homeokinetics is a term so used because regularities in inanimate and animate systems are the result of cycles of energy dissipation and replenishment (so-called thermodynamic engine cycles). Form and function are sustained as limit cycle processes (e.g., Iberall, 1977, 1978; Iberall & Soodak, 1987; Yates, Marsh & Iberall, 1972). Like a simple pendulum clock, these processes, when momentarily perturbed to operate at either larger space–time scales (e. g., the pendulum makes bigger and slower swings) or smaller space–time scales (e.g., the pendulum makes smaller and faster swings), habitually converge on characteristic space–time scales (e.g., a particular pendulum amplitude and frequency of swing needed to keep time). The constants that inspired the notion of physiological homeostasis (e.g., a constant body temperature of 98.6°F) are the mean states of oscillatory mechanisms.

In the homeokinetic perspective, an organism is a multitude of biochemical chains with characteristic rate-governing steps that foster, in each case, a limit-cycle process. The fact that an organism's time scales are often lengthy (minutes, days) suggests the prominent roles of endocrinological mechanisms and the chemical messengers—the hormones. The variable operating characteristics of this battery of biochemical oscillators results in the aforementioned behavioral patterning. More specifically, the cyclic processes are motor-sensory-internal organ motions (Bloch, Cardon, Iberall, et al., 1971). A biospectroscopy is implied at the macroscopic scale of the organism-environment system with individual organism–environment systems distinguished, in principle, by the particulars of their spectra. Iberall (1972) summarizes the condition as follows:

> One is hard put not to conclude that in order to attain global stability the large number of only loosely coupled chains must represent an extensive collection of atomistic elements which have to be canonically constrained in accordance with an ergodic hypothesis.
>
> (p. 170)

The key idea of biospectroscopy—namely, homeokinetics—addresses why there are multiple behavioral modes, why the system must ring through these modes, why the modes are coupled largely as a Markov chain, and why switching among the modes must be simple (e.g., Iberall & Soodak, 1987). It does not (as yet) address directly, however, the question as to why the baseline frequencies of the different behavioral modes differ as they do. This limitation aside, the ultimate significance of a recurring ring of behavioral modes is that it allows the organism to balance the entropic (order-reducing) degradations associated with the chains of processes, thereby ensuring persistence of its characteristic forms and functions (Iberall & Soodak, 1987).

2.4.3 Reinforcement Redux

Returning to the concept of reinforcement, it can be seen, therefore, that to restrict any particular activity in which an organism engages is to perturb the distribution of all of the organism's activities—that is, to bring about a global disequilibrium. In this light, increases in instrumental behaviors are by-products of a comprehensive reorganization of behavior due to homeokinetic processes attempting to return the organism–environment system to global equilibrium. Despite its profoundly personal nature, reinforcement may be understandable only in terms that address the organism and its environment in full, that is, as a CES model (minimally). We will have more to say about organism–environment dualism more generally in subsequent lectures (particularly Lecture 22).

Notes

1 In general, binary opposites should be viewed with circumspection (Bunge, 1977; Newell, 1973). That there are any truly opposite things is unlikely. Some advertised polarities arise from merely equating opposite with the absence of a property. Brentano's intentionality is possibly an example: the absence of this property identifies matter in opposition to mind. Many are more properly interpreted as pairs of different things rather than pairs of opposite things. From a strictly materialistic perspective, there are no two things that can be completely different, no two things for which the degree of similarity can be zero. Patently, every thing is like every other thing in being constituted of parts that satisfy universal physical laws. At best, opposites in scientific discourse can only be relative (Bunge, 1977).

2 In terms of the CES (*composition*, *environment* and *structure*) model of Lecture 1, $C(s)$ is the null set. The system either lacks internal parts or its internal parts are ignored purposely by the observer.

3 Pertaining to a process that is inherently repetitive, with the outcome of each repetition typically depending on the outcome of the previous repetition.

4 For P to *entail* Q means that Q is a logical or necessary consequence of P; it is a relation such that the truth of P (however defined) ensures the truth of Q. An *entailment* is a strict, logical or analytical implication.

5 An automorphism is a transformation that preserves (leaves invariant or unchanged) structure—in this case, "transition between phases."

6 Eventually, we will consider that this holds only for simple systems. For complex systems, we will entertain the possibility that the causal categories become intertwined in such a way as to render inadequate a description in terms of the dualism of states and dynamical laws (Rosen, 1987).

7 Ergodic is the property of a system or process in which averages computed from a data sample over time converge in a probabilistic sense, to ensemble or special averages.

References

Allison, J. (1989). The nature of reinforcement. In S. B. Klein & R. R. Mower (Eds.), *Contemporary learning theories: Instrumental conditioning theory and the impact of biological constraints on learning* (pp. 13–39). Hillsdale, NJ: Erlbaum.

Arnold, V. I. (1990). *Huygens & Barrow, Newton & Hooke*. Boston, MA: Birkhäuser Verlag.

Bloch, E., Cardon, S., Iberall, A. S., Jacobowitz, D., Kornacker, K., Lipetz, D., McCulloch, W., Urquhart, J., Weinberg, M., & Yates, F. (1971). *Introduction to a biological systems science*. NASA CR-1720.

Bohm, D. (1969). Some remarks on the notion of order. In C. H. Waddington (Ed.), *Towards a theoretical biology, Volume 2* (pp. 18–40). Chicago, IL: Aldine Publishing.

Bunge, M. (1977). *Ontology I: The furniture of the world*. Dordrecht, Netherlands: D. Reidel.

Bunge, M. (1979). Causality and modern science (3rd ed.). New York: Dover Publications.

Dennett, D. (1969). *Content and consciousness*. London: Routledge & Kegan Paul.

Dennett, D. (1971). Intentional systems. *Journal of Philosophy*, 68, 87–106.

Dewey, J., & Bentley, A. F. (1949). *Knowing and the known*. Boston, MA: Beacon.

Domjan, M. (1998). *The principles of learning and behavior* (6th ed.). Belmont, CA: Wadsworth.

Fodor, J. A. (1975). *The language of thought*. Cambridge, MA: Harvard University Press.

Gregory, R. (1972). Seeing as thinking: An active theory of perception. *London Times Literary Supplement*, June 23, 707–708.

Iberall, A. S. (1972). *Toward a general science of viable systems*. New York: McGraw-Hill.

Iberall, A. S. (1977). A field and circuit thermodynamics for integrative physiology: I. Introduction to the general notions. *American Journal of Physiology/Regulatory, Integrative, & Comparative Physiology, 2*, R171-R180.

Iberall, A. S. (1978). A field and circuit thermodynamics for integrative physiology: III. Keeping the books – a general experimental method. *American Journal of Physiology/Regulatory, Integrative, & Comparative Physiology, 3*, R85–R97.

Iberall, A. S., & McCulloch, W. (1969). The organizing principle of complex living systems. *Transactions of the American Society of Mechanical Engineers: Journal of Basic Engineering, 19*, 290–294.

Iberall, A. S., & Soodak, H. (1987). A physics for complex systems. In F. E. Yates (Ed.), *Self-organizing systems: The emergence of order* (pp. 499–520). New York: Plenum Press.

James, W. (1975). *Pragmatism and the meaning of truth*. Cambridge, MA: Harvard University Press (original work published 1907–9).

Järvilehto, T. (1998a). The theory of the organism–environment system: I. Description of the theory. *Integrative Physiological and Behavioral Science, 33*, 321–334.

Järvilehto, T. (1998b). The theory of the organism–environment system: II. Significance of nervous activity in the organism–environment system. *Integrative Physiological and Behavioral Science, 33*, 335–342.

Kim, J. (1998). *Mind in a physical world: An essay on the mind-body problem and mental causation*. Cambridge, MA: MIT Press.

Lewontin, M. (1978). Adaptation. *Scientific American, 239*, 213–230.

Lewontin, R. C. (1982). Organism and environment. In H. C. Plotkin (Ed.), *Learning, development and culture* (pp. 151–170). New York: Wiley.

Lewontin, R. C. (1983). Gene, organism and environment. In D. S. Bendall (Ed.), *Evolution from molecules to men* (pp. 273–285). Cambridge, UK: Cambridge University Press.

Mace, W. M. (1974). Ecologically stimulating cognitive psychology: Gibsonian perspectives. In W. B. Weimer & D. Palermo (Eds.), *Cognition and the symbolic processes* (pp. 137–164). Hillsdale, NJ: Erlbaum.

Michaels, C. F., & Carello, C. (1981). *Direct perception*. Englewood Cliffs, NJ: Prentice-Hall.

Newell, A. (1973). You can't play 20 questions with nature and win. In W. G. Chase (Ed.), *Visual information processing* (pp. 283–308). New York: Academic Press.

Premack, D. (1965). Reinforcement theory. In D. Levine (Ed.), *Nebraska symposium on motivation* (pp. 123–180). Lincoln: University of Nebraska Press.

Rosen, R. (1987). Some epistemological issues in physics and biology. In B. J. Hilley & F. D. Platt (Eds.), *Quantum implications: Essays in honor of David Bohm* (pp. 315–327). New York: Routledge & Kegan.

Rosen, R. (1988). Similarity and dissimilarity: A partial overview. *Human Movement Science, 7*, 131–153.

Rosen, R. (1991). *Life itself*. New York: Columbia University Press.

Russell, B. (1927). *The analysis of matter*. London: George Allen & Unwin.

Sekuler, R., & Blake, R. (1994). *Perception*. New York: McGraw Hill.

Shaw, R. E., & Bransford, J. (1977). Introduction: Psychological approaches to the problem of knowledge. In R. E. Shaw & J. Bransford (Eds.), *Perceiving, acting and knowing* (pp. 1–39). Hillsdale, NJ: Erlbaum.

Shaw, R. E., & Turvey, M. T. (1981). Coalitions as models for ecosystems: A realist perspective on perceptual organization. In M. Kubovy & J. Pomerantz (Eds.), *Perceptual organization* (pp. 343–415). Hillsdale, NJ: Erlbaum.

Shaw, R. E., & Turvey, M. T. (1999). Ecological foundations of cognition: II. Degrees of freedom and conserved quantities in animal-environment systems. *Journal of Consciousness Studies*, 6, 111–123.

Soodak, H., & Iberall, A. (1978). Homeokinetics: A physical science for complex systems. *Science*, *201*, 579–582.

Timberlake, W. (1980). A molar equilibrium theory of learned performance. In G. H. Bower (Ed.), *The psychology of learning and motivation* (Vol. 14, pp. 1–58). New York: Academic Press.

Turvey, M. T. (1977). Contrasting orientations to the theory of visual-information processing. *Psychological Review*, *84*, 67–88.

Turvey, M. T., & Shaw, R. E. (1979). The primacy of perceiving: An ecological reformulation of perception for understanding memory. In L-G Nilssen (Ed.), *Perspectives on memory research: In honor of Uppsala University's 500th anniversary* (pp. 167–222). Hillsdale, NJ: Erlbaum.

Turvey, M. T., & Shaw, R. E. (1995). Toward an ecological physics and a physical psychology. In R. Solso & D. Massaro (Eds.), *The science of the mind: 2001 and beyond* (pp. 144–169). Oxford, UK: Oxford University Press.

Turvey, M. T., & Shaw, R. E. (1999). Ecological foundations of cognition: I. Symmetry and specificity of animal-environment systems. *Journal of Consciousness Studies*, 6, 85–110.

Van Valen, L. (1973). A new evolutionary law. *Evolutionary Theory*, *1*, 1–30.

Yates, F. E., Marsh, D., & Iberall, A. S. (1972). Integration of the whole organism: A foundation for a theoretical biology. In J. A. Behnke (Ed.), *Challenging biological problems: Directions towards their solutions* (pp. 110–132). New York: Oxford University Press.

Zajonc, A. (1993). *Catching the light*. New York: Bantam Books.

Lecture 3

Direct Perceiving, Indirect Perceiving

In order to put our upcoming historical survey into perspective, we need to ask: "What should we expect of perceiving?" In addressing this question, key aspects of Lecture 2 will be elaborated.

A reasonable answer, considering what is required for the behaviors of living things at all scales, in all phyla (Turvey, 2013), is that perceiving must provide a reliable means for orienting and adjusting activity to the environment. Patently, perceiving is the basis for the practical success of everyday behavior. It is the basis for flying, swimming, running, jumping, climbing, intercepting, grasping, building, and so forth. When we are observing a dragonfly, chickadee, raccoon, or deer weaving or steering its way through the thickets of a Connecticut forest, and ask, "To what does its perceiving refer?", we should expect the answer, "That to which its activity refers." This is simply to say that we presume that the proper "objects" of perceiving are the same as those of activity (Gibson, 1979/1986; Turvey, Shaw, Reed & Mace, 1981). To be an "object" of activity is to be an aspect of the surroundings that entails activity. Examples might include "a stand on-able surface," "a fly through-able opening," "a cross over-able gap," and so on. Our expected answer, therefore, is that the perceiving of the dragonfly or chickadee or raccoon or deer refers to *activity-specific meanings* of the surroundings.

It would seem to go without mention that, for any activity to be realized the material properties of the organism and the material properties of the environment must fit. This mutuality in material design is the support for activity. For a deer, standing, walking and running are possible if and only if the ground surface can supply reactive forces complementary to those that the deer supplies. This mutuality, of course, is a matter of physics. For a deer to stand, to walk and to run, the mutuality cannot be compromised.

Consider the organism depicted in Figure 3.1. Standing still, walking and running are all relations between the organism and its supporting surface. As the preceding paragraph highlights, the supporting surface is as essential to posture and locomotion as are, for instance, the organism's legs. It also makes evident that, in order to control posture and locomotion, the organism must direct its perceiving toward that same surface (its perceiving must be

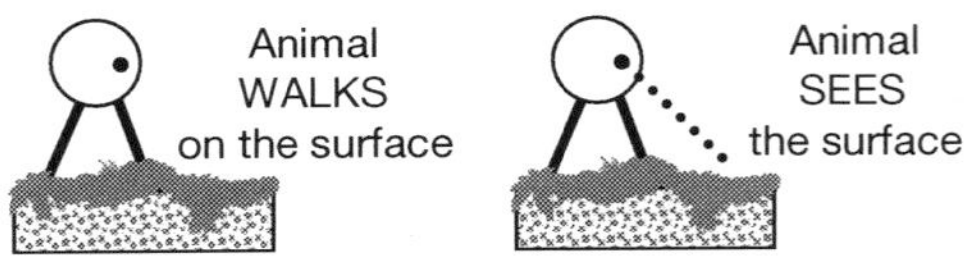

Figure 3.1 A reasonable hypothesis is that the proper "objects" of perceiving are the same as those of activity. For the depicted animal, a two-term relation involving the same surface exists in both cases. There is no other "object" between the animal and the surface. The two-term relation is all that is meant by *direct perception.*

(From Figure 6.1, Turvey, 2013, adapted with permission, MIT Press.)

about the walk on-able surface). Thus, it would seem that a two-term relation involving the same surface or ground can exist in both cases: the organism *walks* on the ground and the organism *perceives* the ground. This much should be common sense. There is no thing *between* the organism and the surface in the relation. This is what is meant by direct perception in Gibson's (1979/1986) ecological approach (Lombardo, 1987; Michaels & Carello, 1981; Turvey, Shaw, Reed & Mace, 1981); and, for future reference—when activity is under discussion—this is also what is meant by direct action (Reed, 1984). The organism in Figure 3.1 sees the relation between itself and the surface and acts by changing the relation between itself and the surface.

As we pursue the history of perceptual theorizing, it will become evident that the common-sense view of perception does not remain so in the face of philosophic and scientific analyses. Conceptual struggles with issues of causality and meaning force the introduction of other types of "objects." In this matter, visual perception has led the way. The objects introduced into the common-sense picture of visual perception conveyed in Figure 3.1 have included the retinal image, retinal patterns, sense data, ideas, percepts, and, most generally, representations. When perception is thought of as mental events, divorced from activity, there is encouragement to interpret an object of the preceding

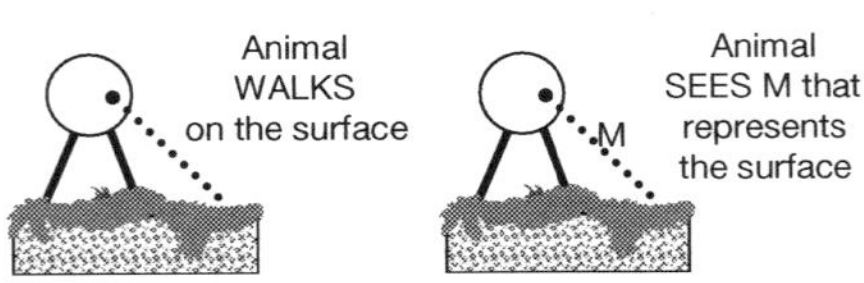

Figure 3.2 The reasonable hypothesis—that the proper "objects" of perceiving are the same as those of activity—has not fared well historically. A three-term relation is commonly proposed in the case of perceiving. For the depicted animal, there is another "object," a representation, between it and the surface. The three-term relation (here, animal to M to surface) is all that is meant by *indirect perception.*

(From Figure 6.1, Turvey, 2013, adapted with permission, MIT Press.)

kind as the object to which perception is directed, an object *between* the organism and the surface. This is portrayed in Figure 3.2. Perception as a two-term relation is replaced by perception as a three-term relation (e.g., Brown, 1992). In Figure 3.2, there is the organism, the surface and an in-between thing designated M.[1] The in-between thing M (for mediator) is a proximal surrogate for the surface (the epistemic mediation suggested in Lecture 2). The content of the organism's perception, what the perception is about, is the surrogate of the surface not the surface. In the simplest of terms, this three-term relation is what is meant by indirect perception.

The contrast between Figure 3.2 and Figure 3.1 can be expressed starkly (Shaw, Turvey, & Mace, 1982). Figure 3.2 is a depiction of perception as *true by force of argument*: perceiving is identified with an inferential conclusion (about perceiver and environment). Figure 3.1 is a depiction of perception as *true by force of existence*: Perceiving is identified with an existential fact (about perceiver and environment).[2]

In both Figures 3.1 and 3.2, we presume that the ground is real. By the use of "real" one typically means that the ground does not depend for its existence on the organism's perception of it. A fundamental question for philosophy is whether perception is metaphysically active or passive (e.g., Kelly, 1986). Does perception create or constitute its own objects, so that the environment perceived by an organism depends on the organism's act of perceiving? Or is the function of perceiving to acquaint an organism with the objects composing its environment as they exist independently of perceiving? In Figure 3.2, the in-between thing is clearly a very different thing from the ground on which the organism stands and walks. Unlike the ground, the in-between thing (at least in most of its incarnations) does depend on, is constituted in, the act of perceiving.

From the perspective of the student of perception and action, combining activity with perception-as-indirect would seem to create a dilemma. Although potentially real (e.g., it could be the retinal image, it could be isomorphic with a brain state), the in-between thing M of Figure 3.2 does not have the requisite physical properties to support standing, walking and running. Very crudely, organisms do not stand or run on images or ideas or representations. Nonetheless, the implication is that walking in Figure 3.2 is expressed, like perceiving, as a three-term relation. To preserve symmetry, the sentence "the organism perceives the surface's surrogate" must be paralleled by the sentence "the organism walks on the surface's surrogate." That, in a nutshell, is the dilemma. The dilemma is underscored by revisiting (from Lecture 1) the point of Brentano's (1874/1973) *direction upon an object*. An organism cannot want without wanting something, perceive without perceiving something, sit without sitting upon something, or walk without walking on something. The point, for Brentano, is that the object in the first two (mental) cases does not exist or need not exist unlike the object in the second two (physical) cases. Preserving the symmetry in Figure 3.2 would mean, contrary to Brentano's point, that a potentially nonexistent object is common to both perceiving and walking.

Historically speaking, the aforementioned dilemma has not figured in debates on theories of perception. The likely reason is because perception has been divorced from action along the lines that perception is of the mind and action is of the body. Tradition has it that whereas perception deals in mental entities, action deals in physical entities: perception is psychology, action is mechanics. For our present purposes, therefore, given our immediate goal of understanding the historical issues shaping theories of perception, we will delay considerations of action. We can achieve a great deal of progress by focusing upon the question: what would make a theory of perception a theory of *direct* perception?[3] What must be supposed about organisms or their environments or both that would permit a theorist to commit to the two-term relation: organism O perceives environment *E*?

3.1 The Information Hypothesis (or InformationL)

Introducing a third thing M between O and *E* suggests that O perceives *E* by means of M. O must do something with M in order to perceive *E* (for example, O might have to use M as a premise from which to infer something about *E*). But we should note that, whereas O's perception of *E* is indirect (via M), O's perception of M is direct. There is no term mediating O's perception of M. Of course, another thing could, in principle, be introduced, inserted between O and M. Then, M would be perceived *indirectly* and the new thing would be perceived *directly*. The important lesson to learn here is that any theory of indirect perception must include direct perception in some form. If it did not, then the mediating things would increase without end (Shaw & Bransford, 1977).

Clearly, therefore, what makes a theory of perception a theory of *direct* perception is not the assertion that there are things that can be directly perceived.[4] Rather, it is the precise assertion that *E* can be directly perceived. In order for that to be possible, there must be something available to O that specifies *E*. One could hypothesize, for example, that patterned energy distributions ambient to O are lawfully generated by properties of *E* and, under conditions to be defined, specific to *E*. Let us call this something *information* in the sense of *information about* (Gibson, 1966, 1979/1986). Better, let us give it the designation *informationL*[5] to distinguish it from the usage in communication theory (Shannon information[6]) and to highlight its grounding in lawful relations (*L*). The lawful relations referred to must be defined at the scale of organisms and their environments—what might be called the ecological scale. We can then say that what makes a theory of perception a theory of direct perception is the hypothesis that *perception is based on ecological information that is specific to its source: InformationL is specific to E*. It then follows that theories of perception that lack this information hypothesis are theories of indirect perception.

It should be clarified immediately that the hypothesis of informationL does not constitute a complete theory of perception. That is to say, the theory of direct perception would not be exhausted by the provision of detailed formal descriptions of informationL available to O. At this juncture, our concerns remain fairly modest and it suffices that we can identify a theory of direct perception as a theory whose distinguishing mark is the informationL hypothesis. Some hints as to what else will be required to fill out a theory of direct perception are provided below.

3.2 What Does a Theory of Direct Perception Negate?

What kind of thing is M? Above, we said that it was, basically, a kind of representation (which is, unfortunately, one of those loose terms anticipated in Lecture 1). Obviously, M is not E but it might be an image of E, or a sketch of E, or a sign of E, or any number of things that can stand for E and do so with greater or lesser thoroughness. Whatever M is precisely, it has to be worked upon by O in order to reveal what it conveys about E. For example, if M is a sign, then it has to be interpreted. The type of work suggested by "interpreting" is traditionally described as psychological in that it involves mental processes of memory, evaluation, judgment, decision and so on. (The modern inclination, of course, would be to describe this type of work as *computational.*) The auspices that this type of work is conducted under would also be described as psychological—for example, O interprets M while motivated to attain a certain goal or while in a particular emotional state. In sum, there is a great deal of psychology implied in a theory of indirect perception and the question should be raised as to what becomes of this psychology in a theory of direct perception.

The informationL hypothesis that distinguishes a perceptual theory as a theory of direct perception does not imply that there are no psychological factors in direct perception but it does imply an important limitation on what they can do: *They cannot alter informationL that is the basis of perception.* To begin with, informationL, grounded as it is in lawful relations at the ecological scale, is not the kind of thing that can be altered willfully. Second, if to the contrary psychological factors could affect informationL, then specificity would be compromised and perception could not be direct. In the three-term account of perception, we can envisage some of the various psychological factors as processing M—that is, treating its content or form as input and producing a different content or form as output. The informationL hypothesis negates such a transforming and producing role for psychological factors but it leaves plenty of room for considering how psychological factors might affect O's exploitation of informationL (for example, O can learn to exploit better, be motivated to exploit, and can exploit selectively; Gibson, 1966 1979/1986). And it makes room for alternatives (e.g., resonating, extracting, optimizing, and symmetricalizing) to the processing and producing metaphors (Gibson, 1966, 1979/1986).[7]

The psychology implied in a theory of indirect perception is primarily in the form of internal states of O. The aforementioned internal states are representations and processes that function as epistemic mediators and operations upon them. Echoing the question above, we should ask what becomes of internal states in a theory of perception as direct. Recalling Lecture 2, the general definition of a state is a specification of what a system is like at a given instant in time. The informationL hypothesis that distinguishes a perceptual theory as a theory of direct perception does not imply that application of Newton's formalism would fail to identify any internal states in an instance of direct perceiving. Any system that has internal DF (such as O) will have internal states in Newton's formalism. What the hypothesis does imply is that *the concept of internal state in an account of perception abiding Newton's formalism must be dissociated from the concept of internal representation.*[8] The difference between a theory of indirect perception and a theory of direct perception is, therefore, not that the former postulates internal states and the latter rejects them. Internal states in Newton's dynamical sense are necessarily aspects of both. In a theory of direct perception, the interpretation of internal states must be considered strictly in respect to informationL. If informationL is specific to its source, as asserted by the informationL hypothesis, then it is reasonable to suppose that perceptual systems evolved to register informationL. In registering informationL, O perceives *E*. So how should the internal (neurophysiological) states of O be interpreted? It is quite likely that providing a satisfactory answer to this question on route to comprehending direct perception will require a willingness to (a) think beyond the familiar linear causal chain and (b) abandon explanation of perception in literal and sensuous[9] terms. A willingness to renounce explanations in sensible form developed reluctantly in the history of science (Cassirer, 1950). It began and reached fruition first in theoretical physics. The challenges of quantum theory provided the final push. Consider Heisenberg on the atom (quoted by Cassirer, 1950):

> *All* its qualities are inferential: no material properties can be directly attributed to it—that is to say, any picture of the atom that our imagination is able to invent is for that very reason defective. An understanding of the atomic world in that primary sensuous fashion . . . is impossible
> (p. 117)

Let us become acquainted with accounts framed as causal chains. The theories of perception that we will encounter in these lectures are, with rare exceptions, modeled as such.

3.3 The Linear Causal Chain

The most common construal of (indirect) perception is the linear causal chain, an example of which is depicted in Figure 3.3. The depicted chain is composed of neurophysiological processes that are obviously in the head of O (when O is a member of the kingdom Animalia) with a mental state, an

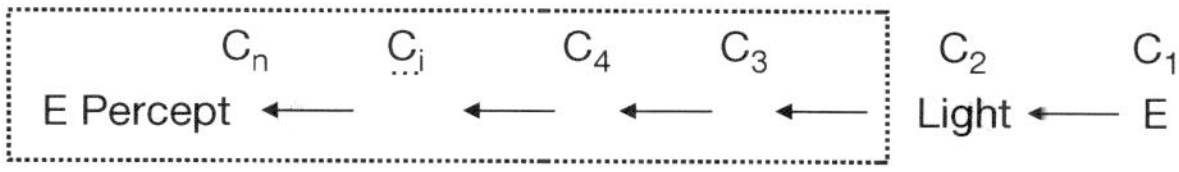

Figure 3.3 Perception depicted as a linear causal chain. Brain states (C_3-C_n) as efficient causes that produce the percept of the environment (*E*). Brain states reside in the organism as does the *E* percept.

E-percept, as the last link in the chain. This terminal link is also inside the head. A foremost expositor of the causal theory of perception, Bertrand Russell (1927/1954), made the observation that,

> Whoever accepts the causal theory of perception is compelled to conclude that percepts are in our heads, for they come at the end of a causal chain of physical events leading, spatially, from the object to the brain of the percipient.
>
> (p. 320)

The favored example of the causal chain is that of billiard balls transferring momentum: a moving ball strikes a second ball, which in turn strikes a third ball, and so on. The physical events in this example are sensible, discrete, and similar in kind. One obvious advantage of this example is that it provides an understanding of causality in "primary sensuous fashion." Recall from Lecture 2 that Newton equated causality with a sequence of state transitions. The contacts between balls, the exchanges of momentum, are the efficient causes (Lecture 2) that produce the effects—the motions of the balls—and also explain them. In the linear causal model of perception depicted in Figure 3.3, brain states are the nominated efficient causes that are presumed to produce and explain the *E*-percept. In Figure 3.3, each cause brings about a transition from an initial state to a new state in the manner defined by Equation 2.1 and each cause is external to the brain subsystem that it affects in the manner expressed in Figure 2.1. The ultimate brain-state (C_n) is the proximal efficient cause of the *E*-percept (or, alternatively, it is that state which is directly perceived).

The linear causal chain, though prominent in perceptual theory and in science more generally, is arguably a defective strategy of explanation. Given that claim, we should duly consider the reasons for the model's prominence. Hanson (1969) suggests that they are three in number: the mathematical-deductive method, the need to design experiments as chain-like as possible, and the successes of mechanical artifacts. Just as the premises and conclusions of a deduction are connected by a sequence of formal steps, so it was intuited by Galileo, and those whom he inspired (Lecture 5), that nature's phenomena were likewise constituted as a series of events, like links in a causal chain. It proved to be a persistent intuition: The causal chain has been consistently construed in perceptual theory as a hypostasis of logical inference. Turning to the second reason, the art of good experimentation is to squeeze a bunch of theoretical notions into a succinct hypothesis that is then tested in an experimental setting that keeps all things constant except the factors of relevance to the hypothesis. If done right, then one experiment leads to another, with circumstances contrived on each occasion to keep the "irrelevant" aspects of nature constant. The upshot is that the set of experiments submits to a summary in terms of "when this happens, that happens, and then . . ." implying a linear causal chain (even though the explanation of the results does not typically fit the mold). Finally, machines and other engineered devices are analogous to an ideal experiment in that they are constrained to operate with wide indifference to exterior conditions. Once started, they proceed in a series of steps and with an apparent single-mindedness that invites thinking about the persistent behavior of the stars, tides, and other natural phenomena in similar machine-like terms (Lecture 13).

Where is the linear causal chain defective? As an explanation of a phenomenon it gives the impression that the explanatory terms, the "causes," and the things to be explained, the "effects," are all at the same logical level, obscuring the fact that the explanatory language is, to the contrary, multi-leveled. A legitimate causal term is impregnated with theory, intelligible only in the context of a pattern of theoretical notions. The "cause x" and the "effect y" do not name links in a chain of events but point to interlocked conceptual structures that place guarantees on the inference from cause to effect. Hanson's (1969) position is that

> Questions about the nature of causation are to a surprising degree questions about how certain descriptive expressions, in definite contexts, coupled together, complement and interlock with a pattern of other expressions. (p. 62)

It is an assertion that linear causal chains are not so self-explanatory as they appear at first blush. What is explanatory is not the links in the chain, but the multiple hypotheses and theories that are the underpinning of the words used to designate the links (Bunge, 1979). Hanson (1969) ventures to claim that, metaphorically (see Figure 3.4, bottom right), causes may be "less like the links of a chain and more like the legs of a table" (p. 52).

The *chain links* or *sequence* analogy (versus the *table legs* or *support* analogy) may only be truly appropriate for accidental happenings, where genuine causal connections cannot be expressed, as in the famous accidental series beginning with "For want of a nail, a shoe was lost."[10] More generally, the linear causal chain—that is typically extracted from phenomena involving linkages among numerous factors (as depicted in Figure 3.4)—expresses a simplicity that is unreal. The strict causal chain does not exist and perfect isolation from surrounding influences is a theoretical myth. Together, however, the causal

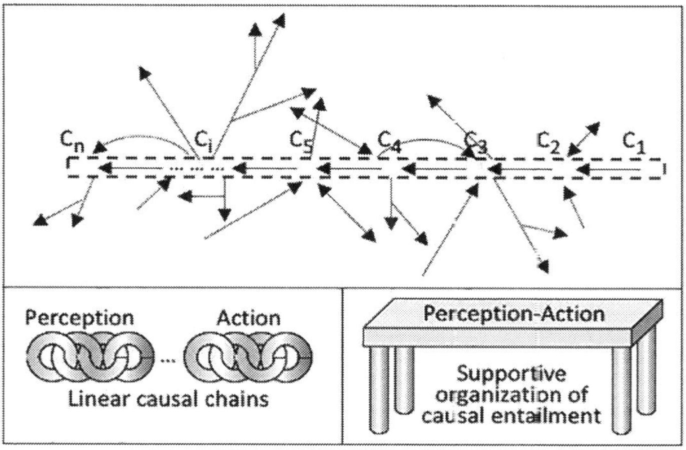

Figure 3.4 (*Top*) The fiction of the linear causal chain (*Bottom*) Isolating a single line of production in what is, factually, a dense network of causal entailments is an unavoidable scientific strategy. It means, however, that the chain is of questionable ontological status. At best, the linear causal chain is a useful fiction.

(Top: from Figure 14, Bunge, 1979, adapted with permission from Dover Publications.)
(Bottom: from Figure 7, Turvey, 2004, adapted with permission, Springer.)

chain and the experimental effort to isolate factors seem to be necessary aids to understanding.[11] They can provide, in limited contexts, an approximation of real "becoming" (Bunge, 1979). They do so, in all likelihood, because the time-evolution of events in reality bears some vague resemblance to a causal chain.

The defense of the linear causal chain on practical grounds does not, however, provide much help to its incarnation in Figure 3.3. There, that which the chain is supposed to *produce and explain* is the *E*-percept. Meaning (e.g., food, haven, or obstacle) is a property of the *E*-percept, the product of the chain of causes, but it is not obviously present in the causes, taken singly or in combination. Any aspirations we might have about hanging the *E*-percept on the same causal line as C_1 to C_n is thwarted by the fact that the *E*-percept is different in kind from the neurophysiological states and on a different theoretical level. The principles of scientific explanation that we hope to buy into by adopting the causal chain metaphor (whatever those principles might be) elude us when the metaphor is applied to perception.

The primary question at hand, of course, is how to refer to the internal states of O in a theory of direct perception. It is of no concern to such a theory that the linear causal model is defective. By definition, the model with one or more causal links as epistemic mediator of the *E*-percept is inappropriate at the outset. We can try to sketch a different picture from that of Figure 3.3, one that is better tailored to the demands of a theory of direct perception, keeping in mind the suggestion above that an explication of direct perception in "primary sensuous fashion" may well be impossible. Figure 3.5 is one such effort. It makes explicit the distinction in theoretical level between the epistemic act of perceiving *E* and registering informationL (Shaw & Bransford, 1977; Turvey, Shaw, Reed, & Mace, 1981). Whereas registering informationL is situated at O, perceiving *E* is a relation in the larger realm comprising O, *E* and informationL. Figure 3.5 portrays the internal states as supportive bases (along with informationL, *E*, and other supports not identified) simultaneous with the function "perceiving *E*" rather than efficient causes antecedent to the entity "*E*-percept" (Ben Zeev, 1983). In terms of the *CES* model (Lecture 1), the idea is that perceiving *E* is a function organized over C(O), *E*(O) and S(O) (see Figure 1.1 with *s* = O) sustained or maintained by the supportive bases. The causal image conveyed by the links of a chain is ideal for questions of the form "Why did the clock stop running?" But the causal image conveyed by the legs of a table is better for questions such as "Why does the clock keep running?" (It is even better for questions of the form "How does the clock keep time?") In respect to Figure 3.3, one construes perception in the spirit of the "stop running" question, as a state that starts and stops in response to momentary causal events. In respect to Figure 3.5, one construes perception in the spirit of the "keep running" question, as a continuous event sustained by an organization of causal entailments. James Gibson (1979/1986) thought about the act of registering or picking up informationL as

> a continuous act, an activity that is ceaseless and unbroken. The sea of energy in which we live flows and changes without sharp breaks. Even the tiny fraction of this energy that affects the receptors in the eyes, ears, nose, mouth, and skin is a flux, not a sequence. The exploring, orienting, and adjusting in these organs sink to a minimum during sleep but do not stop dead. Hence, perceiving is a stream, and William James's description of the stream of consciousness (1890, Ch. 9) applies to it. Discrete percepts, like discrete ideas, are "as mythical as the Jack of Spades."
>
> (p. 240)

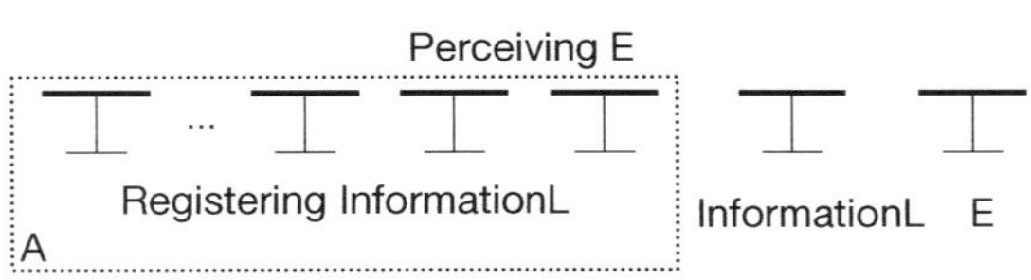

Figure 3.5 Brain states as one of the supportive bases (*legs-of-a-table* rather than *links-in-a-chain* image) of perceiving *E*. Brain states registering InformationL reside (obviously) in A but perceiving *E* does not. Perceiving *E* is a state of affairs of A and *E*; it is a relation in the system comprising A and *E*.

3.4 The Defining Question: "What is Specificity to a Source?"

We have been considering the question of what is required, fundamentally, to make a theory of perception a theory of direct perception. We have come to understand that the answer is not (a) the assumption that *something* is perceptible directly, or (b) the exclusion of psychological factors in perception, or (c) the denial of internal states. Rather, what makes a perceptual theory a theory of direct perception is the assertion of specificity. The position that psychological factors and internal states are not epistemic mediators does not define a theory of direct perception but follows as an implication of specificity. Figure 3.2 is distinguished from Figure 3.1 by the explicit inclusion of M as an entity mediating O's perception of the surface. Yet Figure 3.1 was discussed as a two-term relation that includes implicitly *information*—referred to as informationL and available to O—that is specific to its source. An important question to be addressed, therefore, is this: Why is informationL not an epistemic mediator? For what reasons should one not assume that informationL is that which is perceived directly (rather than *E*) analogous to the very traditional argument in the study of vision that the retinal image is that which is perceived directly (rather than *E*)? What prohibits the interpretation of informationL as another candidate M? Why should we not consider Figure 3.6 as reasonable?

The only retort available is that "Because of the *specificity* of informationL to *E* (the source of informationL) direct perception is of *E* not informationL." This sole retort can be stated more generally in the form of a contrast between representation and specification: Given O and *E*, *X* mediates *E* if it represents *E* to O but not if it specifies *E* to O. These retorts merely defer explaining why informationL is not an epistemic mediator. The desiderata are answers to very fundamental questions that are key to a theory of direct perception: *What is specificity to a source? What entails specificity to a source?*

It will help at this juncture to restore "activity" to our discussion. The minimal requirement for a theory of perception to be a theory of direct perception is the information hypothesis expressed thusly: informationL is specific to the *activity-related meanings* of *E*. What the minimal formulation

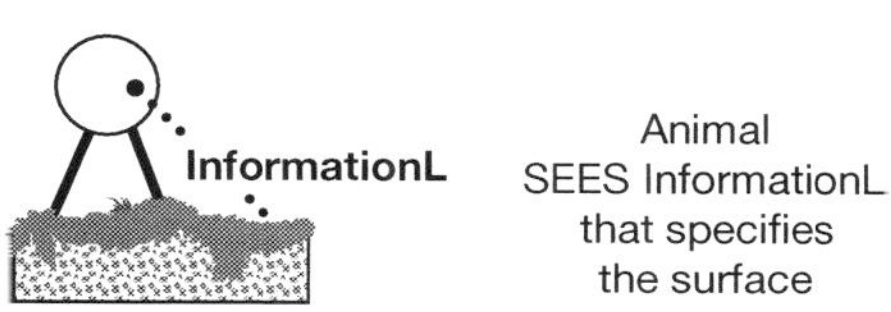

Figure 3.6 InformationL depicted as an epistemic mediator. What prohibits this depiction?

(Adapted from Figure 6.1 in Turvey, 2013, with permission from MIT Press.)

makes precise is that informationL is about meanings—that informationL is intentional and semantic. The questions of specification just posed, therefore, are closely tied to the questions of why some thing *X* can be about another thing *Y* and why some thing *Y* can mean something to another thing *Z*. These questions probe the system of entailments at the scale of living things and their environments. Consider the act of pointing with the index finger to indicate the whereabouts of something, for example, your cat. The intentionality of the pointing finger is that the finger's posture is about something else, namely the cat's whereabouts, not the finger itself. For the intentionality to be realized, the cat must be at the location indicated. But in addition to that, the cat that is referred to (pointed to) must be referred back to the finger that is doing the referring (the pointing). More formally, "*X* is about *Y*" is true only if *X* entails *Y* and *Y* entails *X* are true (Shaw, 2001). There is a closed loop of entailment. We can recognize *specificity* similarly as a closed entailment loop: specificity of *X* to its source *Y* means that *X* entails the source by which *X* is entailed. Stated succinctly in the terms particular to direct perception, *informationL is entailed by E and entails E.*

3.4.1 Impredicativity

Diagrammatically, an entailment (strict implication) can be expressed as X→Y. The primary property of an entailment is that it propagates "truth" hereditarily—Y inherits the "truth" of X (Rosen, 1991, 2000). If X is assumed to be "true" (whatever "true" might be in a given context), then it must likewise be the case that Y is true. Thus, a closed loop of entailment can be diagrammed as X→Y→X and it can be read as saying that truth propagates hereditarily in both directions. Entailments that are closed loop are impredicativities (a term coined by Poincaré; see Kline, 1980) and are counter to the vicious circle principle (Russell, 1903). An impredicative definition of a concept (or entity) is in terms of the totality to which it belongs (Figure 3.7). The following definition of Sue is an example: "Sue is the best ball-handler on her basketball team." In this example, the impredicative loop is that one must know the larger system (the totality of Sue plus teammates) to characterize the smaller system (Sue), but one cannot know the larger system in the absence of a characterization of the smaller system. The vicious circle principle is intended to filter out impredicativities. It disallows any whole that may contain parts that are definable only in terms of that whole. In system terms, it disallows consulting a larger system (a context) when attempting to understand a given system; only simpler subsystems can be invoked, in particular those whose defining properties and behaviors are context-free. The assumption motivating the principle is that any definition or description of a thing in a collection is suspect—not "objective"—if it relies on the use of the collection itself.

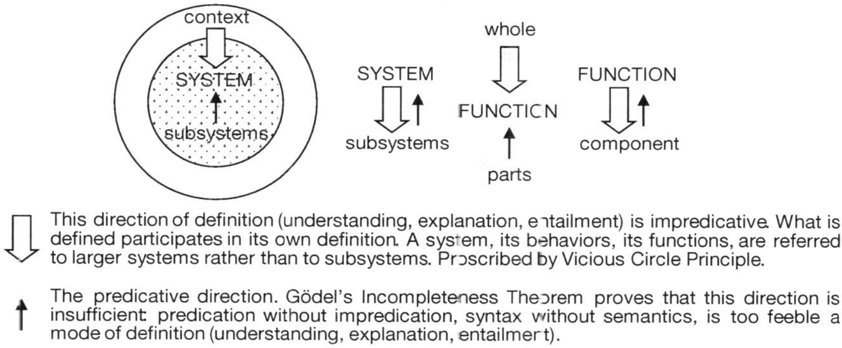

Figure 3.7 Concept of impredicativity.

(From Figure 6, Turvey, 2004, adapted with permission, Springer.)

The immediate goal of the vicious circle principle was to proscribe self-reference in the descriptions and definitions of systems and hence (given that referencing self is an instance of referencing in general) to proscribe semantics. In so doing, argued Russell (1903), all the paradoxes[12] that plagued logic and mathematics could be kept at bay. Consistent (paradox-free) formalisms, could be assured, Russell suggested, by replacing things with impredicative properties by things with predicative properties (those true of individual things only). We will encounter the full significance of the vicious circle principle and its far-reaching consequences in later lectures when we engage the conceptual developments associated with Hilbert, Gödel, and Turing, and the interpretation of perception and action in computational terms. For the time being, we defer to Rosen (1988, 1991, 2000): Complex systems (such as perception-action systems) have inherent impredicative loops.

3.4.2 Problem of Impoverished Entailment

Let us return to Figure 3.3. Causal entailment in the linear causal chain is strictly open (e.g., C_i to C_j) and never closed (e.g., C_i to C_j to C_i). It is strictly from parts to wholes and never from wholes to parts. Historically it has been the case—most certainly since Newton—that only open, parts-to-whole, causal links are "objective" (Rosen, 1991, 2000). Only open, parts-to-whole, causal links can be arrayed in a fixed time frame from this moment to the next. We can be assured that this temporal feature of open entailments has been a further enduring reason (see Section 3.4) for the prominence of the linear causal chain as the model of causality. Paralleling the open aspect of causal entailment in Figure 3.3 is that the entailment is restricted to a single mode: present states can only entail subsequent states. In regard to the primary focus of this lecture—the question of what makes a theory of perception a

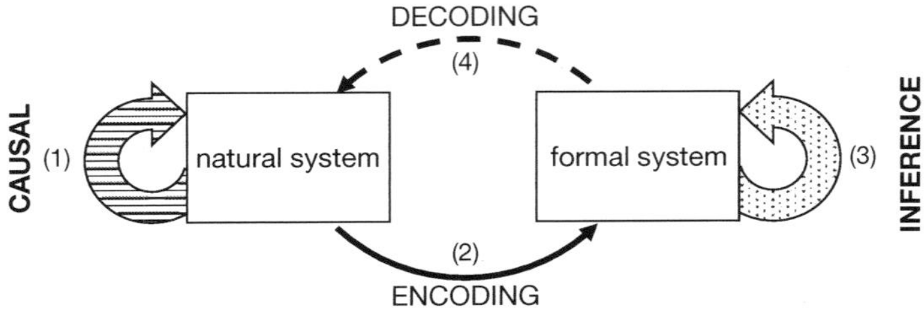

Figure 3.8 Modeling relation between causal entailment in a natural system and syntactic entailment in a formal system. There are two paths: (1) and (2) + (3) + (4). Path (1) is causal entailment in the natural system. In the second path, (2) encodes phenomena in the natural system to propositions in the formal system, (3) generates theorems entailed strictly by the propositions qua hypotheses, (4) decodes theorems as predictions about the natural system. The formal system is a model of the natural system if the same consequences (answers) are reachable by either path. The modeling relation may be viewed as an embodiment of the notion of *natural law.*

(From Figure 3H.2, Rosen, 1991, *Life itself*, adapted with permission, Columbia University Press.)

theory of direct perception—we can now recognize that the entailment structure of the conventional Newtonian framework is insufficiently rich to accommodate a theory of direct perception. We might call this the problem of impoverished entailment (Chemero & Turvey, 2007; Turvey, 2004).[13] A theory of perception is made into a theory of direct perception by the information hypothesis and as far as we can currently discern that hypothesis requires closed loops of causal entailment, the impredicativities that the Newtonian framework disallows.

So, what makes a theory of perception a theory of direct perception? The answer, at its most fundamental level, is an enriched entailment structure. Consider the modeling relation depicted in Figure 3.8 and consider it as embodying law at the ecological scale. Then, a theory of perception becomes a theory of direct perception when the modeling relation between the causal entailment and inferential entailment answers the question of "*Why informationL is specific to E?*" and in so doing the very general questions of "*What is specificity to a source?*" "*What entails specificity to a source?*"

Notes

1 For ease of depiction, M has been literally interposed in Figure 3.2 between the organism and the surface. Think of this M as the image of the surface on the retina.

2 The goal in these lectures on perception is less a matter of demonstrating that perception is direct and more a matter of (a) identifying what must be the case for it to be so, and (b) spelling out the consequences if it were so.

3 This question and the issues to be considered in arriving at an answer follow in significant degree from Reed (1980).
4 As we shall see, that something is perceived directly has been asserted many times in the historical development of theories of perception. Particularly noteworthy are the theories of Descartes (Lecture 6) and Helmholtz (Lecture 11).
5 The term is Millikan's (2000) but present usage follows Gibson's (1966, 1979/1986) more closely than that of Millikan.
6 Shannon information is based on the idea of a close, inverse relation between information and probability (P). It is generally defined as

$$\sum_{i=1}^{N_S} P_i \log\left(\frac{1}{P_i}\right)$$

where N_s is the number of possible states and i designates the individual state, hence P_i represents the entire ensemble of individual probabilities.
7 Although Gibson is likely to figure in most textbooks, his work is "routinely assimilated to theoretical positions he emphatically rejected, e.g., cue theory, stimulus-response psychology, and nativism" Costall & Morris, 2015, p. 1).
8 As Beer (1995) remarks, "But is the mere possession of internal state a sufficient condition for representation? Obviously not, since all physical systems possess internal state" (p. 126).
9 The usage of *sensuous* here is its first meaning: of or relating to the senses or sensible objects; suggesting pictures or images of sense. It is likewise the case for the usage of *sensible*: capable of being perceived by the senses; apprehensible through the sense organs.
10 It continues as follows: "for want of a horse a rider was lost; for want of a rider a battalion was lost; for want of a battalion a battle was lost; for want of a victory a kingdom was lost—all for want of a nail." The lyric suggests a multiplicative (not additive) relation among interdependent (not independent) events.
11 Any scientific experiment is based on the assumption that the studied system can be isolated in some respects and to some reasonable degree from extra-system factors. The necessary working assumption is that the things composing the universe are partially not fully interconnected.
12 The most well-known non-mathematical paradox is the Liar Paradox. Consider statements such as "This sentence is false" or "I am lying." Denote the former statement as S. If S is true, then what it asserts is true, and so S is false. If S is false, then this is what it asserts, and so S is true. A famous mathematical paradox is Russell's paradox of classes. Consider *N*, the class of all classes that do not belong to themselves. (A class of ideas is an idea but a class of books is not a book.) Where does *N* belong? If *N* belongs to *N*, it should not by the definition of *N*. If *N* does not belong to *N*, it should by the definition of *N* (Kline, 1980; see Barwise & Etchemendy, 1987).
13 Indirect theories of perception are often introduced as mandated by the *problem of impoverished stimuli.*

References

Barwise, J., & Etchemendy, J. (1987). *The liar: An essay on truth and circularity*. New York: Oxford University Press.

Beer, R. (1995). Computational and dynamical languages for autonomous agents. In R. F. Port & T. Van Gelder (Eds.), *Mind as motion* (pp. 121–147). Cambridge, MA: MIT Press.

Ben Zeev, A. (1983). Toward a different approach to perception. *International Philosophical Quarterly*, *23*, 45–64.

Brentano, F. (1973). *Psychology from an empirical standpoint*. London: Routledge & Kegan Paul (original work published 1874).

Brown, H. (1992). Direct realism, indirect realism and epistemology. *Philosophy and Phenomenological Research*, *52*, 341–363.

Bunge, M. (1979). *Ontology II: A world of systems*. Dordrecht, Netherlands: D. Reidel.

Cassirer, E. (1950). *The problem of knowledge*. New Haven, CT: Yale University Press.

Chemero, A., & Turvey, M. T. (2007). Complexity, hypersets, and the ecological approach to perception-action. *Biological Theory*, *2*, 23–36.

Costall, A., & Morris, P. (2015). The textbook Gibson: The assimilation of dissidence. *History of Psychology*, *18*, 1–14.

Gibson, J. J. (1966). *The senses considered as perceptual systems*. Boston, MA: Houghton Mifflin.

Gibson, J. J. (1986). *The ecological approach to visual perception*. Mahwah, NJ: Erlbaum (original work published 1979).

Hanson R. N. (1969). *Patterns of discovery*. Cambridge, UK: Cambridge University Press.

James, W. (1983). *The principles of psychology*. Cambridge, UK: Cambridge University Press (original work published 1890).

Kelly, D. (1986). *The evidence of the senses*. Baton Rouge: Louisiana State University Press.

Kline, M. (1980). *Mathematics: The loss of certainty*. New York: Oxford University Press.

Lombardo, T. (1987). *The reciprocity of perceiver and environment: The evolution of James J. Gibson's ecological psychology*. Hillsdale, NJ: Erlbaum.

Michaels, C. F., & Carello, C. (1981). *Direct perception*. Englewood Cliffs, NJ: Prentice-Hall.

Millikan, R. (2000). *On clear and confused ideas*. Cambridge, UK: Cambridge University Press.

Reed, E. S. (1980). *What is direct perception?* Unpublished manuscript, Center for Research in Human Learning, University of Minnesota.

Reed, E. S. (1984). From action gestalts to direct action. In H. T. A. Whiting (Ed.), *Human motor actions: Bernstein revisited* (pp. 157–168). Amsterdam, Netherlands: Elsevier.

Rosen, R. (1988). The epistemology of complexity. In J. A. S. Kelso, A. J. Mandell, & M. F. Shlesinger (Eds.), *Dynamic patterns in complex systems* (pp. 7–29). Singapore: World Scientific.

Rosen, R. (1991). *Life itself*. New York: Columbia University Press.

Rosen, R. (2000). *Essays on life itself*. New York: Columbia University Press.

Russell, B. (1903). *Principles of mathematics*. Cambridge, UK: Cambridge University Press.

Russell, B. (1954). *The analysis of matter*. New York: Dover (original work published 1927).

Shaw, R. E. (2001). Process, acts, and experiences: Three stances on the problem of intentionality. *Ecological Psychology*, *13*, 275–314.

Shaw, R. E., & Bransford, J. (1977). Introduction: Psychological approaches to the problem of knowledge. In R. E. Shaw & J. Bransford (Eds.), *Perceiving, acting and knowing* (pp. 1–39). Hillsdale, NJ: Erlbaum.

Shaw, R. E., Turvey, M. T., & Mace, W. M. (1982). Ecological psychology: The consequence of a commitment to realism. In W. Weimer & D. Palermo (Eds.), *Cognition and the symbolic processes II* (pp. 159–226) Hillsdale, NJ: Erlbaum.

Turvey, M. T. (2004). Impredicativity, dynamics and the perception-action divide. In V.K. Jirsa & J. A. S. Kelso (Eds.), *Coordination dynamics: Issues and trends* (pp. 1–20). Berlin, Germany: Springer Verlag.

Turvey, M. T. (2013). Ecological perspective on perception-action: What kind of science does it entail? In W. Prinz, M. Beisert, & A. Herwig (Eds.), *Action science: Foundations of an emerging discipline* (pp. 139–170). Cambridge, MA: MIT Press.

Turvey, M. T., Shaw, R. E., Reed, E. S., & Mace, W. M. (1981). Ecological laws of perceiving and acting: In reply to Fodor and Pylyshyn (1981). *Cognition*, 9, 237–304.

Lecture 4

Simulative, Projective, and Locality Assumptions

Two questions with a very long history are the departure point for Lecture 4: (1) What illuminates objects so that the mind can experience them? (2) How can illuminated objects at a distance bring about an experience in the mind, localized as it is in the perceiver? Somewhat surprisingly, our efforts to answer them bring us to the forefront of contemporary science.

4.1 The Simulative and Projective Assumptions

An early influential answer to the first question was that light radiating from the sun and light emanating from the eyes, an "outer" and an "inner" light, combined to produce the conditions for vision. The concept of *emanation* is thought to have originated in the 6th century before the current or common era (BCE) with Pythagoras (Ronchi, 1957, 1967). It was championed by Plato and Euclid and would affect theorizing about visual perception for 1,500 years (Zajonc, 1993).

Emanation theory (Figures 4.1a and b) itself identified two phases necessary to the visual perception of an object. In combination, the two phases satisfied the consensus opinion of the time that there could be no "action at a distance" (Lombardo, 1987). First, the rays of light from the eyes contacted the object and, in consequence of this contact, took on the object's form. Second, these impressed forms were returned to the eyes, contacted the eyes and, in turn, contacted the mind of the perceiver. Obviously, integral to emanation theory was the assumption that all causes are local or, similarly, all cause is by contact. This is the *principle of nearby action* (Bunge, 1977, 1979). Given two things, *A* and *B*, *A* must make physical contact with *B* at some moment in time, that is, be contiguous with *B*, if *A* is to cause a change in *B*.

Euclid's contribution to emanation theory was to clarify mathematically the nature of the light as it proceeds from the eye to the object. It was, he suggested, describable rather simply as points and lines. A ray of light was the line that connected one point—say, at the eye—to another point—for example, one belonging to the facing surface of a distal object. The set of rays connecting the apex at the eye with the points composing the edge or base contour of the object formed a visual cone or, better, given that the object need not be circular, a visual solid angle (Gibson, 1979/1986). Euclid was laying the groundwork for geometrical projection as the possible foundation of visual perception (Lombardo, 1987). Laws of perspective for objects were implicated: The solid angle decreases with object distance and is laterally compressed as the object is tilted or turned. Visual hypotheses suggested themselves: if the lengths of visual rays were measurable, then object distance was, in principle, knowable (Ronchi, 1957).

Major elements of emanation theory were brought into sharp focus by the opposing view of the atomists of the 5th century BCE. For Democritus and Leucippus, physical objects, as material complexes of atoms, issue effluxes of finer atoms composing eidola (idols, images) or simulacra (simulations; Figure 4.1c). They do so continuously and independently of perceivers. These faint images that simulate their source objects in the world could, on contacting the eyes, transmit their shapes to the mind's atoms by means of nearest-neighbor interactions of the body's atoms.[1]

The *eidola theory* addressed the physical basis for vision through the principle of nearby action and the *simulative assumption*. This assumption is that the starting point for vision is a simulation (copy, replica, simulacrum) of the environment (Boring, 1950; Lombardo, 1987). With the emphasis upon light (as in emanation theory), rather than on atoms (as in eidola theory), the simulative assumption addresses the essential question of "What is the optical support for vision?" The answer, simply, is "replicas or copies contained in the light of things in the environment." A closely allied assumption, implicit in

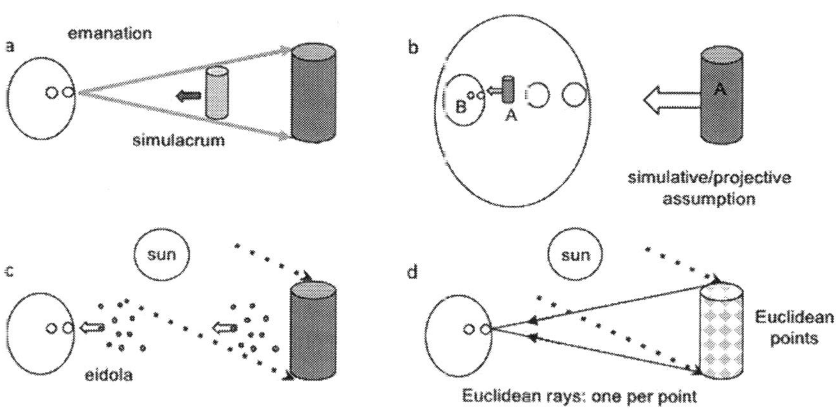

Figure 4.1 (a) and (b) The emanation theory of Pythagoras, Euclid and Plato and the principle of nearby action. (c) The eidolon theory of Democritus and Leucippus. (d) A single theory combining the mathematical (emanation) and physical (eidolon) approaches as advanced by Alhazan.

(From Figures 1 and 2, Turvey, 2015, adapted with permission, Imprint Academic.)

the simulative assumption but worthy of its own identity, addresses the question of what happens to these simulations of the environment. The answer is that they are projected or sent into the mind. This should be called the *simulative, projective or intromittent assumption* (Figure 4.1b). This latter assumption incorporates the principle of nearby action, an inner causal chain, and implicates, in addition, a final step analogous to an act of inner observation. Together, the simulative and projective assumptions of the ancient Greeks compose a causal theory of perception and the hypothesis of an internal agent (a human analogue or homunculus). It is not an exaggeration to say that the working premises of modern investigators of perception are, for the most part, these assumptions made 2,500 years ago. Without a significant loss of understanding, the history of the core concepts underpinning the science of visual perception could stop here.

4.2 Alhazen

The adding of scientific detail began most notably around the cusp of the 10th and the 11th centuries with the Arabic scholar Abu Ali al-Hasan ibn al-Haytham, known historically by his Latin name Alhazen (Crombie, 1964). To begin with, there was the matter of light proceeding from the eye. That this conception was still prominent at the time of Alhazen owes much to the prestige of two of its major proponents, Plato and Euclid. Despite his sophisticated geometric treatment of light, Euclid nonetheless adhered to the emanation of visual rays, with apex at the eye, as primary to the visual process. One line of defense was the everyday failure to see things even when looking at them (Zajonc, 1993). Euclid suggests that you should drop a needle on the ground and then wonder why you cannot see it. Given that the needle is illuminated by the sun, and that your field of view encompasses the needle, then the needle's simulacrum ought to be available to the eyes. Yet the needle remains non-visible suggesting that illumination by external light does not suffice for sight. The needle only comes into sight, argued Euclid, when struck by the rays emanating from your eyes. Alhazen would advance a series of logical arguments[2] and conduct a variety of experiments to prove the contrary. He established that sight was based not partly but wholly on external light (Howard, 1996; Lindberg, 1976, 1992; Lombardo, 1987). With this latter conclusion at hand, he proceeded to craft a new version of the eidolon theory that appropriated the visual cone of the emanation theory and, thereby, its mathematical power (Figure 4.1d). That is, he united the physical and mathematical approaches to vision in a single theory (e.g., Lindberg, 1992). Other issues followed from the unification with significant psychological consequence. In respect to the simulative assumption, how good were the simulations? In respect to the projective assumption, what did inner observation entail? Although Alhazen did not address them as such, his answers to these questions, and how he garnered them, were to have extended significance.

He conducted experiments with a dark chamber into which light entered through a small hole (Figure 4.2). Inside the chamber, Alhazen could see an outside scene fully imaged on the wall opposite to the tiny aperture. Its details, however, were upside down and in reverse order. Moreover, the imaged scene changed in size with the distance of the outside scene. Alhazen was experimenting with the *camera obscura*, the forerunner of the modern-day pinhole camera (Hammond, 1981). It permitted him to establish that light traveled in straight lines[3] and that its physics was approachable in the elemental terms of discrete rays connecting discrete points. His thinking followed that of Al-kindi in the 9th century (Islam's first philosopher). Al-kindi had encouraged a thorough-going development of the pointillism implicit in Euclid's treatment of light. For Alhazen, the copies carried by the light to the eye were not environmental forms as such but the collection of points that composed them. The eye was not so much a recipient of images (eidola) but, rather, the recipient of rays from which images could then be formed.

The properties of these images and, therefore, the copies implied by the simulative assumption were suggested by the images of the camera obscura: flat, reversed, inverted[4] and ambiguous. If such were the case, the intromittent copies, the starting point for vision, were less than ideal. Inner observation, Alhazen presumed, could not be a passive inspection of an internal image of the environment. It would have to be more similar to an intellectual act, such

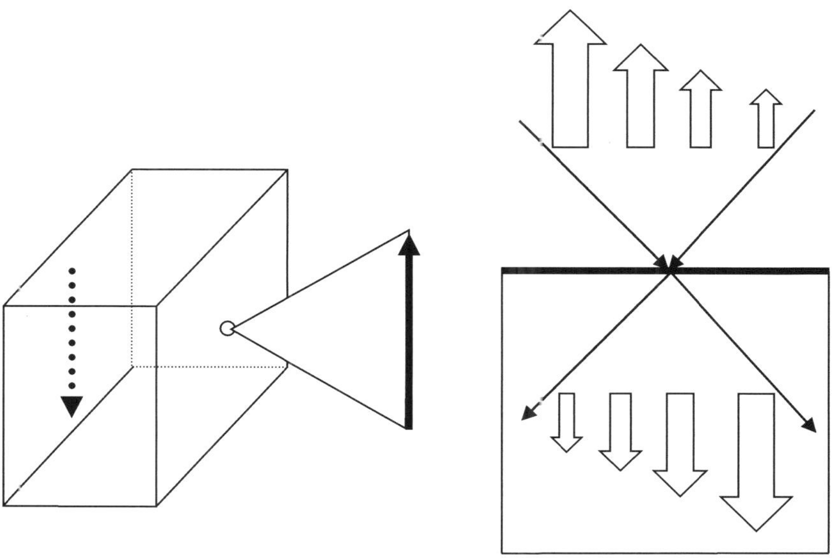

Figure 4.2 Alhazen's *camera obscura*. (*Left*) The up-down inversion of light reflected from an arrow projected through a peep hole of an enclosure. (*Right*) The left–right inversion of several spaced arrows.

as inference, that occurred at speed and without awareness (Howard, 1996; Sabra, 1989). Alhazen's elaboration of the inner observation entailed by the projective assumption was in keeping with Plato's antithesis of body and mind. Alhazen departed from Plato, however, in assuming that this interpretation was based in past experience rather than inherent knowledge.

4.3 Innateness and Properties

C. 380 BCE, Plato provided the original explicit defense of innate knowledge through a learning paradox that has come to be known as "Plato's Problem" (e.g., Landauer & Dumais, 1997; Weimer, 1973). The learning paradox is often discussed in terms of the "Poverty of the Stimulus" argument (e.g., Chomsky, 1965) and is closely linked to the "Problem of Induction" or the "Problem of Projectible Predicates" (e.g., Goodman, 1965). All of these will be discussed in good time. For the present we note that the paradox, roughly speaking, is that a person's knowledge about *X* outstrips or transcends his or her experience with *X*. Language learning provides the prototypical example. For any language, the grammatical rules involve abstract categories and classifications that are ostensibly far removed from the evidential base provided to the child in the form of specific utterances. The rapid (relatively speaking) and complete acquisition of the grammar seem to point to the pre-existence of a set of likely hypotheses about what classes of rules are probable and which are improbable. Plato saw the general resolution of the learning paradox in terms of a process by which episodic experiences unfold universal pre-existing forms. The philosophical framework within which resides this proposed resolution, this innate-ness of knowledge, has had broad appeal over the ages. Conventional perceptual theory bears its imprint.

Plato advanced two different epistemologies (systems of knowledge), each with its own ontology (theory of reality) (see Figure 4.3). Perception, based in the physical senses, was for Plato the source of mere "opinion"

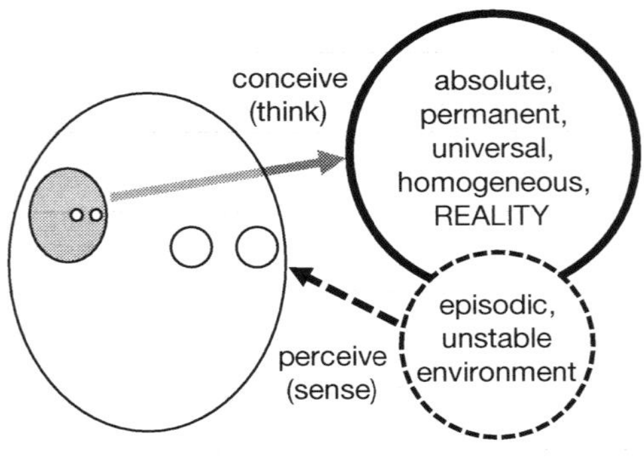

Figure 4.3 Plato's two ontologies and two epistemologies.

about the episodic and unstable conditions of the environment. Reason, embodying abstract and eternal truths, assigned interpretations to the outputs of the senses. By means of reason, an absolute, permanent, universal and homogeneous reality is detected. Humans perceive (sense) the changing facts of phenomenal existence, but conceive (think) the principles of reality. Hence, two distinct ways of knowing are identified corresponding to two different worlds to be known.

The latter of the two ontologies, the world revealed by reasoning but not by perceiving, is the realm of properties. For Plato, properties exist in ideal forms, separate from and external to matter. These Platonic Ideals, the forms of true reality, are transcendent: They are non-sensory and immaterial and, thereby, are beyond the limits of ordinary experience. As universals, these incorporeal forms precede matter; they become realized in, or exemplified by, particular material things. In other words, there are universal properties that are "thing-less" and there are particular things in the world that are "property-less" (or "bare") in which these abstract universal properties become instantiated (Loux, 1970). Plato's doctrine of properties is realized in his perceptual theory as an opposition between abstract and concrete. Paraphrasing the description above, abstractions are restricted to the intellect and reason—that is, the mind; in contrast, the presentations of the body's senses are, as it were, bare particulars (Lombardo, 1987).

By Plato's insistence, leading ontological questions concern properties: How real are properties and what is their relation to the individual things that compose the world? The contemporary student of perception and action will encounter three major opinions as to how these questions are to be answered. Fortunately, they submit to a simple classification.

- *Properties without things*. Plato's view, as we have just seen, is that properties are the ultimate reality and that the individual things that make up the clutter of the environment only exemplify them. Individual things serve as the carriers of universal properties.
- *Things without properties*. This is the very opposite of Plato's view. Sometimes referred to as nominalism, it regards properties as conceptual (intensional) and not real. The claim is that there are only individual things composing the world—that is, only individual things are real, and that any given property is no more than a name (hence the label "nominalism") or concept attached to a set of particular things. A property is identical with its extension—for example, *stand on-able* is identical with *all surfaces and objects that can support the upright posture of a given animal*. The mental conjunction of attributes associated with *stand on-able* is the intension of *stand on-able*. Intension determines extension; or, mind ascribes properties.
- *Things with properties*. This view opposes both Platonism and nominalism. In respect to its anti-Platonism it follows the argument of William of

Ockham[5] in the 14th century that properties should not be detached from particulars—for example, one should discuss and analyze perceiving, thinking, acting things rather than the detached abstraction "mind." Likewise, one should discuss and analyze living things rather than the detached abstraction "life." It is then a small step to the claim that neither properties nor individual things are real independently of each other. Arguably, this is the ontological position that most readily conforms to the assumptions of most working scientists (Bunge, 1977): there are only propertied things.

4.4 Principle of Local Causality

To bring closure to our select discussion of the origins of the simulative and projective assumptions, and to set the stage for subsequent developments, we would be well served by reflecting further on the matter of action at a distance. This hypothesis, so distasteful to the early perceptual theorists, will be regarded with even greater disdain by the scholars of the 17th century—the founding fathers of the mechanistic approach to perception and action. Here, we trace the evolution of the discourse on the necessity of contact and catch a glimpse of current thinking on what persists as one of the most central ontological issues.

Consider two distinct things, A and *B*, at two different places (Figure 4.4). Logic allows that A can act upon *B* directly, the principle of action at a distance, or that A can act upon *B* through a third thing C that is intermediate between A and *B*, the principle of nearby action. For either case, A's effect on *B* could occur instantaneously or after some delay. Ancient Greek scholars, for the most part, presumed that action by contact was the more logical than action without contact. They also presumed, for the most part, that cause antecedent to effect was more logical than cause simultaneous with effect—that is, they presumed what Bunge (1977, 1979) has referred to as the *principle of antecedence*.

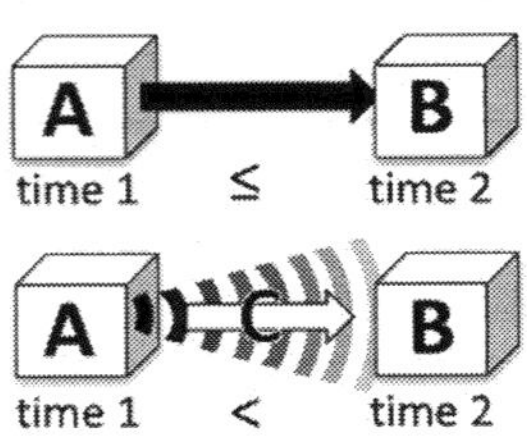

Figure 4.4 (*Top*) Action at a distance, with or without antecedence: Thing A acts directly upon thing *B* instantaneously or at some delay. (*Bottom*) Nearby action with antecedence: Thing A acts upon thing *B* through thing C with some delay.

Despite its logically inferior status, the principle of action at a distance was enshrined in Newton's inverse square law of gravity and, a century later, in Coulomb's inverse square law of electric forces. Ambiguity in regard to the action principles of Newton and Coulomb was dissolved in the 19th century with the development of the field concept. As Faraday and Maxwell conceived it, *A* exerts an influence on all surrounding space (*C* in Figure 4.4), with the force on *B* being exerted directly by the condition of space at the point of *B*'s position (Maxwell, 1890; see Lecture 14). That condition in the case of the electric field, for example, varies as the inverse square of the distance between *A* and *B*.

Ambiguity in regard to the antecedence principle was dissolved to the satisfaction of most scientists of the early 20th century by (a) the success of field theories, (b) the determination that physical actions are propagated with finite velocities (light travels at a constant non-zero speed), and (c) the related development of Einstein's relativistic physics. Special relativity identifies the restriction that the antecedence principle imposes on the interaction of *A* and *B*. In space-time, *A* cannot affect *B* if *A* cannot be tied to *B* by the fastest (known) chain of events (light) (Bunge, 1979). In relativistic physics, separation defined only in spatial terms is insufficient. The coordinates pinpointing *A* and *B* are space-time coordinates.

The resolution of these ambiguities for known physical actions yields the *principle of local causality*: No instantaneous action at a distance; or, every action of *A* on *B* satisfies both the principle of antecedence and the principle of nearby action (Bunge, 1977). Locality is the keystone of science, passé and contemporary. If locality did not hold, then past and future would contaminate the present. If locality did not hold, then no system or system component could be disengaged from the rest of the universe.

4.5 Nonlocality

At the present time, a particular experiment (the Einstein–Podolsky–Rosen or EPR experiment) and its falsification of a particular theorem (Bell's theorem) imply *nonlocality*. The motivation for the experiment and the theorem is quantum mechanics. Whereas an apparently sound working assumption for science, from its earliest beginnings to the present, would be that to measure something is to gain knowledge about a preexisting state, quantum mechanics teaches that some things have no specific states until they are measured. The lesson of quantum mechanics is not that measuring can affect things that are measured—that is, the lesson is not that measuring perturbs a particular thing from a definite but unknown state (that it happens to be in) to some other state. Rather, quantum mechanics teaches that measurement gives definition to a thing's quantities that were indefinite prior to measurement. A previously indeterminate thing is forced (as it were) by measurement to assume a definite appearance (Lindley, 1996).

Experiments by Stern and Gerlach in 1922 make explicit what is at issue. The essential format and results of these experiments are shown in Figure 4.5. Stern and Gerlach sent a beam of atoms through a magnetic field (see Lecture 14) produced, for example, by a larger magnet positioned above a smaller magnet. The atoms themselves can be thought of as extremely tiny magnets that will be pulled upward or pushed downward depending on the degree to which their poles are aligned with the north–south direction of the magnetic field (on the principle that like poles repel, unlike poles attract). Now if the atoms are randomly oriented on entering the magnetic field, *that is, have preexisting states*, then they should also be oriented randomly when leaving the magnetic field, albeit with each individual atom oriented differently when exiting than when entering. To the contrary, Stern and Gerlach found that the atoms exited either parallel or anti-parallel to the magnetic field (right Figure 4.5). They found that this restriction to two possible outcomes held whether the magnetic field was vertical or horizontal or, for that matter, at any inclination in between.

Two major generalizations follow from experiments of the kind conducted by Stern and Gerlach. The first is that the definition of something's (real) nature requires not only a description of the something under study, but it also requires, in equal degree, a description of the measurement that is made on it. The second is that it is improper to suggest what that nature might be prior to the making of the measurement. Thus, in the left panel of Figure 4.5 it was improper to assume that the atoms were, initially, randomly aligned, a mistake that is rectified in the right panel (by introducing question marks).

We can come to terms with another major feature of quantum physics (implicit in our discussion thus far) by a simple extension of the experiment depicted in Figure 4.5. In rough-and-ready terms, an electron is a spinning top with spin restricted to up or down relative to an external magnetic field (Figure 4.6). Now, let us send a beam of electrons through two Stern–Gerlach magnets in succession as shown in Figure 4.7. The first is oriented vertically and the second is oriented either vertically or horizontally. As above, the vertical Stern–Gerlach magnet will split the beam into "ups" and "downs." Focusing on the "up" electrons, think of them (again) as tiny bar magnets aligned parallel to the device's magnetic field. If now passed selectively through

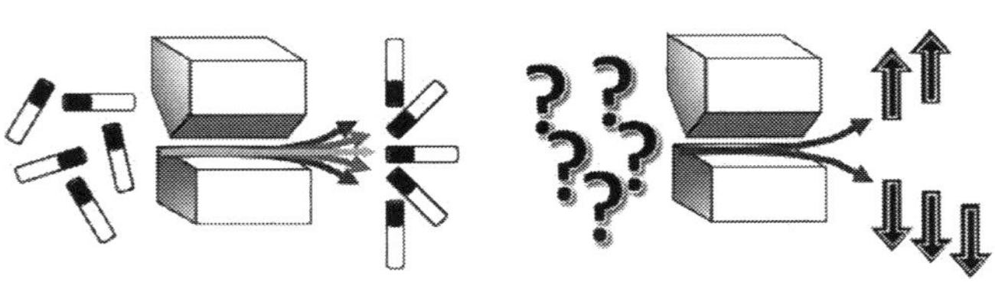

Figure 4.5 The basic Stern and Gerlach experiment.

(From Figure 1, Lindley, 1996, *Where does all the weirdness go?* Adapted with permission, Artellus.)

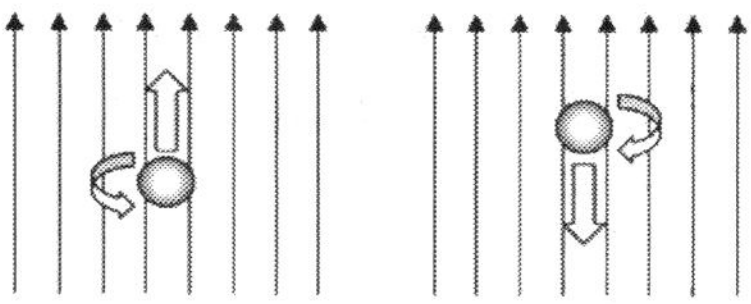

Figure 4.6 Along a given spatial direction, the measured spin of an electron can have only two values: spin "up" (parallel to magnetic field), spin "down" (anti-parallel to magnetic field).

a second vertical Stern–Gerlach magnet, these vertical "up" electrons should (we might intuit) get a further nudge to align parallel and should exit the second device in the same alignment as they entered. These vertical "ups" should not split into "ups" and "downs." Indeed, experiments show that electrons that are defined as "up" by the first measurement stay "up" (top Figure 4.7). The surprising fact is that for a given electron that is definitely "up" on exiting the vertical Stern–Gerlach device, its status in terms of "up" and "down" prior to entering the horizontal Stern–Gerlach magnet is indeterminate. An "up" electron passing through the horizontal device will come out as either "left" or "right" with 50–50 probability.

Let us dwell on this latter observation. We might suppose (mistakenly, improperly) that an "up" electron exiting the vertical magnet possesses just this definite parallel orientation to the magnetic field (Figure 4.7) prior to entering the horizontal magnet and should pass through the horizontal magnet

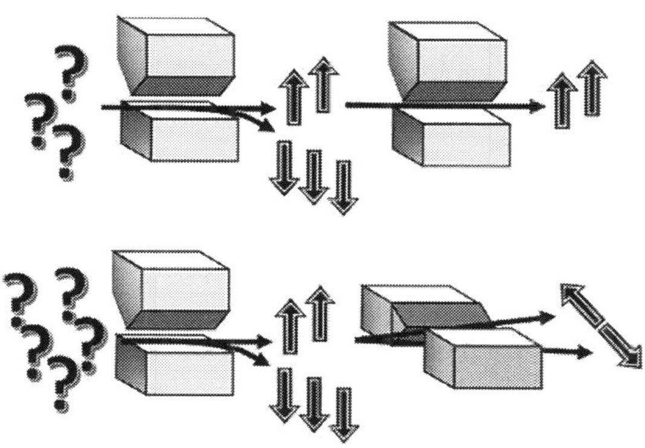

Figure 4.7 Stern–Gerlach magnets with a means of selectively passing "up" electrons from the first to the second magnet. (*Above*) Each magnet stack is vertical; (*below*) the first is vertical and the second is horizontal. An electron's "up" status is retained 100 percent in the above setting but changed (from vertical to horizontal) in the setting below

(From Figure 2, Lindley, 1996, *Where does all the weirdness go?* Adapted with permission, Artellus.)

with its "up" status intact. We are assuming the obvious: having just measured the electron's spin we know its state exactly and, therefore, can predict the outcome of future measurements. But our assumption is wrong for the very fundamental reason identified above. The electron is in a definite state only with respect to the measurement by a vertical Stern–Gerlach magnet. In respect to the upcoming measurement by the second and horizontal Stern–Gerlach magnet the state of the electron is as indefinite as it was prior to the first measurement. "Definite" and "indefinite" are relative designations, not absolute. They are relative to the specific measurement being made.

In a nutshell, Figure 4.7 depicts the *uncertainty principle*. Despite having obtained a measure of one property of the electron (its spin relative to a vertical magnetic field) we remain completely in the dark, completely uncertain, about another closely related property of the electron (its spin relative to a horizontal magnetic field). The uncertainty principle is a very general feature of quantum mechanics. The traditional exposition in terms of the inability to measure a particle's position and velocity simultaneously captures but one instance; it does not exhaust the principle's scope. The uncertainty principle is simply an expression of the fact that the nature of a thing in quantum physics is defined by the system composed of the thing and the measure performed upon it. A thing is defined in terms of the whole of which it is a part. Referring to Figure 3.7, it is defined *impredicatively* (Lecture 3) and, therefore, its definition is context dependent. Change the whole of which the thing is a part—that is, change the meter—and the thing's nature changes. System *P* composed of a position meter and a thing with no particular properties is different from System *V* composed of a velocity meter and a thing (the same thing) with no particular properties (Figure 4.8). Consequently, the propertied thing defined impredicatively by *P* is not the same propertied thing as that defined impredicatively by *V*. The *P*-measure that yields a definite

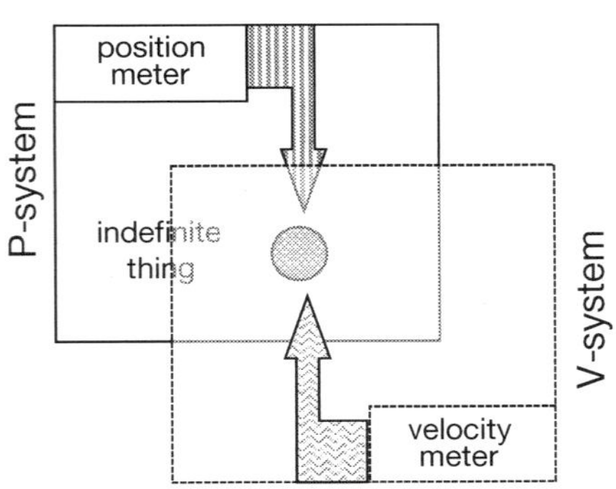

Figure 4.8 An indefinite quantum thing defined simultaneously and impredicatively by a position measuring system *P* and a velocity measuring system *V*.

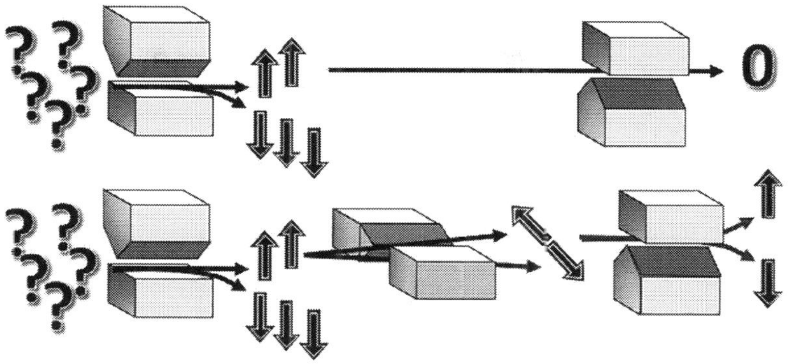

Figure 4.9 (*Above*) Electrons defined "up" by a vertical Stern–Gerlach magnet fail to exit a second Stern–Gerlach magnet that inverts the magnetic field direction of the first magnet. (*Below*) Some "up" electrons exiting from a vertical magnet can pass through an inverse magnetic field if an intermediate magnet redefines them.

(From Figure 2, Lindley, 1996, *Where does all the weirdness go?* Adapted with permission, Artellus.)

thing has no bearing on the *V*-measure that yields a different definite thing, and vice versa.

The uncertainty principle invokes concerns about "objectivity" because, as was just highlighted, in quantum physics one cannot avoid defining a thing that is part of a system in terms of the system. The traditional and conventional hope of science is predicative definition—to proceed strictly from parts to whole. Figure 4.9 provides a nice example of the uncertainty principle/impredicative definition that characterizes quantum physics. The lower panel shows electrons being passed through three Stern–Gerlach magnets. Without the intermediate magnet that changes the definition of "up" no electrons exiting from the first magnet will emerge from the third magnet, as is made clear by the sequence depicted in the upper panel.

4.5.1 The EPR (Einstein–Podolsky–Rosen) Experiment

We will call a Stern–Gerlach magnet so modified as to pass only spin "up" electrons (as in Figures 4.7 and 4.9), a Stern–Gerlach *filter*. It can be represented simply as a cube with an attached arrow that indicates the "up" direction. We can use Stern–Gerlach filters, electrons, and the uncertainty principle to set up a *gedanken*[6] EPR experiment. The experiment is sketched in Figure 4.10.

We begin by imagining a pair of electrons X and Y originating from a common source and moving oppositely at the same speed, each toward a vertical Stern–Gerlach filter at some distance from the source. We imagine further that the total spin of the two electrons is zero. Let "up" have the value

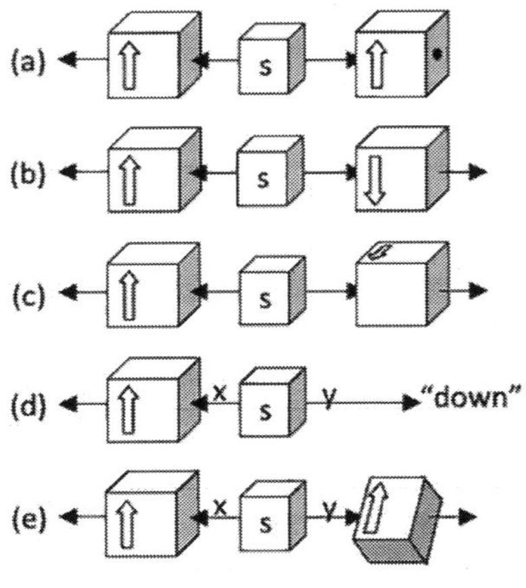

Figure 4.10 The EPR experiment and the experimental test of Bell's inequality (*s* is the source of the two electrons X and Y with total spin of zero).

+1 and "down" have the value −1, then if electron X is measured "up" electron Y must be "down" to satisfy the total sum of 0. Very simply, when the two filters have the same orientation—that is, the relative angle α between the filters is 0°—if one filter passes an electron, the other does not (Figure 4.10a). The correlation between the X and Y measures is zero. Conversely, if they have opposite orientations, α = 90°, then either both filters pass electrons or neither filter passes an electron (Figure 4.10b). The correlation between them is 1.0. The implication is that if only one electron, say X, is measured, the state of Y is known (Figure 4.10c). It will be the case that, despite the claim for the indefiniteness of Y until it is measured, if an experimenter measures X the experimenter will have definite knowledge of Y without measuring Y. The significance of this gedanken outcome for Einstein, Podolsky and N. Rosen (1935) is evident from the following famous quotation:

> If, without in any way disturbing a system, we can predict with certainty (i.e., probability equal to unity) the value of a physical quantity, then there exists an element of physical reality corresponding to this physical quantity.
>
> (p. 777)

In a phrase, the point of the EPR experiment is to show that electrons possess objective (context-independent, measurement-independent) reality. The counter from quantum mechanics—from the collection of experimental results depicted in Figures 4.4–4.7 and the inferences drawn from them—should come as no surprise. It is that the two electrons form a single quantum whole and until a measurement is made, whether it be on X or Y, it is improper to conceptualize the two things as existing separately from and independently of each other. The major implication of this counter to the objective reality interpretation of the EPR experiment is, however, scientifically disturbing. The measurement of either electron has an instantaneous effect on the other. In Figure 4.10d, the measurement of Y (the rightward moving electron) is achieved remotely, without an ostensible link between the thing measured and the thing doing the measuring. There is instantaneous action at a distance (Figure 4.4 top with $t_2 = t_1$).

4.5.2 Bell's Inequality

The two interpretations of the EPR experiment can be distinguished. The basis for the distinction is Bell's inequality (Bell, 1964). At the outset, it should be recognized that his inequality, its proof and its experimental tests, have nothing to do with quantum mechanics. Bell's inequality is simply an embodiment of a particular, commonly attested to, view of reality. The governing assumptions are that (a) propertied things exist independent of (prior to) observation, (b) inductive inference is valid, and (c) the principle of local causality holds (d'Espagnat, 1979).

Let A, B, C be three relatively independent two-valued parameters of some class of objects and let N designate number, for example, the number of objects with parameter A. Then, Bell's inequality reads (Harrison, 1981):

$$N(A, \text{not } B) + N(B, \text{not } C) \geq N(A, \text{not } C).$$

Here is an example of an object class and associated parameters. Let the class be "toy blocks" (paralleling an example of Harrison (1981)). For this class, A is wood and not-A is plastic; B is yellow and not-B is blue; C is cube and not-C is cone. Then Bell's inequality is that the number of wood objects that are blue plus the number of yellow objects that are cones is equal to or greater than the number of wood objects that are cones. If there are 20 objects (or 378 objects or one million objects), then no matter how many are wood and how many are plastic, how many are yellow and how many are blue, how many are cubes and how many are cones, it will always be the case that Bell's inequality is satisfied. A simpler example is a typical class of students with the parameters of A is male, B is height over 173 cm, and C is blue eyes. Whatever the composition of the class, it will always be true that the number of men less than 173 cm plus the number of students (men and women combined) taller than 173 cm with non-blue eyes will be equal to or greater than the number of men with non-blue eyes. Bell's inequality is an ingenious arrangement of parameters and their combinations. The inequality is ensured indifferent to the specific numbers composing the relationship.

Before addressing how the inequality is brought to bear on the interpretation of the EPR experiment, we need to take a moment to consider that any inference to be made from a failure to satisfy the inequality rests on the logic of negation. Of the three assumptions behind the inequality, a violation of the inequality means that *at least one* of them is wrong. Assumption (a) and assumption (b) above—of the necessity of realism and the validity of logic—seem far too foundational to the enterprise of science to be discarded. Only slightly less foundational is the locality assumption (c), the conjunction of the principles of antecedence and nearby action. The best bet, in the view of some scholars, is that if anything has to be given up, it must be locality (e.g., d'Espagnat, 1979). Science as an enterprise could, perhaps, live with that.

Let us return to Figure 4.10. We will build the experimental implementation of Bell's inequality using three pairs of Stern–Gerlach filters, one that is identical to Figure 4.10c, and two that are in the format of Figure 4.10e. The latter format defines a more complicated and telling case: that in which the two filters are oriented at 45° to each other. As the relative angle between the two filters changes, the correlation changes smoothly as the square of sin ($\alpha/2$). It was an element of Bell's genius to recognize that $\alpha = 45°$, with a correlation between "ups" of 14.6%, was an especially useful case for prizing apart the two interpretations of the EPR *gedanken* experiment (Lindley, 1996). For the EPR arrangement of Figure 4.10e, an "up" state for X does not inform with certainty about the state of Y but neither does it deliver a strictly random 50–50 outcome. Let θ stand for the inclination of a Stern–Gerlach filter to upright and identify the three parameters composing the inequality as follows: A is "up" for $\theta = 0°$ and not-A is "down" for $\theta = 0°$; B is "up" for $\theta = 45°$ and not-B is "down" for $\theta = 45°$; C is "up" for $\theta = 90°$ and not-C is "down" for $\theta = 90°$. Bell's inequality is then written as:

N("up" 0°, not-"up" 45°) + N("up" 45°, not-"up" 90°) ≥ N("up" 0°, not-"up" 90°).

Stated in the above form, the inequality is not experimentally testable. The Uncertainty Principle rules out simultaneous measures—for example, "up" 0° and "not up" 45°, of the same electron. However, situating the inequality within the EPR paradigm circumvents the Uncertainty Principle. In respect to Figure 4.10e, we can determine whether X is ("up" 0°, not-"up" 45°) by measuring X's spin at 0° and Y's spin at 45°. The experimentally testable form of the inequality is written:

N(X "up" 0°, Y "up" 45°) + N(X "up" 45°, Y" up" 90°) ≥ N(X "up" 0°, Y "up" 90°).

According to the quantum mechanical rule:

N(X "up", Y "up") = $1/2 \sin^2 [(\theta_X - \theta_Y)/2]$,

the testable form of Bell's inequality instantiated in Figures 4.10c and 4.10e should yield 0.146 ≥ 0.250 (Harrison, D., 1981). The violation predicted by quantum mechanics has been confirmed many times, with varied and typically more demanding versions of the testable form than presented here (e.g., Aspect, Dalibard, & Roger, 1982; Lanyon, Zwerger, et al., 2014; Rowe, Kielpinski, Meyer et al., 2001), and with the filters at (relatively) vast separations measured in miles (e.g., Tittel, Brendel, Zbinden, & Gisin, 1998). These experiments are taken as proof that nonlocality is a feature of nature, that the principles of nearby action and antecedence do not apply to all things, that locality may not be science's keystone (e.g., d'Espagnat, 1979; Nadeau & Kafatos, 1999).

4.6 The Problem of Perception by Scanning: Does Perception as a Two-term Relation Assume Nonlocality?

The student of perception and action should wonder what forms nonlocality might take, if any, in the phenomena that compose the student's domain of experimental inquiry. The student need not suppose that nonlocality in perception and action must necessarily cleave to the form manifest in the EPR situation. Nonlocality may be expressed in less exotic (but no less surprising and intellectually challenging) ways in the ordinary activities of organisms. We can try to identify a potential case by way of concluding this lecture. As will become apparent, the case in question suggests that whether one thinks that nonlocality is relevant to perception or not depends on the class of theory, direct or indirect (Lecture 3), that one adheres to.

In Figure 3.1 we expressed direct perception as a two-term relation between organism O and environment *E*. The figure was then amended to include a third, mediating term M in order that we might express the notion of indirect perception. The amendment produced Figure 3.2. We will reconsider the two figures in light of the local versus nonlocal issue.

Consider an organism (with frontal eyes such as ourselves) scanning its environment, that is, looking at parts of the environment in succession. Typically, scanning involves eye movements, head movements, and locomotion. For simplicity, imagine a cat exploring a novel enclosure such as a room in a new home. The issue at hand is the cat's visual perception of the simultaneous layout of the surfaces composing the room. How does it achieve the perception of the room as a constant unchanging entity on the basis of a succession of different optical samples? The principle of local causality requires that the cause of the "unitary room perception" be contiguous with the "unitary room perception." It mandates a process of integration by which samples earlier and later in the sequence are retained as memory traces and collected into a simultaneous whole within short-term memory (Neisser, 1967; Turvey, 1977)—the "unitary room stimulus" (Figure 4.11). The local causality principle mandates that each perceptual sample must be brought forward into the present for unitary perception in the present to occur. If we were to generalize Figure 3.2 to the current example of perception by scanning, then M in this new figure would be the simultaneous whole produced by integrating the series of samples. The integrated whole ($\Sigma\tau$ in Figure 4.11) is the epistemic mediator between the exploring cat and the unchanging spatial layout of the room.

Patently, a very different approach to the problem of perceiving by scanning is required by the theory of perception as a two-term relation. The theory proscribes the construction of a simultaneous composite from the sequence of samples—that is, it proscribes a mediating "unitary room stimulus." Figure 3.1's perceptual panel must remain the same under the substitution of *room* for *surface*. The temporally extended sequence as such, therefore, must specify the simultaneous layout of the surfaces composing the room, as Gibson (1966; see also Shaw & Pittenger, 1978) has tried to argue: "if the sequence contains the scene . . . it does not have to be converted into one" (p. 262).

Nonlocality *in some form* is implied. The foremost historian of psychology reached this conclusion in a review of the ideas of the foremost proponent of direct perception. Edwin Boring (1967) wrote of James Gibson (1966):

> As to causality, Gibson tells us that the perceptual composite, its parts distributed in both simultaneity and time, need not be cumulated into a simultaneous whole in order to function; it is nonsense, he says, to think that successive events have to be preserved as traces for the sequence to act as a totality (p. 251). Well, Newton got away with action at a distance,

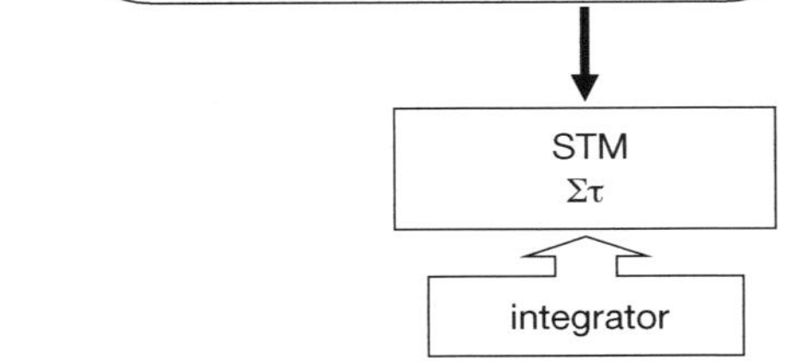

Figure 4.11 The solution to the scanning problem in a three-term theory of perception (STM: short-term memory; τ: memory trace of a sample).

(From Figure 1, M. T. Turvey, Contrasting orientations to the theory of visual-information processing. *Psychological Review*, *84*, 67–88, 1977, APA, adapted with permission.)

preposterous as it seemed, and perhaps Gibson could ultimately win our assent to a temporal vacuum between a cause and its effect *but it would require revolutionary thinking.*

(p. 152, italics added)

Notes

1 Democritus brought the theories of eidola and emanation into convergence. If an eidolon's atoms contacted atoms emanating from the eyes, then the object simulated by the former could be transmitted to the latter. This way of thinking generalized to the relation between the inner and outer light of original emanation theory. The light proceeding from the eyes and that radiating from the sun coalesce, forming a single homogeneous body of light and, thereby, a link between the environment's objects and the mind (Lindberg, 1976). This would become, essentially, Plato's view.

2 For example, he asked how it would be possible, when a person views the sky, for the eye to be the source of a material emanation that could fill all space up to the stars (Lindberg, 1992).

3 He positioned five lanterns outside the room and observed five lanterns imaged in the room. If he placed an obstruction between a lantern and the room, then a lantern image would disappear if and only if the lantern, obstruction, and aperture lay on a straight line.

4 Alhazen was sufficiently perturbed by the fact of inversion to seek a mechanism in the eye that ensured against it occurring. He proposed that, by refraction, the lens modulated the light rays in such a way as to preserve the image's upright orientation.

5 Ockham held that the base of all knowledge was the direct experience of individual things and particular events. He advanced a radical empiricism and realism and introduced nominalistic analysis of the language used to describe knowing. The hallmark of his nominalism was an "extreme economy of ontological commitment (Moody, 1969.p. 307)." He sought the systematic elimination of abstract or intensional entities that were not linguistically constrained through the logical analysis of language (Moody, 1969).

6 An experiment carried out by proposing a hypothesis in thought only, a "thought experiment."

References

Aspect, A., Dalibard, J., & Roger, G. (1982) Experimental tests of Bell's inequalities using time-varying analyzers. *Physical Review Letters*, *49*, 1804–1807.

Bell, J. S. (1964). On the Einstein, Podolsky Rosen paradox. *Physics*, *1*, 195–200.

Boring, E. G. (1950). *A history of experimental psychology*. New York: Appleton-Century-Crofts.

Boring, E. G. (1967). Review of 'The senses considered as perceptual systems'. *American Journal of Psychology*, *80*, 150–154.

Bunge, M. (1977). *Treatise on basic philosophy*, *Vol. 3*. (*Ontology I: The furniture of the world.*) Dordrecht, Netherlands: D. Reidel.

Bunge, M. (1979). *Causality and modern science* (3rd ed.). New York: Dover.

Chomsky, N. (1965). *Aspects of a theory of syntax*. Cambridge, MA: MIT Press.

Crombie, A. C. (1964). Early concepts of the senses and the mind. *Scientific American, 210* (No. 5, May), 108–116.

d'Espagnat, B. (1979). The quantum theory of reality. *Scientific American, 241*, 158–181.

Einstein, A., Podolsky, B., & Rosen, N. (1935). Can quantum-mechanical description of physical reality be considered complete? *Physical Review, 47*, 777–780.

Gerlach, W., & Stern, O. (1922). Der experimentelle nachweis der richtungsquantelung im magnetfeld. *Zeitschrift für Physik A Hadrons and Nuclei*, 9, 349–352.

Gibson, J. J. (1966). *The senses considered as perceptual systems*. Boston, MA: Houghton Mifflin

Gibson, J. J. (1986). *The ecological approach to visual perception*. Mahwah, NJ: Erlbaum. (Original work published 1979)

Goodman, N. (1965). *Fact, fiction and forecast*. Indianapolis, IN: Bobbs-Merrill.

Hammond, J. H. (1981). *The camera obscura: A chronicle*. Bristol, CT: Hilger.

Harrison, D. (1981). Bell's inequality and quantum correlations. *American Journal of Physics*, 50, 811–816.

Howard, I. P. (1996). Alhazen's neglected discoveries of visual phenomena. *Perception, 25*, 1203–1217.

Landauer, T., & Dumais, S. T. (1997). A solution to Plato's problem: The latent semantic analysis theory of acquisition, induction, and representation of knowledge. *Psychological Review, 104*, 211–240.

Lanyon, B. P., Zwerger, M., Jurcevic, P., Hempel, C., Dür, V., et al. (2014). Experimental violation of multipartite Bell inequalities with trapped ions. *Physical Review Letters, 112*, 100403.

Lindberg, D. C. (1976). *Theories of vision from Al-Kindi to Kepler*. Chicago, IL: University of Chicago Press.

Lindberg, D. C. (1992). *The beginnings of western science*. Chicago, IL: University of Chicago Press.

Lindley, D. (1996). *Where does the weirdness go?* New York: HarperCollins.

Lombardo, T. (1987). *The reciprocity of perceiver and environment: The evolution of James J. Gibson's ecological psychology*. Hillsdale, NJ: Erlbaum.

Loux, M. J. (1970). *Universals and particulars: Readings in ontology*. London: University of Notre Dame Press.

Maxwell, J. C. (1890). *The scientific papers of James Clerk Maxwell*. Cambridge, UK: Cambridge University Press.

Moody, E. A. (1969). William of Ockham. In P. Edwards (Ed.), *Encyclopedia of philosophy, Vol.* 8 (pp. 306–317). New York: Macmillan.

Nadeau, R., & Kafatos, M. (1999). *The non-local universe*. Oxford, UK: Oxford University Press.

Neisser, U. (1967). *Cognitive psychology*. New York: Appleton Century Crofts.

Ronchi, V. (1957). *Optics: The science of vision*. New York: New York University Press.

Ronchi, V. (1967). *The nature of light*. Cambridge, MA: Harvard University Press.

Rowe, M. A., Kielpinski, D., Meyer, V., Sackett, C. A., Itano, W. M., Monroe, C., & Wineland, D. J. (2001). Experimental violation of a Bell's inequality with efficient detection. *Nature*, 409, 791–794.

Sabra, A. I. (1989). Form in ibn al-Haytham's theory of vision. *Zeitschrift für Geschichte der Arabisch-Islamischen Wissenschaften*, 5, 115–140.

Shaw, R. E., & Pittenger, J. (1978). Perceiving change. In H. L. Pick & E. Saltzman (Eds.), *Modes of perceiving and processing information* (pp. 187–204). Hillsdale, NJ: Erlbaum.

Tittel, W., Brendel, J., Zbinden, H., & Gisin, N. (1998). Violation of Bell Inequalities more than 10km apart. *Physical Review Letters*, *81*, 3563–3566.

Turvey, M. T. (1977). Contrasting orientations to the theory of visual information processing. *Psychological Review*, *84*, 67–88.

Turvey, M. T. (2015). Quantum-like issues at nature's ecological scale (the scale of organisms and their environments). *Mind & Matter*, *13*, 7–44.

Weimer, W. B. (1973). Psycholinguistics and Plato's paradoxes of the Meno. *American Psychologist*, *28*, 15–33.

Zajonc, A. (1993). *Catching the light*. New York: Bantam Books.

Lecture 5

The Mechanistic Hypothesis

We are now well prepared for the questions that identify the next stop in our brief historical tour. Are the ways that things appear to be, the ways things really are? What is the proper domain of physics? How is the principle of local causality implemented in living things?

5.1 Appearance and Reality

The perspective on how the world could be known by sight was redirected and sharpened by the scholarship of the 17th century.[1] In answering the foregoing questions, it would lay the foundations for a program of investigation that has continued to the present. As will become apparent in the next two lectures, this program should be referred to as the *Cartesian Program* (Turvey & Kugler, 1984).

The issue of the fidelity of optical simulacra or eidola had been raised by the investigations of Alhazen. Those who followed Alhazen's lead and sought to explain image formation by the chambered eye would further emphasize the deficiency of optical simulation. Once the design of the chambered eye common in the kingdom Animalia was properly understood, primarily but not exclusively through the efforts of Kepler (Crombie, 1964; Lombardo, 1987), the limits of simulation became more obvious. The image on the retina did not simulate object distance and, perforce, could not simulate solid shape. The corresponding mental experiences would have to be achieved through the inner observation aspect of the projective assumption, however construed. Requiring inner sight to complete the resemblance that was incompletely provided by outer sight (eidola) allowed the possibility of slippage between the way things looked and the way they really were. Could forms in the mind be at odds with the forms of the world? Would providence allow such discrepancy?

In 1543, some 61 years prior to Kepler's explanation of the eye, these questions had been answered with a resounding "yes!" What seemed the most prosaic of visual experiences, the daily rotation of the sun around the earth and the smallness of the sun in comparison to the earth, had been exposed as mere appearances, not facts. Copernicus's heliocentric (sun-centered) theory of the universe made evident that the daily motions of the heavens was an illusion due to the earth's rotation about an internal axis. Also illusory was the annual motion of the sun relative to the constellations of the Zodiac and the peculiar wandering of certain "stars" (the planets). Both kinds of motions were the consequences of the slow orbit of the (small) earth around the (very much larger) sun.

The way the heavens looked to a human observer, therefore, bore no resemblance to actual fact. The optical copy sent to the eye simulated nothing real. The year 1543 is taken as the birth date of modern science (Cohen, 1985). It might also be regarded as the birth dates of the dichotomy of appearance and reality, and the accepted superiority of reason over perceptual experience as the means of "knowing about."

Copernicus's theory, centering astronomical events at a static sun rather than a static earth, turned medieval science on its head, demanding a new unimaginable physics. Peculiar questions had to be addressed, such as why, given a translating and rotating earth, birds were not blown from their perches, detached objects did not whirl away, objects thrown straight up did not land in some distant place. And what now were the locations of heaven and hell? It does not surprise that the Copernican view was adopted grudgingly, by scholars, and lay people alike. The slow pace of approval ended abruptly in 1609, however. From that point on Copernican ideas rapidly assumed the status of orthodoxy. In 1609, scientists, particularly Galileo Galilei, began to use the telescope to make systematic studies of the heavens. From the compelling fit of the new facts of observation to the heliocentric system came the motivation to pursue a physics that would apply with "equal validity on a moving earth and throughout the universe" (Cohen, 1985, p. 54). The laws of inertia, force and gravitation were in the offing.

5.2 Nature is Inherently Mathematical

Galileo engaged the pursuit of the new physics through a commitment to mathematics as the right tool. His applications of geometry were novel and abstract. Lines typically used to represent simply lines or distances were used to represent any physical variable—for example, time or velocity. Remarkably, Euclid's deductive system, designed to serve the analysis of geometric forms, was incorporated by Galileo to serve the analysis of object motions. From this analysis followed his law that the distance traveled in free-fall is proportional to the squared time and his proof that a projectile's path is parabolic based on assuming independent horizontal and vertical components of motion (Cohen, 1985; Dugas, 1988).

Galileo's innovative use of mathematics was to have two major consequences for how scientists and philosophers would think about the workings of the mind. The first consequence followed from his famous methodological canon: "[T]he book of nature is written in mathematical characters, without a knowledge of which men cannot understand it."

Individual phenomena were knowable to the extent that (a) nature's language of mathematics was known and (b) the language could be used to address them. Any aspect of nature that did not lend itself to mathematical analysis was, therefore, of questionable status. Smells, colors, tastes and sounds fell into this latter category. They were, argued Galileo, mere appearances, qualities ascribed by mind, subjective rather than objective, secondary rather than primary. They were not like size, shape, number and motion. These were amenable to mathematical description, purely objective, and, therefore, candidates for understanding in terms of physical laws.

The need to distinguish and to keep separate the two classes of properties, the primary and the secondary, was encouraged by other 17th-century scientists—most notably, Boyle and Newton. The consequence of the separation was the exclusion from natural science of a particular class of relational properties, the psychological phenomena, which are the hallmarks of organism–environment interactions. Whatever might be systematic about those relations would have to be understood through principles other than those by which the world (including the body) was to be understood.

Oddly enough, Galileo's innovative use of mathematics suggested one form the special mental principles might take. Galileo's interpretation of *motion as geometry* was transmuted by Thomas Hobbes into the interpretation of *thinking as computation* (Haugeland, 1985). The act of thinking for Hobbes (1651/1968, Chapter V, Part 1) consisted of symbolic operations, internal variants of talking aloud or calculating using pen and paper. The operations were not conducted in respect to spoken or written symbols but, rather, in respect to special brain tokens referred to by Hobbes as "phantasms." Simply, he equated thought with the movements of some substance in the head. The phantasms or thought "parcels" were moved about by the rules of reason, as if a mental abacus was being manipulated. Ratiocination, the process of exact thinking, was mechanical. Hobbes preoccupation was the possibility of explanation by mechanism as was that of his contemporary, René Descartes, whose own theorizing would invoke the rational manipulation of symbols.

5.3 Inert Matter, Passive Machine

Despite substantial conceptual differences, a common aim of 17th-century scientists (mainly Galileo, Descartes, Boyle and Newton) was to give a thoroughgoing account of any natural phenomenon by demonstrating the mechanical processes by which it was realized (Toulmin, 1967). The unifying assumption was that all genuinely physical processes, those reflecting properties of matter, should ultimately prove explicable in mechanistic terms. A particular version of this *mechanistic hypothesis*—namely, the idea that the body is a mechanism, was successfully exploited by Kepler to explain the workings of the eye (Crombie, 1964). On extension, the mechanistic hypothesis would clarify the right kinds of questions to ask of the senses and perception—answerable physical questions as opposed to unanswerable metaphysical questions (Crombie, 1964). Three questions in particular were identified. First, what are the mechanisms by which external physical motions are transformed into internal physical motions of the sense organs, nerves and brain? Second, in what manner do the physical motions of the sense organs, nerves and brain produce sensory experiences? And third, what physical and physiological cues or clues are necessary for perception?

Behind these questions manifesting the mechanistic hypothesis were the 17th-century views of matter, machine and mechanism (Toulmin, 1967). By *matter* was meant those things that have length and width and thickness, and which offer resistance to touch. By *machine* was meant a device that allowed a person or persons to lift a weight or displace a heavy object or overcome a resistance, achievements that would not be possible without its aid. The examples of machines were the six basic simple machines known since the time of Archimedes: lever, wheel and axle, pulley, inclined plane, wedge and screw. Significantly, both matter and machines were just instruments permitting the transmission and/or modification of actions that were impressed upon them from the outside. As convention had it, and as part of Aristotle's continuing legacy, matter cannot put itself into motion. Self-motion or self-cause was anathematized (Juarrero, 1999)

By *mechanistic*, the 17th-century scientist meant an explanation, therefore, in which a physical system was interpreted through the known actions of the known machines, singly or in combination (Toulmin, 1967). The heart of the explanation was the principle of local causality, not as sophisticated as it would become in the 20th century, but nonetheless the essential idea of subsequent events following preceding contiguous events. If the explanation was not exhaustive in terms of implementing local causes at every step of the way, then the explanation was suspect and its author was viewed as delving into the occult (Toulmin, 1967).

The prohibition against self-cause, allied as it was with the concept of matter and machines as inert, exaggerated further the polar opposition between mind and matter. There was a long-standing strategy for avoiding any self-reflexive paradox such as the infamous Liar Paradox (e.g., "All Copernicans are liars; I am a Copernican"; Lecture 3). It was, simply, to devolve the force of the paradox on distinct parts. Thus, the argument goes, when the Copernican deceives himself by telling himself a lie, one part of the Copernican does the deceiving and another part is deceived. Likewise, if a system causes itself to move, then one part does the moving whereas another part is moved. In his famous mechanical treatise *On the Movement of Animals* (1680/1989), Giovanni Borelli described biological movement in these terms:

> [M]uscles are instruments and machines by which the motive faculty of the soul moves the limbs and the parts of the animal. . .muscle by itself is a dead and inert machine in the absence of an external motive faculty. The latter orders, stimulates the muscle from its lethargy and forces it to move.
>
> (pp. 7–8)

Because muscles were no more than passive material instruments, Borelli and fellow proponents of the mechanistic hypothesis had to seek the origin of animal movement elsewhere, outside of matter (Toulmin, 1967).

The mechanistic hypothesis fashioned in the 17th century presented, therefore, a curious mix for future students of perception and action. The body was identified as a machine, a passive physical instrument through which mind and the material world interacted. The mind, however, had to be self-causing, self-moving, and so on. The mind, therefore, could not be a machine and, synonymously, could not be material.

5.4 Pragmatic versus Absolute Truth

Before proceeding further, perhaps we should adopt a more circumspect perspective on the central ideas that shaped the thinking of the era in which the mechanistic hypothesis arose. To begin with, we might need to take a more tempered view of the implications of the Copernican revolution. A useful question to raise is this: Do presumed differences between the appearances of things and the descriptions of them as determined by physics and human reason actually make a difference in regard to the fit between organism and environment? The modest behavior of a simple arboreal vine, *Monstera gigantea*, provides some illumination on this matter (Turvey & Shaw, 1979).

The seeds of *Monstera gigantea* germinate on the ground subsequent to falling from the parent plant. Shortly after germination, the seedling grows in the direction of the nearest tree. Following contact, it climbs the tree, losing its roots in the process. The seedling's adaptive behavior is a refinement of the tendency to move toward darkness (skototropism); the seedling in fact moves in the direction of the darkest sector of the horizon (Strong & Ray, 1975).

In the seedling's environment, the darkest sector invariably corresponds to a tree that can be reached with a minimum of horizontal growth. A tree is a climbable object. That means it must satisfy certain minimal strength, rigidity and texture requirements in order to support the vine's mode of climbing. These defining properties of a climbable object, those that would be identified by science, do not, however, have to be detected by the seedling. Given the aforementioned invariant, it suffices that the seedling detects the darkest sector.

The issue of appearance versus reality is brought to center stage by an experiment in which the ecological relation between light distribution and tree location is eliminated. With the open end of an opaque tube on the horizon going proxy for a tree as a producer of a dark sector, the seedling grows into the open end (Strong & Ray, 1975). How a tree appears in the vine's ecology, and not what a tree is under scientific description, is the constraint on the adaptive behavior of *Monstera gigantea*.

From an evolutionary perspective, it seems injudicious to claim that the vine's sensitivity erred in this experimental setting. The vine did, after all, detect and grow toward the darkest sector of its horizon, the behavior that it had evolved to enact. Facts of this kind are suggestive that the description of reality relevant to any given organism is not likely to be a description that is true in any absolute or metaphysical sense. It is perhaps a description that is true in a pragmatic, context-dependent sense (Shaw, Turvey & Mace, 1982; Turvey & Shaw, 1979).

In one of the earliest discussions of the pragmatic doctrine that truth is what is *useful* (Dewey, 1916; James, 1907/1975), Plato suggested that correct opinion or *doxa* could often serve just as well as knowledge (Ryle, 1967). Correct *doxa* is not idle opinion that is true by luck. Rather, it is efficacious opinion that is valid and is so for the right reason—namely, it conforms to environmental facts to a degree sufficient to motivate useful action. The sensitivity of *Monstera gigantea* to the darkest sector on the horizon is an example of correct *doxa*. It motivates pragmatically true (useful) action that leads to success as relatively defined in the semantic context of the vine's niche (Shaw et al., 1982).

5.5 The Right Degrees of Freedom

Circumspection is also called for in respect to another cornerstone of the mechanistic hypothesis, the division between primary properties as the topic of physical science and secondary properties as the topic of a very different form of inquiry. We should try, at this juncture, to get as clear as possible on this division and its interpretation because a thorough-going account of perception and action may well be, at bottom, a theory of properties that are mutual to organism and environment, properties that have the look of secondary properties.

It is extremely important to appreciate exactly what was at issue in drawing the distinction. A modern interpretation of "doing physics" will be very helpful in this regard (Krieger, 1992). A handle onto the world is a *degree of freedom*. As Krieger (1992) remarks colorfully:

> A degree of freedom is a direction for potential action, once we figure out how to take hold of that handle in an effective way. One needs to shake the handle with just the right energy, and in just the right direction, and one will hear the music of Nature in its purest tones.
>
> (p. xii)

If the right degrees of freedom are chosen, the physics is more tractable and more revealing than if the wrong degrees of freedom are chosen. The *right* degrees of freedom lead to theories of wide applicability. This is how one 20th-century physicist (Weinberg, 1983) has described the situation:

> You may use any degrees of freedom you like to describe a physical system, but if you use the wrong ones, you'll be sorry.
>
> (p. 16)

Finding the right degrees of freedom, the right handles onto the world, is precisely what 17th- century scientists were attempting to do. Distinguishing primary from secondary qualities or properties was part of the search for the right degrees of freedom, those that would sustain a truly explanatory science (Smith, 1990).[2]

For the most part, science since Galileo has been comfortable with the notion of *intrinsic* property. On examining a substantial thing in the environment—say, a stone—the scientist presumes that it has properties that are internal to it, traits that have nothing to do with how they will be observed and measured. When an intrinsic property of the stone has been isolated to satisfaction, it is represented in the scientific formalism by a *concept*, *attribute* or *predicate*. A predicate is something that is affirmed or denied of the substantial thing. Predication may be right or wrong, may serve a useful purpose or be a hindrance. Keeping the distinction between a thing and its predicates—that is, between its substantial as contrasted with its formal properties—is essential to scientific progress.

In the framework of classical mechanics, when we predicate "mass" of the stone (using the word predicate now as a transitive verb) we intend to identify a substantial property intrinsic to the stone that is the same whenever and wherever the stone is observed. To predicate "velocity" of the stone when the stone is a projectile is slightly more complicated. The property in question is of a pair of substantial things, the moving stone and a reference frame—that is, the predicate "velocity" picks out a *relational* or *mutual* property (Bunge, 1977). For Galileo, and science since his time, relational properties qualify along with intrinsic properties as *primary* properties under the following proviso: The property of any substantial thing A is expressed by, but not actualized in, its relation with another substantial thing B (Gomatam, 1999). If the *actualized in* clause prevails, then the property is *secondary*. Thus, to predicate "velocity" of the stone is to refer to a primary property but to predicate "gray" of the stone is to refer to a secondary property. The stone's color is actualized in the stone's relation to a perceiver.

Importantly, a stone enters into other relations, not involving perceivers, in which a property of the stone, one might argue, is both expressed and actualized (Gomatam, 1999). For example, when a stone is placed on a pile of papers, we predicate "paperweight" of the stone. Similarly, when the stone is positioned at the foot of a door, we predicate "doorstop" of the stone (Figure 5.1, top panel). Prior to setting up the appropriate spatio-temporal relations between the stone and the pile of papers and between the stone and the door, "paperweight-ness" and "doorstop-ness" are, respectively, potential properties of the stone. They become physically real only when the spatio-temporal relations are in place (Gomatam, 1999). It should be iterated that, from a conventional viewpoint, these relational properties of the stone might still qualify as objective properties in that they are expressed in relation to non-living things.

There are other relational properties of like kind, however, which do engage living things. For example, when a stone is grasped and brought down hard and repetitively on another object, we can predicate "hammer" of the stone. Similarly, when a stone is grasped and scraped across the surface of another object, we can predicate "scraper" of the stone (Figure 5.1, bottom panel). Patently, these predications implicate a perceiver-actor. But is subjectivity also implicated? The requirement "graspable" for the stone to be a hammer or scraper means that a primary property of the stone—namely, its size—must be commensurate with the same primary property of the perceiver-actor's grasping system. Objectivity, not subjectivity, is implicated.

Conceivably, there are many relational properties that a stone might have by virtue of its relation to either other objects or perceivers-actors, but they are, at best, indefinite properties until a particular spatio-temporal relation is effected. When that happens, one of the many potential relational properties of the stone is actualized without compromising the others. For example,

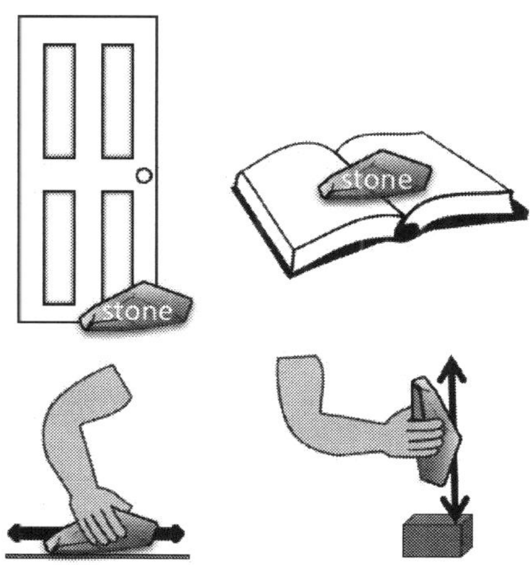

Figure 5.1 Clockwise, predicate grey stone as doorstop, book weight, hammer, scraper. (From Figure 15, Turvey, 2015, adapted with permission, Imprint Academic.)

when a stone becomes a "hammer," it is still potentially a "scraper," just as when an electron (recalling Lecture 4) becomes an "up" electron, it is still potentially a "down" electron. We can imagine that Galileo, Boyle and Newton would have asked the following methodological question: In what settings do relational properties of the kind identified above arise in such a way that they could be of significance to the development of physical science? As highlighted in Lecture 4, physicists in the 20th century encountered phenomena in relational settings that forced them to consider a possibility that would have been unthinkable to their 17th-century predecessors: *nothing is real until it is measured* (i.e., placed into a particular spatio-temporal relation with a meter or measurement device). If an object with its primary properties of mass, position and velocity is always in only one of its logically possible states, and all variables composing a state have determinate values at all times, whether measured or not (see Lecture 2), then the aforementioned possibility is unthinkable. What made that possibility thinkable were the discoveries and interpretations that constitute quantum mechanics, the pinnacle of 20th-century physics. At this juncture, it is recommended that Lecture 4, Section 4.5, be revisited. It is also recommended that you anticipate linking the themes of the present lecture to those that will be introduced much later in Lecture 22.

Notes

1 The major scholars were: Galileo (1564–1642), Kepler (1571–1630), Hobbes (1588–1679), Borelli (1608–1679), Descartes (1596–1650), Boyle (1627–1691), Locke (1632–1704), Newton (1642–1727).

2 Consider how difficult it was to make this distinction. Hume (1739–40/2000, 1.4.2.13, p. 128) gave expression to the challenge: "whatever may be our philosophical opinion, colours, sounds, heat and cold, as far as appears to the senses, exist after the same manner with motion and solidity, and that the difference we make betwixt them in this respect, arises not from mere perception." Further: "as far as the senses are judges, all perceptions are the same in the manner of their existence."

References

Borelli, G. (1989). *On animal motion*. Berlin, Germany: Springer Verlag (original work published 1680).

Bunge, M. (1977). *Treatise on basic philosophy*, Vol. 3. (*Ontology I: The furniture of the world.*) Dordrecht, Netherlands: D. Reidel.

Cohen, I. B. (1985). *The birth of a new physics*. New York: Norton.

Crombie, A. C. (1964). Early concepts of the senses and the mind. *Scientific American, 210* (No. 5, May), 108–116.

Dewey, J. (1916). *Essays in experimental logic*. Chicago, IL: University of Chicago Press.

Dugas, R. (1988). *A history of mechanics*. New York: Dover.

Gomatam, R. V. (1999). Quantum theory and the observation problem. In R. Núñez & W. J. Freeman (Eds.). *Reclaiming cognition: The primacy of action, intention and emotion* (pp. 173–190). Thorverton, UK: Imprint Academic.
Haugeland, J. (1985). *Artificial intelligence: The very idea*. Cambridge, MA: MIT Press.
Hobbes, T. (1968). *Leviathan*. London: Penguin Books (original work published 1651).
Hume, D. (2000). *A treatise of human nature*. D. F. Norton & M. J. Norton (Eds.). Oxford, UK: Oxford University Press (original work published 1739–40).
James, W. (1975). *Pragmatism and the meaning of truth*. Cambridge, MA: Harvard University Press (original work published 1907–9)
Juarrero, A. (1999). *Dynamics in action*. Cambridge, MA: MIT Press.
Krieger, M. H. (1992). *Doing physics: How physicists take hold of the world*. Bloomington: Indiana University Press.
Lombardo, T. (1987). *The reciprocity of perceiver and environment: The evolution of James J. Gibson's ecological psychology*. Hillsdale, NJ: Erlbaum.
Ryle, G. (1967). Plato. In P. Edwards (Ed.), *The encyclopedia of philosophy, Vol. 5*. New York: Macmillan.
Shaw, R. E., Turvey, M. T., & Mace, W. M. (1982). Ecological psychology: The consequence of a commitment to realism. In W. Weimer & D. Palermo (Eds.), *Cognition and the symbolic processes II* (pp. 159–226). Hillsdale, NJ: Erlbaum.
Smith, A. D. (1990). Of primary and secondary qualities. *The Philosophical Review, XCIV*, 221–254.
Strong, D. R., & Ray, T. S. (1975). Host tree location of a tropical vine (*Monstera Gigantea*) by skototropism. *Science, 190*, 804–806.
Toulmin, S. (1967). Neuroscience and human understanding. In G. C. Quarton, T. Melnechuk, & F. O. Schmitt (Eds.), *The neurosciences: A study program* (pp. 822–832). New York: Rockefeller University Press.
Turvey, M. T. (2015). Quantum-like issues at nature's ecological scale (the scale of organisms and their environments). *Mind & Matter, 13*, 7–44.
Turvey, M. T., & Kugler, P. N. (1984). An ecological approach to perception and action. In H. T. A. Whiting (Ed.), *Human motor actions: Bernstein reassessed* (pp. 373–412). Amsterdam, Netherlands: North Holland.
Turvey, M. T., & Shaw, R. E. (1979). The primacy of perceiving: An ecological reformulation of perception for understanding memory. In L.-G. Nilssen (Ed.), *Perspectives on memory research: In honor of Uppsala University's 500th anniversary* (pp. 167–222). Hillsdale, NJ: Erlbaum.
Weinberg, S. (1983). Why the renormalization group is a good thing. In A. Guth, K. Huang, & R. Jaffe (Eds.), *Asymptotic realms of physics*. Cambridge, MA: MIT Press.

Lecture 6
The Cartesian Program

No scholar of the 17th century expressed the mechanistic hypothesis and its implications for perception and action as completely as the French philosopher, cosmologist, physicist, biologist and mathematician, René Descartes. His ability to bring the mechanistic hypothesis to the forefront was based on two major conceptual strategies. The first strategy was combining and exploiting two dualisms, that between mind and matter, and that between human and animal. Whereas the human possessed an active self-causing mind over and above the passive body, the animal (he contended) was solely inert matter, a mere automaton set into motion by external causes. The study of animal perception-action, in contrast to that of human perception-action, had the advantage, therefore, of being the study of physical processes abiding the principle of local causality without the involvement of mind. The second strategy was insisting that the distinctively sensory aspects of our experience could not inform us about the nature of physical reality. In the *Meditations on First Philosophy*, Descartes (1641/1911) asked that we consider "the commonest matters, those which we believe to be the most distinctly comprehended, to wit, the bodies which we touch and see" (p. 154).

Upon such consideration Descartes (1641/1911) leads us to the conclusion that "even bodies are not properly speaking known by the senses or by the faculty of imagination, but by the understanding only" (p. 157).

It is a conclusion that spotlights the primacy of reasoning (as opposed to sensing) in knowing about the world and marks the position of *Rationalism* (as opposed to *Empiricism*). It is reflected in Figure 4.3.

6.1 A One-time Proponent of a Two-term Relation?

Descartes' first work was the never-completed treatise *Rules for the Direction of the Mind*, written about 1628 but not printed until 1701 (Williams, 1967). One reading of the *Rules* suggests that Descartes might have begun his investigations as a direct realist (O'Neill, 1974; see also Yolton, 1975). He presumed fundamental units of reality, which he called "simple natures," and emphasized that these were known directly and immediately. That is, in respect to Lecture 3 and the figures depicting direct and indirect perception, it can be suggested that Descartes opted originally for perception as a two-term relation. There was no third thing mediating organism as the thing that knows and the environment as the thing known. This unmediated view, however, would not be his eventual epistemological stance, the one that defines the modern-day Cartesian Program for perception and action. Quite possibly, this proclivity for a dyadic rather than triadic relation persisted during Descartes' career but receded into the background as the difficulties of developing a direct realism consistent with his larger scheme became evident (O'Neill, 1974). The hypothesis of direct awareness of states of the world was whittled down to one of the most influential hypotheses in all of science: there is only direct awareness of states of the body and any awareness of things in the world is by means of the body. We will refer to this central hypothesis of Descartes as the *hypothesis of corporeal ideas* (Reed, 1982).

6.2 The Discovery and Conceptual Implementation of the Retinal Image

As will become apparent, the major barrier (both historically and contemporary) to implementing a two-term relation in (monocular) visual perception is Descartes' variant of the simulative assumption: The basis of vision is an image at the back of the eye (conventionally, a two-dimensional image *on* the retina). In this variant of the simulative assumption, the retinal image is intermediary between the things that constitute environment and the viewer's visual perception of that environment. It is the basis for the thesis that visual perception is indirect (inferential, computational) and, perforce, the major conceptual barrier to the thesis that visual perception is direct (non-inferential, non-computational). To acknowledge the image is to commit to a three-term relation as constitutive of the act of seeing. The relata are: (a) environment and one's body, (b) two-dimensional images of environment and one's body,[1] and (c) inferences about the three-dimensional natures of the environment, and one's bodily movements and orientations in respect to them, with (c) derivative of (b).

Of singular importance to the investigation of the image was the intuition of the astronomer Kepler that to comprehend the functioning of a single eye requires two retinas—one retina to be looked at and one retina to do the looking. Boring (1942, p. 223) expressed Kepler's insight in these terms: An eye's retina could be made visible if there were a means for "another eye to see it." The grounds for such a means was provided through the investigations by Scheiner and subsequently Descartes in the first third of the 17th century. They identified the retina to be made visible as that of the eye of a dead animal (removed from its embedding capsule by a process referred to as *enucleation*) and they identified "another eye to see it" as that of a living human. Whereas a live retina is transparent, a dead retina is opaque (translucent).

This opaqueness is manifest within minutes of the animal dying (Duke-Elder, 1932; Kawashima, Hatake, Kudo et al., 2015). Descartes summarized how the requisite additional image is produced and observed in *Optics* (Discourses Five and Six; 1637/1985). As depicted in Figure 6.1, "a hole is created in the back of the enucleated eye and covered with some white body thin enough to let light pass through (e.g., a piece of paper or an egg-shell)" (p. 166).

The enucleated eye is then so fixed as to face illuminated objects in an otherwise dark room. If an observer looks at the white body *qua* screen at the rear of the enucleated eye, he or she will, in Descartes' words "see there, not without wonder and pleasure, a picture representing in natural perspective all the objects outside" (p. 167).

For Descartes (1637/1985), the images so formed in the back of the eye in the preceding way are images that pass beyond the retina and enter into the brain. Figure 6.2 provides a pictorial summary, with Figure 6.2c the functional equivalent of Figure 6.1.

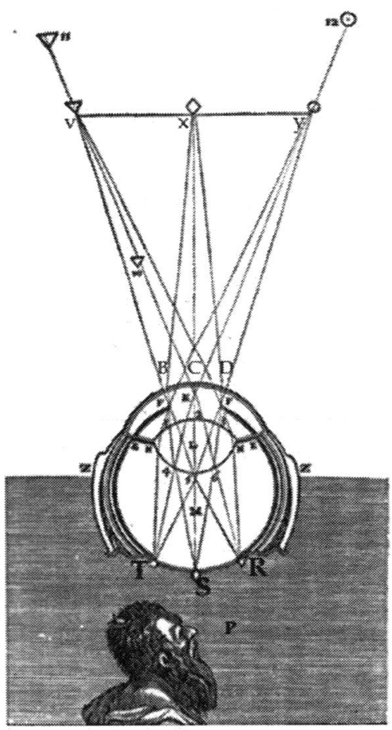

Figure 6.1 Retina *qua* window ("white body") as depicted in Descartes' *La dioptrique* (1637). The retinal region ablated and covered with transparent material extends to the left of and to the right of the region marked by the letters T, S, R.

(Adapted with permission from Wellcome Library, London.)

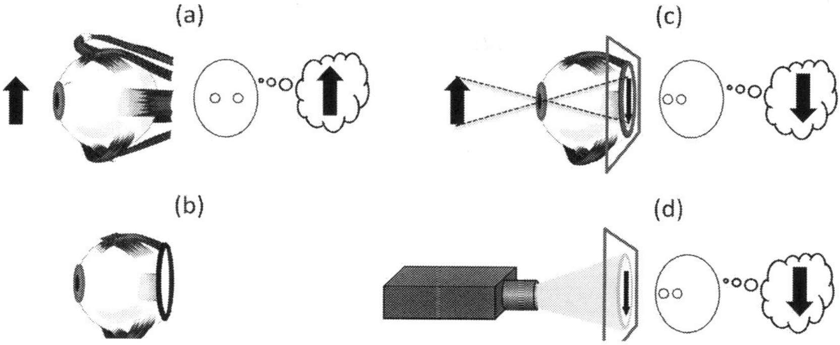

Figure 6.2 (a) Retina as "window." In natural seeing, upright things in any direction from the viewer are seen upright. (b) Scheiner and Descartes scrape off retina and rear coatings of enucleated eye. (c) With "white body" attached to rear of enucleated eye and with viewing of the "white body," upright things are seen inverted. (d) Surgery in conjunction with viewpoint created a new visual system: retina as a "rear projection screen" (cf. Campbell, 1817).

6.3 Rethinking the Simulative and Projective Assumptions

One difficulty in implementing the previously noted two-term relation resided in the simulative assumption. Notwithstanding the aforementioned "wonder and pleasure," the retinal image was not a replica of the scene that was its source, and could be likened to a two-dimensional engraving, with strokes suggestive of aspects that were not strictly visual. Descartes (1637/1985) emphasized that

> in no case does an image have to resemble the object it represents in all respects, for otherwise there would be no distinction between the object and its image. It is enough that the image resembles its object in a few respects. Indeed the perfection of an image often depends on its not resembling its object as much as it might.
>
> (p. 165)

In few words: The image was incomplete at best and ambiguous at worst. The impression was already established among 17th-century proponents of the mechanical philosophy that the light at the eye, the starting point for vision, was imperfect or defective in respect to distal objects (Pastore, 1971). Whatever might be the internal methods for managing the retinal image (in order to access its source in the environment), those methods would not be straightforward.

For Descartes, those internal methods for managing light should be rigorously mechanical as far as logic allowed. He rejected (for the most part) the interpretation of the projective assumption as simply the simulative assumption internalized. That is, he rejected the idea that an object's replica contained in the light, and available in the image at the eye, was transmitted as such to the Theater of the Mind, the *sensorium commune*.[2] Kepler had pressed for the continuity of the simulative and projectives assumptions (Lecture 4). As quoted in Crombie (1964), Kepler wrote:

> To see is to feel the stimulation of the retina, however it is stimulated. The retina is painted with the colored rays of visible things . . . But this picture does not complete the act of vision until the image so received by the retina passes through the continuity of the spirits to the brain, and there is delivered to the threshold of the faculty of the soul.
>
> (p. 115)

The principle of local causality, combined with notions of inert matter and externally driven passive machines, provided Descartes with his version of the projective assumption: physical motions caused by contiguous antecedent physical motions. The retinal image caused motions in the material fiber or tube that was the optical nerve and these, in turn, caused further motions inward to the depths of the brain. These motions did not resemble the retinal image but followed from it, as effect from cause. A human's visual sensations, therefore, did not arise from an inner act of observing a simulacrum but as the effect of an inner mechanical motion. As Descartes stated in his *Optics* (1637/1985):

> [W]hen this picture thus passes to the inside of our head, it still bears some resemblance to the objects from which it proceeds [. . .] however, we must not think that it is by means of this resemblance that the picture causes our sensory perception of these objects—as if there were yet other eyes within our brain with which we could perceive it. Instead, we must hold that it is the movements composing this picture, which acting directly upon our soul insofar as it is united to our body, are ordained by nature to make it have such sensations.
>
> (p. 167)

This particular implementation of local causality involving matter (as cause) and mind (as effect) was not of the same logical kind as implementations in which only matter was involved. One can argue that, for Descartes, this latter dilemma was unavoidable for three fundamental reasons. First, a motive faculty or self-causal agency was required that could not be material, by definition. Second, there could be no action at a distance; the principle of local causality could not be violated. Third, the motive faculty or causal agency had to have direct contact with or awareness of something in order to meet the locality principle and to avoid an infinite regress. Reed (1982) expressed the matter succinctly:

> In Descartes' world there are bodies in motion and there are thinking things. Contact between bodies, *choc*,[3] was the cause of all motion, and there was no action at a distance. However, thinking only exists by being embodied (except for God), so there is also no action at a distance in thinking: All objects of awareness must be in contact with the mind.
> (p. 735)

One can appreciate the methodological benefits of adopting human–animal dualism. In an animal automaton, the causal chain proceeds linearly from light to physical response via the eyes, nerves, brain, nerves again,[4] muscles and skeletal links. The only questions that need to be addressed in order to explain the automaton's perception-action are questions of the mechanics of its physiology. Admittedly, such questions would be challenging but the challenges are technical and, in principle, manageable. In sum, by treating animals as mindless, lacking thought, Descartes was able to clarify the distinction between questions for science—questions of physiological causal chains (see Lecture 5)—from questions for philosophy and psychology—questions of the matter–mind relation (Crombie, 1964).

6.4 The Three Grades of Sense

But what should be assumed, then, of the human? How should this member of the human–animal dualism be approached? To begin with, a human, unlike an automaton, would pass the following tests: using speech appropriately in response to queries and acting appropriately in indefinitely many novel settings (Haldane & Ross, 1911).[5] Second, a human, unlike an automaton, would operate in modes involving awareness, consistent with the hypothesis of corporeal ideas. In common with an automatism, the human possesses a mode of functioning that is purely mechanical. Involuntary human behavior ("thoughtless movements" or "reflexes," one might say) reveals an underlying system of physical reactions to external impressions upon the body. They are brought about by the felicitous (machine-like) manner in which the organs of the body are arranged. This mode of functioning, which involves no awareness, is Descartes' first grade of sense (Reed, 1982).

Both the second and third grades involve awareness, but they are of fundamentally different kinds (Haldane & Ross, 1911; Reed, 1982). It is in respect to Descartes' third grade of sense that the human–animal distinction is primarily made. The second grade of sense involves subjective awareness of states of the body. There are multiple forms of this latter kind of awareness, each associated with an organ of sensing. They are the sensations of brightness, color, sound, smell, taste, touch, and so on.[6] They are, in short, Galileo's secondary qualities. The sensory awareness in each case is the consequence of the body's nearby action on the mind; in each case, the awareness serves to unite mind with matter. The third grade of sense involves objective awareness of states of the environment as a result of the mind's rational operations on the states of the body. It is a mode of judgment directed at ascertaining Galileo's primary qualities—the initial physical causes of the sensations—rather than the sensations themselves.

Together, the second and third grades of sense constitute the hypothesis of corporeal ideas: awareness of the world (as might be obtained through vision, for example) is based in awareness of body states. Together, the first, second and third grades constitute a new ontological hypothesis, a *trialism* rather than dualism (Robinson & Garratt, 1998). Whereas the first grade is essentially material and the third is essentially mental, the second is neither essentially material nor essentially mental (Reed, 1982). The second grade of sense is at the interface of matter and mind, a kind of physical–mental hybrid. On Descartes' trialist view, when Descartes looks at a cat, then certain physical processes occur in his eyes, optic nerves and brain (Grade 1). His sensory experiences of the cat will tell him the cat's color and what kinds of noises it makes (Grade 2). His mind, which is purely mental, will then make judgments about the cat's shape, size, weight, and so on (Grade 3). We should let Descartes speak for himself, as he did so well on this matter in his *Reply to the Sixth Set of Objections* (Haldane & Ross, 1911):

> In order rightly to see what amount of certainty belongs to sense we must distinguish three grades falling within it. To the first belongs the immediate affection of the bodily organ by external objects; and this can be nothing else than the motion of the particles of the sensory organs and the change of figure and position due to that motion. The second comprises the immediate mental result, due to the mind's union with the corporeal organ affected; such are the perceptions of pain, of pleasureable stimulation, of thirst, of hunger, of colours, of sound of savour, odour, cold heat, and the like, which in the Sixth Meditation are stated to arise from the union and, as it were, the intermixture of mind and body. Finally, the third contains all those judgements, which on the occasion of motions occurring in the corporeal organ, we have from our earliest years been accustomed to pass about things external to us.
>
> (p. 251)

6.5 Thought as Mathematical Notation

The operations of the third grade of sense underwrite a truly remarkable human achievement: every person knows about the world and behaves felicitously despite being directly aware of nothing more than the activity in his or her own brain. What could possibly be the form of such operations and how could they be so competent? Descartes' answer to this twofold question was fashioned, in part, by his appreciation of how abstract was mathematics and how broad in scope was its application. His discovery that algebra could encode geometry and his recognition that both notations could represent, in addition to numerical and spatial relations, physical facts and physical laws, led Descartes to two primary realizations (Haugeland, 1985). First, that the notational systems used in mathematics could be extended to cover all meaningful things, including the thought processes implicated by the third grade of sense. Second, that a notational system bore no intrinsic relation to its subject matter (e.g., Euclid's geometry dealt equally with octagons and velocities)—that is, symbols were logically distinct from that which they symbolized. If the thoughts implicated in the third grade of sense were merely symbolic representations, like the symbols of mathematics, then what they represented was equivocal. They could represent with equal force any one of a number of very different topics, or they could represent nothing at all.

To put the mental notational system on a sound footing, to ground it and rid it of ambiguity, Descartes appealed to divine providence. God ensured that, for a conscientious mind, the symbols did indeed symbolize and that what they symbolized was reality—that is, Descartes both recognized and offered a solution to *the mystery of original meaning* (Haugeland, 1985) or the *grounding problem* (Von Eckardt, 1993). This mystery or problem is identifying those relations in virtue of which the relation of a symbol to the thing symbolized holds—for example, why it is that the symbol "cat" in one's thinking has the specific content of being about a cat. Whereas some meanings can be parasitic on other meanings, not all meanings can be parasites; some meanings must be original meanings. Descartes' solution was a special form of innate knowledge (a symbol's ground was an endowment of God's) and this innate knowledge is one major key to the success, the competence, of the operations of the third grade of sense. Other kinds of innateness contributed further to the competence—most particularly, the rules of logical reasoning. To take a single example, Descartes suggested that because no person, regardless of experience, will accept a self-contradictory proposition (such as, nothing at the same time can be black and white, alive and dead, etc.), understanding of the principle of contradiction is an innate given.

6.6 The Highest Grade of Sense: Problems and a Paradox

In sum, the kind of operation that characterizes the third or highest grade of sensing is a rule-governed, quasi-mathematical process of reasoning. It is a kind of inference performed upon the data of the senses made possible by two types of innate knowledge: that of logical and mathematical principles and that of the composition of the world. Descartes was suggesting that perceiving is a species of thinking. In perceiving their surroundings, humans use a knowledge-constrained process that is similar to the process by which they think or reason about ideas. As we may recall from Lecture 5, Hobbes had identified reasoning with the methodical application of rules to symbols, as in writing. If writing words using the letters (symbols) of the alphabet is a good model for reasoning, then Hobbes's account is circular. Just as public writing implies a writer, so private thinking implies a thinker. On Hobbes's account, therefore, the reasoning done by a person presumes a person (but, presumably, not the same one) who is doing the reasoning. This is the *problem of the inner person* or, more traditionally, the *problem of the homunculus*. In Descartes' third grade of sensing, an unexplained homunculus (Latin for "little man") is at work.

The necessity of the homunculus is underscored by the difficulty of mechanizing reasoning in the manner hoped for by Hobbes. Mechanization would be possible if the homunculus attended only to the symbols and the rules (which themselves could be expressed as finite sequences of symbols). If, however, he attended additionally to symbol meaning, then the principle of local causality would be compromised—and, perforce, machine-like behavior would be ruled out—because a meaning is not the kind of thing that exerts a physical force (Haugeland, 1985). In order to reason, in order to determine what is reasonable, requires more than the rules and symbols. It requires heeding what the rules and symbols represent—that is, what they mean. But as we have seen in Descartes' symbol-symbolized (sub)dualism, meanings are not enshrined in symbols but granted by God. Although we might identify symbols with Descartes' corporeal ideas or with Hobbes's brain packets, we cannot do likewise with meanings. Simply put, meanings are purely in the mental realm. Herein lies the *paradox of mechanical reason* (Haugeland, 1985): "[I]f a process or system is mechanical, it can't reason; if it reasons, it can't be mechanical" (p. 39).

We can state the paradox in the terms introduced in Lectures 3 and 4: "[I]f a process or system is strictly predicative, it can't reason; if it involves impredicativities, it can't be mechanical" (p. 39).

The immediate upshot of the paradox is that it will not be a simple matter to discharge the human analogue from within Descartes' third grade of sense. The rule-governed, quasi-mathematical process of reasoning that characterizes perception requires an intelligent inner person to supervise the various processes. Or, to phrase it better (but in a less picture-able form), it requires a solution to the problem of impoverished entailment (Lecture 3).

An additional challenge, intimately connected to the aforementioned paradox, is posed by the origin of the inner person's intelligence. Adopting an economics perspective, one might say that Descartes built the third grade of sense by taking out "loans of intelligence" (Dennett, 1971, 1978). Imagine a bank that transacts its business in intelligence rather than money. When intelligence is needed for a particular purpose, one goes to the intelligence bank, makes an application, and takes out a loan. Of course, like a regular money bank, the intelligence bank expects to be repaid. In Descartes' case, he went to The Manager at The Bank. There are no indications that Descartes planned to pay back his loans (or that The Manager expected him to do so) and there is no possible way in which we can understand how Descartes would have fulfilled his duty if he had so intended.

To appreciate what is at issue here with regard to the inner person, we need to say a little more about the notion of intentionality, or aboutness, introduced in Lecture 1. Philosophers of the 20th century (e g., Chisholm, 1957; Quine, 1960) sought to clarify Brentano's 19th-century thesis by focusing on the logical definition of *intentional idioms* (e.g., decides [that], hopes [that], and recognizes [that]). That is, rather than attempting to define the states or events constituting intentional phenomena they focused on how ordinary language describes or alludes to intentional phenomena (Dennett, 1969). A frequently cited logical definition is that an intentional sentence that is true can be falsified by substituting one term in the sentence by another that denotes the same thing.[7] For example, while it is true that Oedipus hoped that he could marry Jocasta, it is certainly not true that Oedipus hoped that he could marry his mother (where, in Oedipus's tragic case, Jocasta and his mother were, unbeknown to him, one and the same person). The truth of Oedipus's hope is not preserved over coextensive substitution. It turns out that not only do the familiar mental terms satisfy the preceding test, but so do terms that we would associate with the computation-like reasoning processes implied by Descartes' third grade of sense—for example, "storing information *that* corporeal idea *x* was accompanied by corporeal idea *y*" or "assigning the priority *that* processing corporeal idea *x* should precede processing corporeal idea *y*," and so on.

For present purposes, what is important here is that whenever and wherever an intentional idiom is used in explanation, the taking out of a loan of intelligence is implicated. This is similarly true whenever and wherever a term is used in explanation that endows a state with meaning or content or significance. For example, referring to a state as a "signal" or a "message" or a "command," implicates, respectively, a "signal-reader," a "message-interpreter" and a "commander" (Dennett, 1971). Obviously, in constructing the third grade of sense, Descartes used intentional idioms. He presupposed rationality in the form of intelligence loans. If he wished to avoid such loan taking, he would have had to find a way of extending the mechanistic hypothesis that he so actively promoted for the first grade of sense to the second and third grades of sense. But that, obviously, was not an option, as can be emphasized by a further consideration of ordinary language usage. The mechanistic hypothesis is expressed in *extensional* sentences. The truth or falsity of these sentences, unlike that of intentional sentences, is preserved when one term in the extension of a concept is substituted by another term in the extension of the same concept. The sentence "The stone weighed approximately 0.45 kg" preserves the truth of the sentence 'the stone weighed 1 lb." Simply, extensional sentences are non-intentional and a conclusion consonant with Descartes' substance and property dualism (that holds mind and matter distinct) is that intentional sentences cannot be reduced to extensional sentences (Dennett, 1969). It is simply not possible to convert intentional, rational language (intentional sentences) into mechanical language (extensional sentences). We should give this general problem a name. Let us call it the *problem of non-repayable loans of intelligence.*

6.7 The Cartesian Program Defined

We have taken a lengthy and cluttered path to get here, but we are now ready to define the *Cartesian Program* for perception and action (and for cognition more generally). It can be expressed as three injunctions. First, develop as thoroughly as science and mathematics permit a mechanical account of the first grade of sense—that is, explain the workings of the senses in generating secondary qualities and the motor system in generating bodily motions through strict adherence to the principle of local cause using only the extensional language provided by chemistry, physiology, and physics. Second, identify the kinds of knowledge with which the third grade of sense must be endowed a priori—that is, identify what principles governing the workings of the world are known independent of any experience with the world and give expression to the formal structure of the abstract and productive representations that embody this knowledge. Third, discover and explicate the symbol-manipulating procedures employed by the third grade of sense in using the secondary qualities (the second grade of sense) and the endowed knowledge to make successful inferences about the world.

Notes

1 Image formation is common in nature. It is often regarded as an achievement of animals that requires minimally a light source (or an illuminated environment), a chamber with a projection surface, and a lens-fitted aperture. Stoffregen (2013) argues to the contrary in words and photos. The inverted optic image in its multiple forms can be manifest and is made manifest in the absence of members of Animalia. The sufficient conditions for inverted image formation (an illuminated environment, an aperture, and a projection surface) pre-date the origins of life. The image is more properly understood as a fact of physical optics rather than as an invention of evolution.
2 Latin for "common sense," it refers broadly to an inner sense that receives and coordinates the sensations from the five senses.
3 French for "shock."
4 Descartes did not distinguish clearly between sensory and motor nerves (Fearing, 1930/1970).
5 By "appropriately" is meant putting words or movements together in a productive (rule-governed) way. Descartes wished to emphasize that the uttered sentences and demonstrated actions of humans are typically novel and stimulus-independent

organizations of their constituents rather than habitual sequences (see the *Discourse*, pp. 116–117, in Haldane & Ross, 1911).

6 Initially, in his earlier dualist model, Descartes excluded sensation from his description of the animal machine. Not only were they lacking thought, but they were also lacking any kinds of sensory experiences and feelings, such as pain. They were truly non-conscious automata, differing from rocks only in their degree of mechanical complexity. The later trialist model, aimed at explaining sensations, allowed that animals, like humans, have sensations. They simply (*sic*) lack the reasoning process that operates on the sensations.

7 Referred to as the failure of substitutivity of coextensive terms *salva veritate* (Latin for "with truth saved"; Audi, 1999).

References

Audi, R. (1999). *The Cambridge dictionary of philosophy*. Cambridge, UK: Cambridge University Press.

Boring, E. G. (1942). *Sensation and perception in the history of experimental psychology*. New York: Appleton-Century-Crofts.

Campbell, J. (1817). On vision. *Annals of Philosophy*, *10*, 17–29.

Chisholm, P. (1957). *A philosophical study*. Ithaca, NY: Cornell University Press.

Crombie, A. C. (1964). Early concepts of the senses and the mind. *Scientific American*, *210* (No. 5, May), 108–116.

Dennett, D. (1969). *Content and consciousness*. London: Routledge & Kegan Paul.

Dennett, D. (1971). Intentional systems. *Journal of Philosophy*, 68, 87–106.

Dennett, D. (1978). *Brainstorms*. Montgomery, VT: Bradford Books.

Descartes, R. (1985). Optics. In J. Cottingham, R. Stoothoff and D. Murdoch (Trans.), *The philosophical writings of Descartes, Vol. 1* (pp. 152–175). Cambridge, UK: Cambridge University Press (original work published 1637).

Descartes, R. (1911). *Meditationes de prima philosophia/The philosophical works of Descartes, Vol.1*. Cambridge, UK: Cambridge University Press (original work published 1641).

Duke-Elder, S. (1932). *Textbook of ophthalmology* (Volume 1). London: Kimpton.

Fearing, F. (1970). *Reflex action: A study in the history of physiological psychology*. Cambridge, MA: MIT Press (original work published 1930).

Haldane, E., & Ross, J. (1911). *The philosophical works of Descartes, Vols. I and II*. Cambridge, UK: Cambridge University Press.

Haugeland, J. (1985). *Artificial intelligence: The very idea*. Cambridge, MA: MIT Press.

Kawashima, W., Hatake, K., Kudo, R., Nakanishi, M., Tamaki, S., et al. (2015) Estimating the time after death on the basis of corneal opacity. *Journal of Forensic Research*, 6, 269.

O'Neil, B. E. (1974). *Epistemological direct realism in Descartes's philosophy*. Albuquerque, NM: University of New Mexico Press.

Pastore, N. (1971). *Selective history of theories of visual perception, 1650–1950*. Oxford, UK: Oxford University Press.

Quine, W. V. (1960). *Word and object*. Cambridge, MA: MIT Press.

Reed, E. S. (1982). Descartes's corporeal ideas hypothesis and the origin of scientific psychology. *Review of Metaphysics*, *35*, 731–752.

Robinson, D., & Garratt, C. (1998). *Introducing Descartes*. New York: Totem Books.

Stoffregen, T. A. (2013). On the physical origins of inverted optic images. *Ecological Psychology*, *25*, 369–382.

Von Eckardt, B. (1993). *What is cognitive science?* Cambridge, MA: MIT Press.
Williams, B. (1967). Descartes. In P. Edwards (Ed.), *The encyclopedia of philosophy*, *Vol. 2* (pp. 344–354). New York: Macmillan.
Yolton, J. (1975). Ideas and knowledge in seventeenth-century philosophy. *Journal of the History of Philosophy*, *13*, 145–165.

Lecture 7

Empiricism and the Man in the Inner Room

Historically, Descartes' influence has been wide and enduring (Williams, 1967). Most of the developments in theories of perception and action subsequent to Descartes can be considered as occurring in relation to the Cartesian system of grades of sense and as responses to, or accommodations of, the Cartesian Program. Similarly wide and enduring has been the influence of the mechanistic philosophy introduced by Descartes and fellow 17th-century scholars. We can summarize the five main suppositions of their mechanistic philosophy (identified in Lectures 2, 5 and 6):

1 Matter is inert, passive, and changeless (the only permissible transformation is one of location).
2 Matter is organized and patterned by (perfect and immutable) mathematical laws.
3 Matter can be fully understood by mechanics (the applied mathematics of motion).
4 Matter is always in only one of its logically possible states and its state variables have determinate values at all times.
5 Mind is distinct from matter but linked to matter through sense and reason.

The goal of the present lecture is to identify the contributions (to how one knows about the world by sight) of the British Empiricists: John Locke (1632–1704), George Berkeley (1685–1753) and David Hume (1711–1776). Empiricists hold to a system of philosophy (*Empiricism*) that takes the ultimate basis for knowledge to be experience rather than logical reasoning. Whereas Rationalism asserts the primacy of reason in respect to knowing about, Empiricism asserts the primacy of the sensory experience. Locke (1689/1997, II.i.2) stated the position thus:

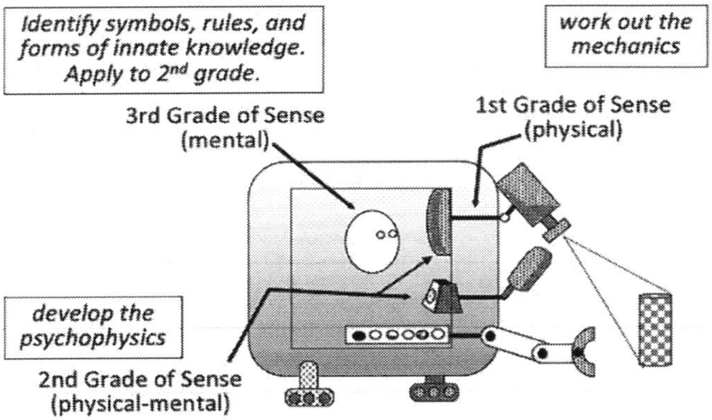

Figure 7.1 The Man in the Inner Room, and the trialism and scientific program of Descartes.

(From Figure 1, Turvey, 2004, adapted with permission, *Ecological Psychology*.)

> Let us then suppose that the mind be, as we say, white paper, void of all characters, without any ideas; how comes it to be furnished? Whence has it all the materials of reason and knowledge? To this I answer, in one word, from *experience*: in that all our knowledge is founded; and from that it ultimately derives itself.
>
> (p. 109)

We can quickly introduce ourselves to the differences among the British Empiricists and their connection to Descartes' views. We can do so by means of Figure 7.1—that is, in terms of the Man in the Inner Room (Toulmin, 1967). For the purpose of being inclusive of action, the inner room is in a mobile home. For the purpose of stage setting, Figure 7.1 is a synopsis of the Cartesian Program.

7.1 Three Perspectives on the Man in the Inner Room

Imagine a man who spends his entire life inside an inner room of a house. What he knows about the world outside his home, the world in which he can be said to live, is based on the pictures and sounds provided by a television set inside the room that receives inputs from cameras and microphones attached to the exterior of the house. This recluse in the inner room may ponder the relation between what he is aware of directly—namely, the TV images and sounds, and the world outside. He may ponder the extent to which the images and sounds represent things in the world, and the extent to which they are artifacts of the system of communication with no real-world counterparts (Toulmin, 1967).

7.1.1 Locke's Perspective

Let us suppose that the man in the inner room is a "realist"—that is, he believes that there is a world outside and that it can be known, at least in part. He also believes that some aspects of the TV displays do represent things in the outside world. He likes to consider himself a "representational realist." In deciding which aspects of the images do resemble things in the world, he conjectures from first principles that the reliable aspects are likely to be geometric and kinematic. He draws up a list of primary qualities: form, size, position, duration, motion and solidity. Critical reflection has revealed to him that these qualities are constantly present in the images on the screen. Apparently, these qualities are transmitted by the principle of local causality with such fidelity that he is willing to claim that what he sees is each quality's resemblance in the transmitted images. Other aspects of the transmitted images, however, such as their colors and degrees of lightness, are rejected as qualities of the objects outside the house.[1] (He notices that by fiddling with the control knobs of the TV he can, for example, remove color and sound, and change brightness while leaving the primary qualities intact.) He identifies color, lightness and sound as secondary qualities, caused somehow by the interaction of the primary qualities with the communication channels. His surmise is that these latter qualities represent and resemble nothing in the outside world, although caused by things in the outside world. Like the primary qualities, they can be sources of his ideas about the outside world, albeit of questionable reliability. He is fully appreciative that these various qualities of the TV images are the ultimate foundations of what he can know about the world beyond the house. At the same time, however, it is evident to him that whatever knowledge he might currently have or subsequently obtain about the outside world depends on his faculties of reason and understanding. How he brings these faculties to bear on the primary and secondary qualities determines his knowledge; it is not the result of simply observing the images.

7.1.2 Berkeley's Perspective[2]

We can give the man in the inner room a different persona. Suppose that he decides that there is no basis for distinguishing between properties of the TV displays that do and do not correspond to real things in the world beyond the walls of the house. He makes this decision on the grounds that there is simply no way in which he can compare the various images and their aspects with the supposed things outside the house that could have caused them. After all, locked in the inner room since birth, he has only ever been in contact with the images on the screen. The only "reality" that he is directly acquainted with at any moment, either in the past or in the present, is that of the ideas resulting from the TV images. To assume another reality, one outside the inner room and one that is constituted by anything other than ideas, is empty speculation. Better to recognize that all of his knowledge came from his experiences in the inner room and to assume that whatever he can experience in the room exists and whatever he cannot experience in the inner room cannot exist.[3] There are presumably many experiences to be had in the inner room, a world of ideas, as it were, of which, at the present time, he has had just a sample. What he can experience, what there is to know, is distinct from his experiences as the one who knows. He supposes that these latter facts, in conjunction with a notion of self, give him no other recourse than to adopt the stance of an "idealist" rather than a "realist" or a "solipsist."

7.1.3 *Hume's Perspective*

There is a third persona of the man in the inner room. It is that of the "skeptic." Given that he is limited to the experiences provided by the TV, he is willing to accept that all that he can know is confined to those experiences in the inner room.[4] He is also, on the same grounds, willing to doubt that anything exists beyond the house, a consequence of which is that he expresses little concern for the processes by which the TV images and sounds get to the inner room. Despite his announced skepticism, however, he finds it very hard to be a true and comprehensive disbeliever. There is something about the ways that his impressions and ideas pattern or organize that invoke in him a belief in the existence of durable objects outside the house. This belief seems to be at odds with the images on the screen. They are typically not durable but, rather, discontinuous in time and not singular (as if a single persisting object) but multiple. There are mechanisms at work, however, that connect his memories of the TV images without his volition and do so, apparently, according to resemblance, closeness in time and space, and as cause–effect pairings. There are also other automatic mechanisms at work, based on the former, that bring to his notice a constancy and a coherency in certain sets of images. He notices that some images assume the same form at each observation and when they change from earlier to later observations, they do so in familiar and patterned ways. It is this constancy and coherency of images that lead him to believe, in the face of his skepticism, that some images are produced by objects that exist outside the house independently of their images on the screen.

7.2 Locke's Intelligence Loans

Each view of the inner man is intended to be a description of the human experience (*we* are the inner man). Each reflects Descartes' trichotomy. The house with its attachments and causal connections from cameras and microphones is a person's body and sensory nerves (first grade of sense). The inner room of the house is the *sensorium* and the inhabitant is the person's mind (third grade of sense). The images and sounds delivered by the TV are the sensory inputs to the *sensorium* and include the secondary qualities of which the person's mind is directly aware (second grade of sense). As versions of empiricism, each view of the inner man necessarily departs in some respects from the strict Cartesian Program, Locke's view (*representational realism*) the least and Hume's view (*skepticism*) the most.

It is evident from the inner man parable that Locke interpreted perception as a three-term relation—namely, a perceiver, an environment and a layer of mental representations, referred to as ideas, that mediates perceiver and environment. Locke's empiricism was marked by a strong denouncement of the possibility that the mediating ideas could be innate. For Locke, the content of each and every thought is traceable back to experience. Certain abstractions, such as the law of non-contradiction (that it was impossible for the same thing to be and not to be; Lecture 6), held no special status for Locke. Such abstractions were not innately given first principles. Rather, they were merely the consequence of applying reason to the ideas derived from experience. In this respect, Locke may not have been at odds with Descartes. In Comments on a Certain Broadsheet (1648/1985) Descartes argued that

> The mind has no need of ideas, or notions, or axioms which are innate: its faculty of thinking is all it needs for performing its own acts. Thus all common notions which are engraved in the mind have their origin in observation of things or in verbal instruction.
>
> (p. 295)

However, where Descartes might have vacillated at times in his opposition to the innateness of ideas, Locke was steadfast. It was in regard to the variety of intellectual operations ascribed to the third grade of sense that the two philosophers were consistently in step. Like Descartes, Locke endowed the highest grade of sense with natural faculties and innate powers to think and reason. He was very appreciative of the challenge that thinking imposed, suggesting (1689/1997, IV.iii.6, pp. 480–481): that God might have chosen to "superadd to matter a faculty of thinking" (p. 480) just as he had "annexed effects to motion, which we can in no way conceive motion able to produce" (p. 481).

Loans of intelligence are similarly evident in Locke's important distinction between simple and complex ideas. All qualities, both primary and secondary, corresponded to *simple* ideas. These single, indivisible qualities were taken by Locke to be the right degrees of freedom for addressing the mind (1689/1997, II.iii.2):

> When the understanding is once stored with these simple ideas, it has the power to repeat, compare and unite them to an almost infinite variety, and so can make at pleasure new complex ideas. But it is not in the power [. . .] of understanding [. . .] of thought, *to invent or frame*

> *one new simple idea* [. . .] nor can any force of the understanding *destroy* those that are there.
>
> (pp. 121–122)

All complex ideas are derived from these immutable simple ideas by the mental operations of combining, comparing, and abstracting. The derivations cannot be arbitrary, however, given that the complex ideas must have some bearing upon the objective reality (the world outside the house in which the inner room and its inhabitant reside). The combining, comparing and abstracting must be rationally constrained. In summary, Locke's empiricism is not pure; it incorporates, in significant degree, rationalism and nativism. His claim that a certain motion in the body produces the idea of a particular color was befitting the mechanical hypothesis but was, nonetheless, very puzzling. When faced with such difficulties, Locke would regularly visit The Bank. He would take out a loan in the form of God's omnipotence and wisdom and in the form of the observation that human knowledge suited human purpose (Clapp, 1967).

7.3 Correspondence, Coherence and Pragmatic Theories of Truth

In Locke's perspective on the man in the inner room, the man must confront the issue of whether his perceptions are true. The common-sense strategy would be for him to accept as true any idea, simple or complex, which is in correspondence with a fact of the world outside the house—the objective reality. The *criterion of correspondence* is simply this: an idea that agrees with its fact is necessarily true. The difficulty lies in applying the criterion. Given his seclusion, Locke's man in the inner room has no direct contact with the outer world and, therefore, no way to assess the fit between idea and fact.[5] Even if he did have such contact, it is not clear that the criterion of correspondence would suffice. To determine that a perceived primary quality (one displayed on the TV in the inner room) does indeed correspond to a primary quality in the world requires the use of an additional criterion which when satisfied specifies correspondence. But any appeal to another test of truth reduces the criterion of correspondence to a mere definition of the truth of an idea ("current idea of primary quality q is true if and only if the primary quality q is present") rather than a decisive test.

If determining correspondence were not possible, then the man in the inner room would be forced to assess the truth of an idea in a substantially different way. For example, he might abide the criterion that an idea is true provided it stands in a suitably strong relation of coherence to other ideas. This is the *criterion of coherence* (e.g., Bradley, 1914). It transforms the common-sense notion that an idea is true if and only if it copies reality into the doctrine that an idea is true if and only if it coheres with another idea or set of ideas. By this criterion of coherence, the validity of an idea depends entirely on its relations internally within the system comprising simple and complex ideas—the current and past arrays of TV images. The internal relations that determine a given idea's coherence include much more than the pattern of consistencies between it and other ideas; they include, in addition, the pattern of inferences and explanations to which the idea gives rise. We can imagine the man in the inner room seeking to arrange his available ideas relative to the given idea so as to evaluate whether they relate consistently and cohesively as parts of an integrated system.

Coherence as a theory of truth is characteristic of rationalist metaphysics (White, 1967). Patently, the adoption of the coherence criterion by Locke's man in the inner room rests on his natural faculties and innate abilities to think and reason. It is also fairly obvious, however, that the coherence criterion would seem to be far more compatible with Berkeley's idealism than with Locke's representational realism. For the man in the inner room, verification by coherence promises, in and of itself, no insight into the composition of the external world.

There is another way to think about what is true, aside from the two traditional theories of correspondence and coherence, but it has no applicability to the man in the inner room. It is the pragmatic perspective encountered briefly in Lecture 5 (precisely, Section 5.4). We can call it the *criterion of workability*. Roughly, if an idea works, it must be accepted as true; it is the workability of an idea that determines its validity. Accordingly, one must look at the consequences that issue from a given idea. An idea's truth is obtained from or measured by its outcomes (James, 1907/1975):

> The truth of an idea is not a stagnant property inherent in it. Truth *happens* to an idea. It *becomes* true, is *made* true by events. Its verity *is* in fact an event, a process: the process namely of its verifying itself, its veri-*fication*. Its validity is the process of its valid-*ation*.
>
> (p. 97)

The criterion of workability implies action, either in the sense of performance or exploration conducted in, and relative to, the world outside the house. It is, therefore, inapplicable to the problem of discerning true ideas faced by the man in the inner room because, in all strictness, the parable of the man in the inner room is a parable about perception. There is no action. More to the point, perception within the Cartesian Program resides in the third grade of sense whereas action resides in the first grade of sense. Distinct and separate theories of perception and action are implicated.

7.4 Hume's Problem, Hume's Solution, and Hume's Touchstone

Hume's empiricism is radical. By this is meant that he sought to account for perception by (a) maximizing the contributions of the senses and (b) minimizing the loans of intelligence and the rational involvement of the inner man. Indeed, the story of the inner man told above from Hume's perspective is somewhat misleading. Hume replaced the human-analogue by a bundle of ideas (sensations) and impressions (roughly, memories of sensations) related by resemblance, contiguity and causation—that is, by associative principles.

We might reconstruct the motivation for this radicalism as follows. Thinking and reasoning should not be presumed as innate mental operations, already supremely organized, but as mental phenomena in need of explanation. To endow the inner man with intentional traits, with the abilities to comprehend and supervise ideas and impressions, is to leave unexplained the very properties of mind that, ideally, one's theory is designed to explain. Hume's problem, therefore, was how to discharge the intelligent homunculus without, at the same time, discharging intelligence. If one is unwilling to take out a loan of intelligence, as was Hume, then one must face squarely the challenge of how to get intelligence from non-intelligence. Minimally, one must get the ideas and impressions, which are the least intelligent mental entities possible, to "think for themselves" (Dennett, 1981, p. 122).

Hume's solution to this problem was to regard the ideas and impressions as analogous to the physical particles that figure so prominently in the mechanics of Newton. Just as physical particles subject to Newton's laws of motion could, in principle, produce the endless variety of the universe, so mental particles subject to the laws of mental mechanics could, in principle, produce the endless variety of the mind. These mental laws were the association laws. Hume (1739/2000, 1.1.4.1 and 1.1.4.6) contended that each association law[6] should be construed as "a gentle force, which commonly prevails" (p. 12), "a kind of ATTRACTION, which in the mental world will be found to have as extraordinary effects as in the natural, and to show itself in as many and as various forms" (p. 14).

It is worth underscoring that, in pressing his mental mechanics, Hume was criticizing the adequacy of the Cartesian Program, in particular the treatment of the mental as a fundamentally ratiocinative or logical process. If, contrary to Descartes, the mind is not organized by principles of logic, then other principles—non-logical principles—must be sought to explain how it works. Hume's associative principles were of the right non-logical kind.

Of some significance, the lawful mechanical nature of these principles suggested that they were not proprietary of humans but, rather, the common property of all animals. The proposed mental mechanics should be universal with respect to things capable of perceiving just as Newton's mechanics were universal with respect to things incapable of perceiving. In short, Hume rejected Descartes' human–animal dualism. Given the opposite doctrine, that put humans and animals on equal footing, he could avail himself of a criterion for distinguishing promising theories from bogus theories of mental process (Massey, 1993). Hume (1739/2000, 1.3.16.3) defined this touchstone as follows:

> This doctrine is as useful as it is obvious, and furnishes us with a kind of touchstone, by which we may try every system in this species of philosophy [. . .] When any hypothesis, therefore, is advanc'd to explain a mental operation, which is common to men and beasts, we must apply the same hypothesis to both; and as every true hypothesis will abide this trial, so I may venture to affirm, no false one will ever be able to endure it.
>
> (p. 118)

Stated broadly, Hume's touchstone identifies as counterfeit any account of perception (and, presumably, action) that does not apply even-handedly to human and non-human animals.[7]

In summary, we can see that Hume's radical empiricism, fashioned within the framework of the three-term relation characterizing indirect perception (Lecture 3), disposed of the related problems of the homunculus and non-payable intelligence loans. It can be argued, however, that in so doing Hume's radical empiricism falls prey to the paradox of mechanical reason (Haugeland, 1985). There is no meaning in Hume's mechanical mind, calling into question whether the mind so constructed can be considered as truly mental. How can the meaningless associative relations among meaningless ideas and impressions induce intentionality? They should, if perceiving is *about something*. Hume, it seems, is caught on the second horn of the dilemma: If meanings do not matter to the processes of perception, then those processes are not truly rational, not truly intelligent (Haugeland, 1985). They are merely the meaningless processes characteristic of a machine. In brief, Hume's mental mechanics do not yield what he aspired: rationality from non-rationality, intelligence from non-intelligence.

7.5 A Mystery and a Glimpse Ahead

The parable of the man in the inner room makes transparent the paradox that emerged in the 17th and 18th centuries. A scholar committed to the mechanistic hypothesis had no options but to separate the mental from the physical and, thereby, no options but to explain perception in terms of the man in the inner room. A difficult scientific problem was replaced by an insoluble mystery (Ryle, 1949; Toulmin, 1967). The scientific problem was how a complete human can know about the world by sight. The mystery was how a mind within a *sensorium*, within a brain, within a complete human, can know about the world by sight given only direct awareness of states of the sensory nerves, the inputs to the *sensorium* (Toulmin, 1967).

The traditional epistemological problems reflect this mystery. The modern student of perception and action would be justified, therefore, in asking the question of what becomes of the mystery and the attendant epistemological problems if the theory of perception were to be built on the physical science of the 21st century rather than that of the 17th century. The question is most certainly warranted. *In the physical science of the 21st century, each of the five presuppositions of the mechanical philosophy of the 17th century identified at the outset of this lecture is rejected.* As a preliminary step toward an answer, two contemporary themes of physical science can be looked at here, if only briefly. The first is the notion that the inertness and passivity of nature can be challenged on at least two fronts. The second theme gives some insight, perhaps, into the reason that the paradox of mechanical reason (unsolved by Hume) is either inevitable or impossible to resolve in the absence of a dramatic rethinking of the logic of dualisms.

7.5.1 Active Matter

Two strands of modern physics have given rise to the comprehension of matter as active agency. One strand is labeled self-organizing physics and includes non-linear thermodynamics and non-linear dynamics. It provides images of matter as continua that spontaneously order themselves when certain circumstances prevail. The other strand is labeled nonlocality—the consequence of the juxtaposition of the EPR experiment and Bell's inequality that was encountered in Lecture 4. It provides images of matter as particles that are aspects of a single nonlocally connected process distributed in space and changing in time according to quantum laws. Common to both strands is the dismissal of the image of matter as inert and passive, as lacking intrinsic power and moved only by external forces (Lecture 2).

Given that we have already been introduced to the notion of nonlocality we can focus here on acquiring some familiarity with the notion of self-organization. A sketch of one well-known phenomenon will suffice. It is a paradigmatic instance of what are referred to as *excitable media.*

Near the middle of the 20th century, an unexpected observation was made in chemistry: When certain substances are mixed in a petri dish (a very shallow, flat dish) and left alone, spatial-temporal patterns of exquisite beauty emerge spontaneously (Figure 7.2). A mixture of organic and inorganic (i.e., carbon-less) chemicals produces concentric rings that propagate outwards from centers that emerge spontaneously throughout the petri dish. The concentric rings are formed at regular intervals, with an encounter between any two or more rings leading to mutual annihilation (unlike the ripples on a pond originating from different sites that pass through each other). The repetitive pattern-formation, pattern-degradation process just described is known as the Belousov–Zhabotinsky, or BZ, reaction (e.g., Winfree, 1987).

There are two key processes in the BZ reaction. The first is a process by which a substance stimulates its own production—a positive feedback effect or autocatalysis. Imagine substance A mixed with substances B, C and D that, in reaction, generate 2A and substances E and F—that is, in the dish, A starts to produce more of itself. As the concentration of A increases, the production of A in neighboring regions is stimulated, resulting in a spreading wave of

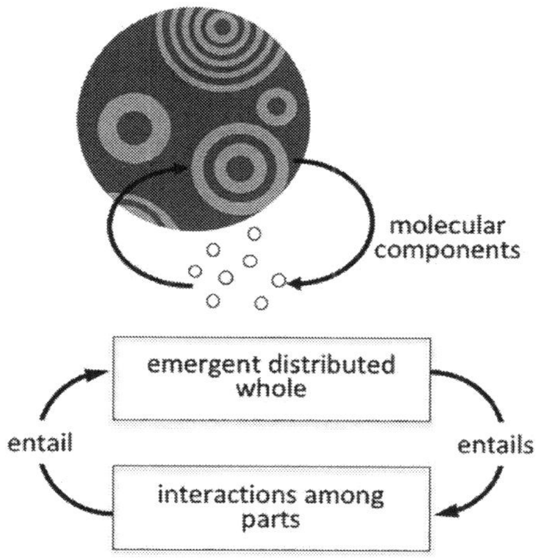

Figure 7.2 A schematic of the Belousov–Zhabotinsky, or BZ, reaction. See text for details.

production of A. At this juncture, the second key process comes into play: an inhibitor of A's synthesis. In many analogous settings, the autocatalysis of a substance is balanced by the rate at which its inhibitor is produced and the mixture settles on a steady state. But the complexity of the BZ recipe is such that production and inhibition of A cannot balance and the mixture oscillates between their competing effects.

7.5.2 Generalized Complementarity Principle

One particularly hard lesson of the current era is that formally incompatible descriptive modes may be necessary for explanation and understanding (Nadeau & Kafatos, 1999; Pattee, 1977, 1978, 1982, 1987). This is, more precisely, an epistemological strategy that generalizes Bohr's (1934, 1937) complementarity principle. The origin of this principle lies in the epistemological challenges posed by quantum mechanics (Jammer, 1974). As typically defined, complementarity applies to what would appear to be mutually exclusive descriptions, such as wave and particle, or mutually exclusive measures, such as those of position and momentum. The two descriptions cannot be applied at the same time. The two measures cannot be made at the same time. For neither pair, however, can one member define the world at the quantum scale in the absence of the other. Both members are required. Consider radiation. It can be viewed as a wave or a collection of particles according to the experiment. Bohr regarded the choice of one mode of thinking versus the other as dictated completely by the experimental environment. Radiation lacks a unique conceptual framework, but one conception or the other must be used in each case: waves when using one particular measuring instrument (a receiving antenna), particles when using another, distinctively different, instrument (a photomultiplier).

Instead of attempting to resolve a dualism (e.g., wave-particle as only wave, mind-matter as only matter) the strategy is to accept it as an irreducible aspect of reality. Bohr (1937) remarked that the quantum of action, defined through the mutually exclusive measures of position and momentum, "forces" acceptance of complementarity as the proper epistemological framework. This is because the quantum of action is one of nature's four constants (the speed of light, Boltzman's constant and the gravitational constant being the others; Cohen-Tannoudji, 1993). *If an incontrovertibly real aspect of nature requires complementarity for its understanding, then complementarity must be an incontrovertibly necessary strategy for investigating nature.* In short, the complementarity principle should be generalized. Bohr (1937) was of the impression that "the lesson taught us by recent developments in physics [. . .] leads us to a general epistemological attitude which might help us to avoid apparent conceptual difficulties in other fields of science as well" (p. 289).

One should not interpret this necessity of two formally disjoint modes of description as implying either a contradiction (which can only occur in a single formal mode) or that the system under observation is composed of polar opposites (Pattee, 1978). This latter point is highlighted in the comparison of explanation by the complementarity principle of the 20th century and explanation by the orthodox or classical means established in the 17th century (Pattee, 1978). Complementarity, it has been suggested, addresses systems that are conceptually unified by their functional coherence (e.g., a cell and an organism) and achieves explanation through two disjoint modes of description. In contrast, orthodox explanation is directed at systems that are conceptually disjoint (e.g., stars and pendulums) and is achieved by means of a single, unified and coherent mode of description, namely, Newton's laws of motion.

The strategy of a generalized complementarity principle is, therefore, not simply a matter of tolerating the polar opposites as if they are merely different perspectives on the same thing. Rather, the strategy (it has been suggested) sharpens the paradox (Pattee, 1982). In respect to the mentalese and physicalese of mind–body dualism or the polarities of any other dualism of equivalent force, it can be argued (Pattee, 1982) that: "Both modes of description, though formally incompatible, must be a part of the theory, and truth is discovered by studying the interplay of the opposites" (p. 28). By this admonition, the problem of non-repayable loans of intelligence (Lecture 6, Section 6) should encourage efforts to understand the relation between extensional and intensional descriptions rather than invite attempts to translate the latter into the former.

We can usefully summarize generalized complementarity as follows: it is a logical framework for addressing binary opposites that (a) preclude one another in a description of the aspect of nature to which they apply and (b) taken together constitute a complete description of that aspect (Nadeau & Kafatos, 1999; Pattee, 1987). The difficulty with this framework is twofold (Pattee, 1978). First, it has undergone little development outside of quantum theory and even there it is hampered by unresolved epistemological problems of measurement. Second, it is limited to the internal consistency of models of observational situations. It has little to say to the scientist expressing a normal interest in *predicting* natural phenomena, such as those of perception and action. At this juncture, complementarity is no more than an epistemological principle, albeit one inspired by the physics of so-called elemental matter. In later lectures, we will encounter substantive reasons for doubting its authenticity.

Notes

1 Locke (1689/1997, II. Viii. 15, p. 136) noted that "whatever reality we by mistake, attribute to them, are in truth nothing in the objects themselves, but powers to produce various sensations in us . . ."

2 Here, we consider the perspective as presented by Berkeley (1710/1998) in *A Treatise Concerning the Principles of Human Knowledge*. A somewhat different perspective, but one that presages the idealism in the *Principles*, could be given based on Berkeley's (1709/1948) *Essay Towards a New Theory of Vision*. The development of the perspective from the *New Theory* is the main task of Lecture 8.

3 As Berkeley phrased it: "To be is to be experienced" (in Latin, *esse est percipi*).

4 Hume (1739/2000, Book 1, Part 2, Section 6, p. 49) wrote: "[N]othing is ever really present with [or to] the mind but its perceptions or impressions and ideas, and that external objects become known to us only by those perceptions they occasion." Similarly, (Hume 1739/2000, Book 1, Part 4, Section 5, p. 157): "[N]o external object can make itself known to the mind immediately, and without the interpolation of an image or perception."

5 To reiterate, the absence of unmediated access to reality was the basis for Berkeley's idealism and Hume's skepticism. Simply, given that perception is indirect, how can any claims about the nature of reality be justified?

6 In using the terms "gentle force" and "attraction," Hume was drawing parallels with the forces of gravity and magnetism by which one object is drawn to another object at some distance from it.

7 An intimation of the preceding lectures is that Hume's touchstone does not go far enough. It will need extending to living things in general, all 96 Phyla.

References

Berkeley, G. (1948). Essay towards a new theory of vision. In A. A. Luce & T. E. Jessop (Eds.), *The works of George Berkeley, Bishop of Cloyne*. London: Thomas Nelson (original work published 1709).

Berkeley, G. (1998). *A treatise concerning the principles of human knowledge*. J. Dancey (Ed.), Oxford, UK: Oxford University Press (original work published 1710).

Bohr, N. (1934). *Atomic theory and the description of nature*. Cambridge, UK: Cambridge University Press.

Bohr, N. (1937). Causality and complementarity. *Philosophy of Science*, *4*, 293–294.
Bradley, F. H. (1914). *Essays on truth and reality*. Oxford, UK: Oxford University Press.
Clapp, J. G. (1967). Locke. In P. Edwards (Ed.), *The encyclopedia of philosophy*, *Volume 4* (pp. 487–503). New York: Macmillan.
Cohen-Tannoudji, G. (1993). *Universal constants in physics*. New York: McGraw Hill.
Dennett, D. (1981). *Brainstorms*. Cambridge, MA: MIT Press.
Descartes, R. (1985). Comments on a Certain Broadsheet. In J. Cottingham, R. Stoothoff, & D. Murdoch (Trans.), *Philosophical writings of Descartes*. Cambridge, UK: Cambridge University Press (original work published 1648).
Haugeland, J. (1985). *Artificial intelligence: The very idea*. Cambridge, MA: MIT Press.
Hume, D. (2000). *A treatise of human nature* (D. F. Norton & M. J. Norton, Eds.). Oxford, UK: Oxford University Press (original work published 1739–40).
James, W. (1975). *Pragmatism and the meaning of truth*. Cambridge, MA: Harvard University Press (original work published 1907–9).
Jammer, M. (1974). *The philosophy of quantum mechanics*. New York: Wiley.
Locke, J. (1997). *An essay concerning human understanding*. London: Penguin Books (original work published 1689).
Massey, G. J. (1993). Mind–body problems. *Journal of Sport and Exercise Science*, *15*, S97–S115.
Nadeau, R., & Kafatos, M. (1999). *The non-local universe*. Oxford, UK: Oxford University Press.
Pattee, H. H. (1977). Dynamic and linguistic modes of complex systems. *International Journal of General Systems*, *3*, 259–266.
Pattee, H. H. (1978). The complementarity principle in biological and social structures. *Journal of Social and Biological Structures*, *1*, 191–200.
Pattee, H. H. (1982). The need for complementarity in models of cognitive behavior: A response to Fowler and Turvey. In W. B. Weimer & D. S. Palermo (Eds.), *Cognition and the symbolic processes*, *Volume 2* (pp. 21–30). Hillsdale, NJ: Erlbaum.
Pattee, H. H. (1987). Instabilities and information in biological self-organization. In F. E. Yates (Ed.), *Self-organizing systems: The emergence of order* (pp. 325–338). New York: Plenum Press.
Ryle, G. (1949). *The concept of mind*. New York: Barnes & Noble.
Toulmin, S. (1967). Neuroscience and human understanding. In G. C. Quarton, T. Melnechuk & F. O. Schmitt (Eds.), *The neurosciences: A study program* (pp. 822–832). New York: Rockefeller University Press.
White, A. R. (1967). Coherence theory of truth. In P. Edwards (Ed.), *The encyclopedia of philosophy*, *Volume 2* (pp. 130–133). New York: Macmillan.
Williams, B. (1967). Descartes. In P. Edwards (Ed.), *The encyclopedia of philosophy*, *Volume 2* (pp. 344–354). New York: Macmillan.
Winfree, A. T. (1987). *When time breaks down*. Princeton, NJ: Princeton University Press.

Lecture 8
The Space Enigmas I: Berkeley

The primary test field for theories of how the world can be known by sight has, over the centuries, been overwhelmingly the general problem of space perception, in particular, distance perception. The first step in addressing this problem is a question of the most fundamental kind: What is space? It is not difficult to appreciate that resolution of the scientific problem of how space is perceived depends ultimately on the correctness of the scientific presumption of *what space is* apropos perception and action. The question can be refined: What kind of *concept* is "space"? The most dominant answer is that space is a mathematical concept. A subordinate, but nonetheless influential answer is that space is a physiological/psychological concept. A third answer, hardly ever entertained, is that space is a biological/ecological concept.

8.1 Molyneux's Premise and Malebranche's Bold Question

From the mechanical hypothesis of the 17th century, the interpretation of space as a mathematical concept was a natural consequence of the joint presuppositions that mathematics was true (absolutely certain) and that nature's laws were mathematical (Cassirer, 1950; Kline, 1980). The notion of extension as a primary quality (matter has size and shape) was combined with the mathematical theory of extension—Euclidean geometry. Space was thus characterized in terms of points, lines, angles and planes.[1] More abstractly, it was conceived as *continuous* (infinitely divisible), *isotropic* (no intrinsically preferred direction), *homogeneous* (the same everywhere), and *infinite*. Perhaps no assumption expresses the hold that empty Euclidean space had on perceptual theorists as profoundly as *Molyneux's premise* (Pastore, 1971) advanced in 1692: "For *distance* of it self, is not to be perceived; for 'tis a line (or a length) presented to our eye with its end toward us, which must therefore be only a *point*, and that is *invisible*" (p. 68).

Molyneux was assuming that no impression about the third dimension could be obtained by use of a single eye because the third dimension consists of the line of sight itself. Any external point on the line of sight would be optically identical to any other point with nothing to indicate whether it was near of far, or even external to the eye (Gibson, 1950).[2]

Efforts to address the perception of this geometrical space have mostly followed the simple logic of the simulative assumption: whatever aspects of space are inadequately copied in the light but are adequately present in perception must, therefore, be supplied by the mind. Said differently, the degree to which the simulative assumption is fulfilled (how thoroughly and faithfully light copies the spatial character of the world) dictates the scope of the projective assumption (how extensive are the mental processes that elaborate and rectify the spatial character of the received copies). The imperfections and defects in simulation were evident to the scholars of the 17th and 18th centuries from both geometric analysis and the equating of retinal images with the images of camera obscura (Lombardo, 1987; Pastore, 1971).

1 The image is flat.
2 The image is ambiguous in respect to size and form (with variations in distance from and orientation to the image plane, multiple different objects can produce the same sized image with the same form and the same object can produce multiple different sized images with different forms).
3 The image is ambiguous in respect to the relative sizes and forms of component parts (with variations in distance and orientation, a larger or smaller object part can produce, for example, a smaller or larger image part, respectively).
4 The image is inverted and reflected.

Given these inadequacies of a retinal image relative to its source object in combination with Molyneux's premise, the challenge was to explain how we see space as we do—that is, as "out there," solid, with definite shapes. What, precisely, does the projective assumption (Lecture 4) entail?

Within the context of the Cartesian grades of sense, Malebranche in 1678 boldly considered what the answer would be if God were excluded.[3] He saw the seriousness of the challenge posed by the vast complexity of ordinary everyday scenes, the kinds encountered in walking through the countryside or along a busy city boulevard. Such scenes comprise indefinitely many objects of indefinitely many shapes, sizes, orientations, and colors at indefinitely many depths moving in indefinitely many ways. With God excluded, Malebranche saw that the projective assumption would entail not only a complete and precise knowledge of physiology, optics, and geometry but also an ability to perform indefinitely many reasoning processes at an instant (Malebranche, 1678/1997a; Pastore, 1971). Looking ahead, Malebranche's bold question and his recognition of the scope of its answer established a benchmark for the class of explanation that knowing the spatial world by sight will require. In very contemporary terms, solutions to "toy problems" (successful explanations of single overly simplified cases) should be accorded reserved admiration.

8.2 Flatland and Spaceland

If a visual system only encounters two-dimensional images, then the question must be raised as to precisely what kinds of visual experience (what kinds of evidence) would be needed to convince the system of the existence of another dimension. In a non-trivial sense, this was the problem posed by Abbot (1884/1952).[4]

Imagine a two-dimensional world called *Flatland* occupied by two-dimensional creatures—specifically, lines (the women) and polygons (the men) whose status in Flatland society is determined by the number of their sides. Because Flatlanders live, by definition, in a plane, every object (other than the women) in Flatland appears visually as a line. Only by feel—that is, only by circumnavigating an object while maintaining contact—can any Flatlander be fully certain of the form of any Flatland object, animate or inanimate (Figure 8.1, top).

The hero in Abbot's tale is a square Flatlander. He has three primary intellectual experiences. In the first, he tries to convince the inhabitants of *Lineland* of the existence of a second dimension. In the second, an inhabitant of *Spaceland* (three-dimensions) tries to convince the square of the existence of a third dimension by means of two adventures (Figure 8.1, middle, bottom). In both adventures, efforts to produce an understanding of the additional dimension by use of analogy fail, as do all logical and mathematical arguments. In the second intellectual adventure, the square does eventually become

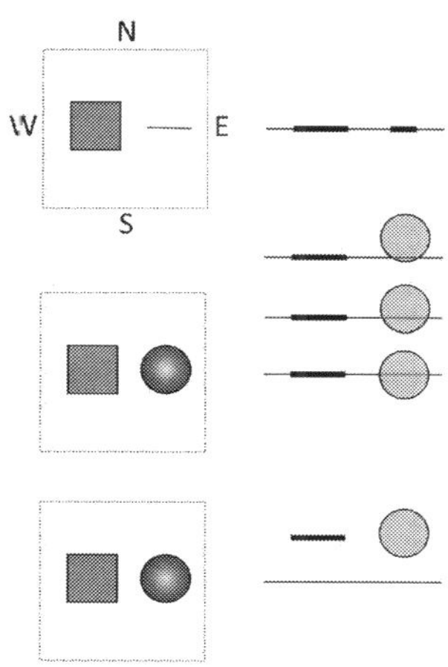

Figure 8.1 Bird's-eye view (*left*) and side view (*right*) of Flatland. (*Top*) Square and a line. (*Middle*) Square visited by a Spacelander (a Sphere), who elevates himself in an attempt to reveal the third dimension. (*Bottom*) Sphere and Square leaving Flatland, and Square's epiphany: There is another dimension.

convinced of a third dimension but only subsequent to a "miracle." He is transported outward from Flatland by his teacher and, thereby, given the opportunity to see Flatland as a Spacelander sees it (a "God's-eye" view).

The third intellectual experience is one of role-reversal. The square tries to convince the Spacelander that, by analogy to the contrasts of Flatland–Lineland and Spaceland–Flatland, and by the authority of the associated mathematics that rationalized the higher dimensional space in each of those cases, there must be yet another land, one of four dimensions, that exists beyond Spaceland. The Spacelander responds querulously and defiantly (Abbott, 1884/1952, pp. 88–89): "Nonsense: what analogy?" "Enough of this trifling." "The very idea of it is utterly inconceivable." As was true of Linelanders and Flatlanders, the Spacelander cannot imagine nor visualize a higher-dimensional reality. He knows not where to point at the direction of the fourth dimension just as they knew not where to point at the direction of the second and third dimensions, respectively.

Likening the retinal image to Flatland and depth perception to Spaceland, Abbott's tale may be taken as a moral lesson for the visual theorist. *If visual experience is limited to two dimensions, then we should expect no three-dimensional visual experience originating from this source* (Politz, 1979). As a Flatlander, the visual system will require the aid of a Spacelander. The Spacelander may be a companion system that is necessarily embedded in three dimensions, such as the movement system, and which provides three-dimensional translations of the Flatlander's two-dimensional visual experiences. Or, the Spacelander may be a very special internal process that continuously reveals the third dimension by transporting the visual system out of Flatland into Spaceland. The first method for aiding vision was promoted by Berkeley (1709/1948). The second method for aiding vision was promoted by Kant (1781/1787/1998). Before we address these two methods, there is the matter of binocular vision.

It is very appealing to consider that the visual system's leap from Flatland to Spaceland originates in the contrast between the two retinal images. In humans and some other animals, the two eyes are at the front of the head with approximately parallel axes. When focused on an object, they yield two different images of the object. Wheatstone (1838/1964) would show that, for fellow humans, two subtly different pictures of the same scene, one viewed by the right eye and one viewed by the left eye, produce a vivid three-dimensional experience (Wade, 1988). A variety of factors, however, caution against over-valuing this phenomenon of stereopsis. It can provide only a temporary escape from the problem of the origin of three-dimensional experience.

Hume's touchstone (Lecture 7) gives reason for skepticism. While two overlapping but different retinal images may be a source of hypotheses about depth perception in humans, these factors cannot function likewise for the vast majority of animals on the planet. In the extreme, if binocular disparity propelled vision from Flatland to Spaceland, then the animal world, with few exceptions, would be forever barred from Spaceland. For those animals that possess two concave (or camera) eyes the location of the eyes is typically lateral rather than frontal and the overlap of images is typically small rather than large (Figure 8.2). For those multitudes of invertebrates that possess convex (or compound) eyes with no overlapping images, we should have to suppose that they are as oblivious to the third dimension as any inhabitant of Abbott's *Flatland*. But it is patently obvious that such a supposition, for either vertebrates or invertebrates, is foolhardy. From the ordinary observation of non-human animals that exploit light—whatever their size and apparent complexity, whatever their habitat, and whatever the nature of their visual systems—it is clear that the behavioral tests of qualification as an inhabitant of Spaceland are passed without exception. A conclusion drawn by Gibson (1966, p. 185) might have satisfied Hume:

> Some [species] have panoramic vision, some frontal. Some have dispersed sensitivity, some concentrated. Some do not fixate the eyes, some do. The primate visual system with compulsory convergence of both eyes on the same detail is a special type. It has its virtues, but the popular notion that our supplementary capacity for binocular depth perception is the only genuine kind of depth perception is a misconception.

There is another kind of reason for concluding that disparity of the two retinal images of human vision cannot be a guarantor of Spaceland. In the absence of disparity, human vision is persistently three-dimensional. Humans deprived of vision in one eye, permanently or temporarily, are not condemned to Flatland, even when permanent deprivation occurs soon after birth (Walk & Dodge, 1962). Their behaviors in everyday settings are appropriate to, and scaled to, the solid distal environment. Furthermore, the absence of disparity when viewing the Ponzo and similar illusions (see Figure 8.3) does not override the human viewer's impressions of differences in relative distance.

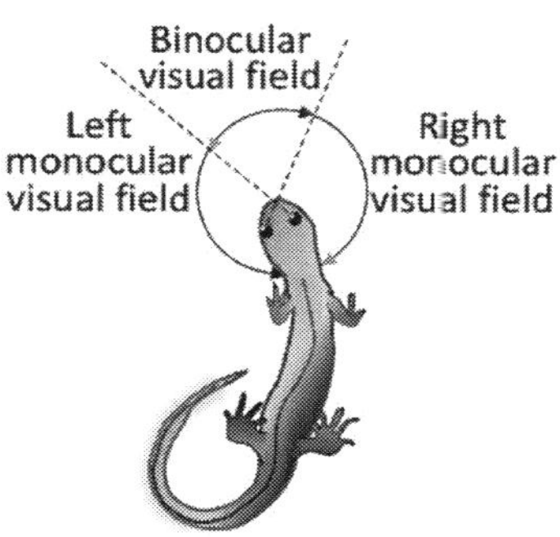

Figure 8.2 For many animals, the two eyes can register nearly the entire array of ambient light, with double registration of the array in front.

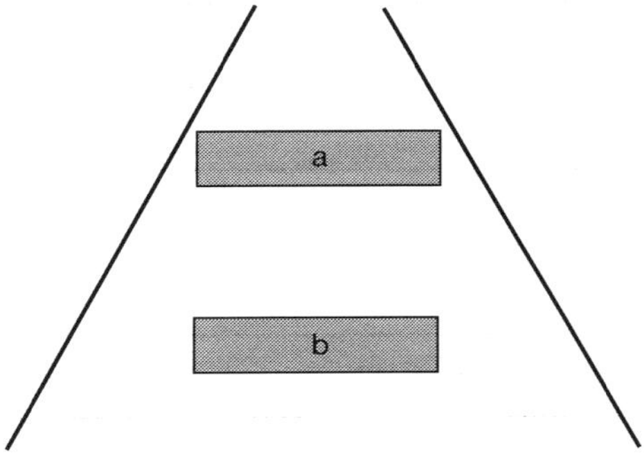

Figure 8.3 The Ponzo illusion: bar *a* seems to be at a greater distance than bar *b*.

8.3 Berkeley's New Theory of Vision

In 1709, George Berkeley (at the age of 24) published *An Essay Towards a New Theory of Vision*. It is arguably the single most influential work in the investigation of how we know about the world by sight. What was "new" about Berkeley's *New Theory* followed from accepting fully the consequences for empiricism of Molyneux's premise. As previewed above, Berkeley took the immediate object of vision to be a two-dimensional extension (a Flatland) with no necessary connection with the third dimension. He expressed Molyneux's premise in stark, psychological terms (Berkeley, 1709/1948, Section 45): "I say, neither distances nor things placed at a distance are themselves, or their ideas, truly perceived by sight" (p. 188).

The immediate object of vision is the psychological consequence of the retinal image (Pastore, 1971). In this respect, Berkeley continues the traditions of the eidolon hypothesis and the projective assumption (Lecture 4). His primary aim in the *New Theory* is to explicate what the projective assumption entails in perceiving the distances, sizes and situations of objects by sight. The explication consists of identifying the contingent relations, the associations of ideas, by which the immediate object of vision is linked to distance, size and situation. His theoretical enterprise is conveyed through an easily grasped everyday example (Berkeley, 1709/1963, Sections 9–10):

> It is evident that when the mind perceives any idea, not immediately of itself, it must be by means of some other idea. Thus, for instance, the passions which are in the mind of another are of themselves to me invisible. I may nevertheless perceive them by sight, though not immediately, yet by means of the colours they produce in the countenance. We often see shame or fear in the looks of a man, by perceiving the changes of his countenance to red or pale. Moreover it is evident that no idea which is not itself perceived can be the means of perceiving any

> other idea. If I do not perceive the redness or paleness of a man's face, themselves, it is impossible I should perceive by them the passions which are in his mind.
>
> (pp. 21–22)

8.3.1 The Geometric Theory of Descartes and Malebranche

The received view at the time was that certain necessary relations were the basis for distance and size perception. Descartes (Optics, 1637/1985) and Malebranche (*Search after truth*, 1712/1997b) had suggested the operation in humans of an innately given "natural geometry." In the case of binocular vision, it took the form of reasoning based on convergence of the eyes similar in kind to a surveyor's calculation when measuring from two different locations. The loan of intelligence here is the knowledge of mathematical optics and its theoretical elements (rays of light, their points of intersection, their angles of incidence to intersecting lines and planes). One must know that object distance necessarily varies in accordance with the angle made at the object by straight lines converging to it from the eyes. When vision is monocular, one must know that the more nearly parallel are the direct rays falling on the eye, the further, necessarily, is the point at which they intersect. The loan of intelligence is further evident in the geometric theory's interpretation of size perception. One must know that for an object of fixed extent, the angle it subtends at the eye necessarily contracts and dilates, respectively, as the object's distance decreases and increases. If distance is known, then the preceding fact of Euclidean geometry enables a reasoning process that yields a constant perception of object size (Malebranche, Elucidation on optics, 1678/1997a).[5]

Berkeley advised against assuming this loan—against the argument that perceivers could be so endowed with knowledge of Euclidean geometry. In his view, the loan was excessive and unjustified. Most telling was the evident fact that the lines and angles of Euclidean geometry are not the kinds of things that the retina can register (simply, they can not be the right degrees of freedom). To reiterate the lessons of Alhazen and Molyneux, what strikes the retina strikes it as a point (Atherton, 1990).

8.3.2 Perceiving Distance and Size through Association, not by Calculation

The dismissal of lines, angles and geometric knowledge from the accounts of distance and size perception has major theoretical outcomes. To begin with, it must be assumed that in visually perceiving distance and size, the visual system's contribution is limited to perceptible qualities present in the immediate object of vision and in the visual system when obtaining the immediate object of vision. One perceptible quality is the confusion or blurring of the immediate object of vision originating in the failure of points on an object to map uniquely to points on the retina. The mixing or confusing of rays from different points occurs when an object, of any size, is very near (inspect your hand when positioned a few centimeters from your face). Another perceptible quality is the faintness or clarity of the immediate object of vision (Figure 8.4). This occurs by reason of the object being at a far distance or because the medium (air or water) is not perfectly transparent. In either case, fewer rays reach the eye. To these purely visual qualities one can add the strain in muscles when converging the eyes upon an object and when trying to focus. It is Berkeley's opinion that the aforementioned perceptual qualities are either consciously available or can become consciously available with a little effort; the same, he argues, cannot be said of pencils of rays and subtended angles. By means of the aforementioned perceptual qualities that vision can register, the perceiver can mentally represent what is happening at and to the eyes.

It has to be emphasized that these mental representations are not—prior to and independent of experience—representations of either distance (in conformity with Molyneux's premise) or size. They can, however, become correlated with non-visual mental representations that are about distance and size, if such representations are available. In dispossessing vision of the mathematical entities to which Euclidean theorems apply, Berkeley dispelled the interpretation of visual spatial perception as a kind of calculation (a rule-governed, quasi-mathematical process of reasoning). Descartes' and Malebranche's computational theory based on necessity (of logical propositions) is replaced by an association theory based on contingency (of ideas or mental representations; Atherton, 1990).

It will serve us well, before progressing much further, to become reasonably clear on what *necessity* and *contingency* mean, together with the related notions

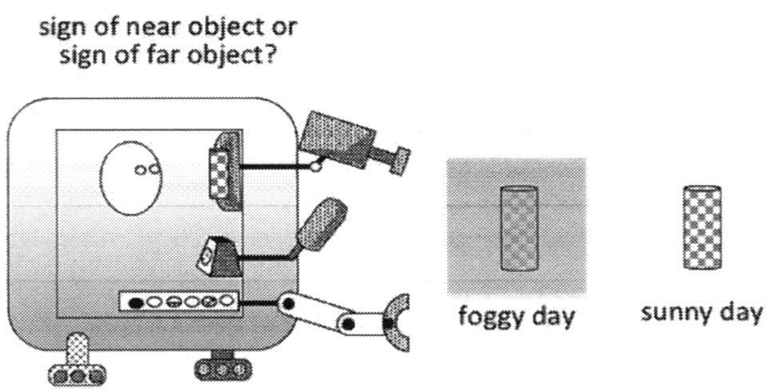

Figure 8.4 "Distance" is an accidental property of faintness. Depending on circumstances it could become a sign for either a near or far object or for nothing at all.

(From Figure 1, Turvey, 2004, adapted with permission, *Ecological Psychology*.)

of *essential* and *accidental* properties. Necessity is attributed to a proposition or state of affairs when it is not possible for the proposition to be false or for the state of affairs to be otherwise. We can say that a proposition (e.g., "with air as the only medium, the angle subtended by a distal object at the eye contracts with increases in the distance of the object") is logically necessary if its denial is formally self-contradictory. A proposition or state of affairs is contingent if it is neither impossible nor necessary; or, said differently, if it is both possible and non-necessary. Although necessity and contingency seem to be opposites, the distinction between them is not captured by "contradictory" (Audi, 1999; Hamlyn, 1967). To develop the contrast between an essential property and an accidental property, consider how one should regard Berkeley's perceptual quality of faintness as a cue to distance relative to Descartes' and Malebranche's convergence angle as a cue to distance. The property that the latter entity has as an index of distance is an essential property. Within Euclidean geometry, the convergence angle cannot exist without necessarily specifying the distance of the point of intersection. In comparison, "distance cue" is an accidental property of faintness (Figure 8.4). Faintness can exist without it being a sign of distance. In Berkeley's scheme, faintness becomes a sign of distance, for example, only subsequent to association with something that does signify distance. To summarize: a property is essential to an entity if, necessarily, the entity cannot exist without being an instance of the property; if the entity can so exist, then the property in question is accidental (Audi, 1999).

8.3.3 *Vision as a Universal Language, Causation as Regularity*

We can now proceed to deepen our understanding of Berkeley's New Theory. In dismissing the possibility of perceptual qualities with essential spatial properties, Berkeley (1709/1963, Section 104) contends that it can always be shown that any spatial property possessed by a perceptual quality is "entirely the result of custom and experience, and depends on foreign and accidental circumstances" (p. 70).

The situation is analogous to that of written and spoken words. The optical and acoustic forms of words are arbitrary in respect to the meanings that the words convey. There is no necessary connection in language between a sign and what it signifies, and there is no necessary restraint on a given sign such that it cannot signify more than one thing.[6] This latter aspect of the contingency versus necessity contrast is at work in Berkeley's argument for the independence of size and distance perception (see Haber & Levin, 2001). Because a given perceptual quality has no necessary connection to distance or size, there is nothing to prohibit it from becoming a sign for both. In principal, the same set of perceptual qualities can enter into contingent connections yielding ideas of object magnitude as they also yield ideas of object distance (Berkeley, 1709/1948, Section 53). "[T]hey have as close and immediate a connexion with the magnitude as with the distance; and suggest magnitude as independently of distance as they do distance independently of magnitude" (p. 191).

In the case of language, with sufficient experience of the contingent connection, the presentation of a word's arbitrary optical or acoustical form is followed at an instant by an appreciation of the word's meaning (e.g., Lukatela, Carello, Savic, et al., 1998). Likewise, suggests Berkeley, when presented with a perceptual quality of the immediate object of vision, the experienced viewer cannot resist an instantaneous and compelling appreciation of its spatial meaning.

Berkeley's language analogy (more precisely, word-recognition analogy) replaces Descartes' and Malebranche's geometric analogy. The issue in respect to vision is not how well vision's representations match the environment's distances, sizes, and situations, but how well vision performs its language function—that is, how well it signifies the means by which behavior relative to the environment can be regulated (Atherton, 1990). This pragmatic, action-oriented twist in Berkeley's theorizing is conveyed by a lengthy but valuable paragraph:

> Upon the whole, I think we may fairly conclude that the proper objects of vision constitute an universal language of the Author of nature, whereby we are instructed to regulate our actions in order to attain those that are necessary to the preservation . . . It is by their information that we are principally guided in all the transactions and concerns of life. And the manner wherein they signify and mark unto us the objects which are at a distance is the same as that of languages . . . which do not suggest the things signified by any like ness or identity of nature, but only by an habitual connexion that experience has made to observe between them.
> (Berkeley, 1709/1948, Section 147, p. 231)

The account of space perception by Descartes and Malebranche is essentialist in nature. In the *New Theory*, Berkeley is opposing this essentialism of vision. His opposition takes the form of a proposal—made via the language analogy—that an account of vision must be framed in terms of laws. A law for Berkeley is a *regularity of succession*, an association or constant conjunction of ideas.[7] Let C stand for cause and E stand for effect. Then, in the manner made popular subsequently by Hume (1739/2000), the law form adopted by Berkeley is *if C, then E always* (Bunge, 1979).[8] It is important to underscore that the preceding formulation is not that of a causal law. It does not state that one thing (or a change in one thing) is *produced* or *engendered* by another thing (or by a change in another thing). It merely asserts that the two things are regularly associated—as the perceptual quality "redness" is, in the case of apples, regularly associated with the perceptual quality "sweetness." "Redness" is a correlate of, not the cause of, "sweetness." It is also important to underscore that the lawfulness of vision that Berkeley proposes is purely with reference to the viewer's experience and knowledge of things and not the things themselves. There are no genetic[9] links among the various things that Berkeley is considering in the *New Theory*: Distances of objects, sizes of objects, faintness of retinal images, tensions in eye muscles, and so on, *just are*. Berkeley (1709/1948, Section 64) did not shy away from the consequence of his fundamental premises (arbitrariness of signs, no genetic links, subjectivity of laws):

> Those ideas that now suggest unto us the various magnitudes of external objects . . . might possibly have suggested no such thing: Or they might have signified them in a direct contrary manner: so that the very same ideas, on the perception whereof we judge an object to be small, might as well have served us to conclude it great.
>
> (p. 195)

That is, he recognized, as Wittgenstein (1921/1961, 5.934) would remark two centuries later, that: "Whatever we see could be other than it is" (p. 58).

The laws of Berkeley's language of vision could be different simply because they are no more than summaries of a viewer's experiences—different experiences, different summaries and, therefore, different laws.

8.3.4 The Exaltation and Incorrigibility of Touch

We must now address the most fundamental aspect of Berkeley's new theory: his solution to the mystery of original meaning (Haugeland, 1985). For the theory to work, visual ideas that are bereft of spatial meaning must be endowed through experience with spatial meaning. There must be a sensory source of ideas that is unequivocal about distance, size and situation. That is to say, there must be a non-visual means of perceiving space that is direct or unmediated in order to furnish vision with mediating ideas of space. In addressing this key issue, Berkeley regarded the perception accompanying mechanical contact with the surroundings as the means by which distances, sizes and situations become known directly (Figure 8.5). The arbitrary associations composing the language of vision are between visual ideas (signs) and tangible ideas (meanings). For what reasons should he have ascribed such exalted status to tactual experience?

Two material things are said to be touching if there is no spatial separation between some point on the surface of one thing and some point on the surface of the other. Touching *is* the principle of nearby action (all cause is by contact; Lecture 4). For this reason, perhaps, when one of the two material things in contact is sentient, it can be supposed that the effect is privileged. Historically, it had been supposed that touch was special among the senses because of its intimate relation to matter; only touch was incorrigible[10] in respect to ascertaining what was material and external to the mind. At the

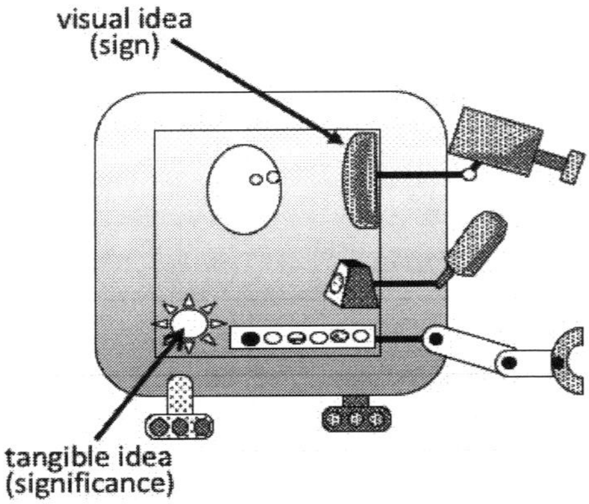

Figure 8.5 Berkeley's man in the inner room resides in a mobile home that ensures mechanical contact with the surroundings. The man can learn what tangible distances experienced through locomotion look like.

(From Figure 1, Turvey, 2004, adapted with permission, *Ecological Psychology*.)

heart of debates on whether experience could reveal necessity, causality, and could resolve objectivity, was the observation of the felt resistance of objects to the touch. In part, due to Berkeley's insistence and, in part, due to the need to escape the epistemological difficulties of the "man in the inner room," the incorrigibility of touch was ascribed to by leading scholars from Berkeley's time well into the 20th century (Pastore, 1971). To name a few: Condillac, Hamilton, Bell, Muller, Helmholtz, Mill, Taine, Bain, Dewey, Sechenov, Höffding, and Ames. Bell (1833/1979) acknowledged the exalted status of touch in these words:

> Whilst this sense is distinct from the others, it is the most important of all . . . touch is necessary to the full development of the powers of all the other organs.
>
> Touch is that peculiar sensibility which gives the consciousness of the resistance of external matter, and makes us acquainted with the hardness, roughness, size and form of bodies. It enables us to distinguish what is external from what belongs to us; and while it informs us of the geometric qualities of bodies, we must refer to this sense also our judgment of distance, of motion, of number, and of time
>
> (pp. 179–180)

And by Helmholtz (1868/1968) in these words:

> [T]he sense of touch is sufficient . . . to develop complete notions of space . . . we are continually controlling and correcting the notions of locality

> derived from the eye by the help of the sense of touch, and always accept the impressions on the latter sense as decisive.
>
> (p. 108)

Berkeley's conception of touch was very general. It included the mechanically based experiences, variously referred to in contemporary science as kinesthesis, proprioception or haptic[11] perception, which accompany motions of the body (notably, walking and reaching). He seemed to have presumed that the extent (or effort or duration or speed) of walking or reaching to an object could be realized as an idea of distance. He would remark (Berkeley, 1709/1948, Section 45) that:

> Looking at an object I perceive a certain visible figure and color, with some degree of faintness and other circumstances, which from what I have formerly observed, determine me to think that if I advance so many paces or miles, I shall be affected with such and such ideas of touch . . .
>
> (p. 188)

His perspective on size perception is precisely the same. To the perceptual qualities of the immediate object of vision, we learn to associate particular kinesthetic experiences of greater or lesser extents generated when we move our hands over objects.

Without question, the truly remarkable nature of this theoretical move to ground vision in touch is the assumption that the two kinds of perceiving are distinguished in the manner depicted in Figures 3.1 and 3.2. Whereas vision must necessarily be mediated (given Molyneux's premise), touch is unmediated presumably because the failings of geometric optics are not shared by contact mechanics (Turvey, 1977).[12] In making this theoretical move in the *New Theory*, Berkeley is following the tenets of the correspondence theory of truth (Lecture 7). The language of vision can be successful (i.e., constrain environment-directed actions felicitously) if, and only if, that which is signified by visual signs corresponds to what is out there. Confidence in the language's ability requires that the correspondence between a tangible idea and its spatial referent be epistemologically unassailable. This latter correspondence is how Berkeley solves the *grounding problem* (Lecture 6): explaining how a symbol can symbolize, how a sign can signify. The problem and the challenge of its solution was described succinctly by William James (1890/1983, p. 798): "If a sign is to lead to *the thing* it means, we must have some other source of knowledge of that thing."

8.3.5 Does Walking or Running Without Seeing Yield a Definite Tangible Idea of Distance?

One can give a reading of Berkeley that suggests the promotion of a truly non-intuitive hypothesis: locomotion measures distance.[13] Consider Berkeley's (1709/1948, Section, 45) assertion:

> what he sees only suggests to his understanding that after having passed a certain distance, *to be measured by the motion of his body, which is perceivable by touch,* he shall come to perceive such and such tangible ideas which have been usually connected with such and such visible ideas.
>
> (p. 188, italics added)

Stated more precisely, the hypothesis implicit in the two preceding quotations is that legged locomotion from one location A to another location B is, in and of itself, specific to the distance from A to B. For this to be so, however, a very special kind of perceptual constancy must hold. A stretch of non-visible ground between A and B can be traversed at different speeds and in different styles of gait. Berkeley's hypothesis requires, therefore, that legged locomotion without vision must yield an unvarying impression of the distance traversed despite variations in the manner of legged locomotion.

That locomotion might yield an invariant measure of distance is suggested by investigations with humans, arachnids, and insects, conducted nearly three centuries after the *New Theory*. Figure 8.6 summarizes experiments in which blindfolded human participants, on any given trial, went from a fixed starting point A to a variable terminus B—signaled during locomotion by the experimenter—and then attempted to return to A (Schwartz, 1999). From A to B,

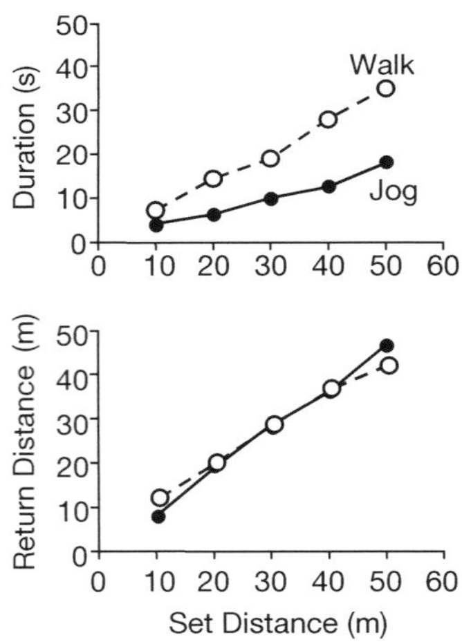

Figure 8.6 (*Top*) The time taken to walk or jog blindfolded as a function of distance. (*Bottom*) Accuracy of return trip where mode of travel was walking blindfolded with the aid of a cane.

(From Figures 2 and 3, M. Schwartz, Haptic perception of the distance walked when blindfolded. *Journal of Experimental Psychology: Human Perception and Performance, 25*, 852–865, 1999, APA, adapted with permission)

the participants either walked with the aid of a long cane to prevent veering from the path or jogged with the aid of a sighted partner, similarly to prevent veering from the path. Additionally, in both modes of travel between A and B, the participant was distracted so as to minimize the use of explicit strategies such as counting the number of steps. From B to A, participants walked alone with the aid of a long cane and without distraction. As Figure 8.6 shows, jogging from A to B took less time (and involved fewer step cycles) than walking from A to B, but the accuracy of the return trip from B to A for each of the distances traversed was the same. Taking the accuracy of the return trip as the index of perceived distance in the outgoing trip, the implication is that distance is perceptible by locomotion and is so indifferently to the duration and style of locomotion. This implication is strengthened by the further observation that perceived distances conform closely to actual distances over combinations of systematic variations in step cadence and step length (Schwartz, 1999; see also Turvey, Romaniak-Gross, Isenhower et al. 2009, and Abdolvahab, Carello, Pinto et al., 2015).

Berkeley's larger hypothesis that walking per se provides definite tangible ideas of space receives support from the behavior of the tropical wandering spider *Cupienius salei*.[14] Proprioception is by sensors in the legs that detect small deformations or strains in the exoskeleton. These sensors, called slit sensilla, function as biomechanical strain gauges[15] (Zill & Seyfarth, 1996). Each is a fine canal (or slit) in the cuticle that is covered by a very thin membrane on its outer surface. On the legs these slit sensilla form organized groups defining a lyriform (harp-shaped) organ (Figure 8.7). Of special significance is the fact that each sensilla in a lyriform organ is oriented slightly differently from its neighbors, providing an array of sensors able to detect different strains in different directions.

The experiment of relevance to Berkeley's hypothesis involves a temporarily blinded spider in a level arena into which is placed a live and humming housefly (Barth, 2002; Seyfarth & Barth, 1972). Once the spider locates and captures the housefly, it is immediately separated from its prey and chased some distance away. Soon thereafter it returns to the fly's original location even though the fly has been relocated. The spider can achieve a successful return even if steered along a curved detour path. It recovers from the momentary detour, not by retracing its curved path, but by assuming another heading toward the original prey location. It is, so to speak, haptically oriented to its surroundings. As Figure 8.8 indicates, this ability (which is not infirmed by the removal of visual, olfactory, and gravitational factors) is infirmed by rendering the slit sensilla non-functional.[16] Not shown is the additional fact that the "blind" spider with intact gauges is capable of controlling the overall distance of the return path (Seyfarth & Barth, 1972; their Figures 4 and 9).

The evidence in humans and arachnids (and ants, Schaefer & Wehner, 1993; Wittlinger, Wehner, & Wolf, 2006, 2007) that locomotion without benefit of vision constitutes an instrument for measuring distance is favorable

Figure 8.7 A tropical wandering spider's lyriform slit sense organ is an array of strain gauges (depicted as black strokes). It is a device for detecting different magnitudes of strain in different directions.

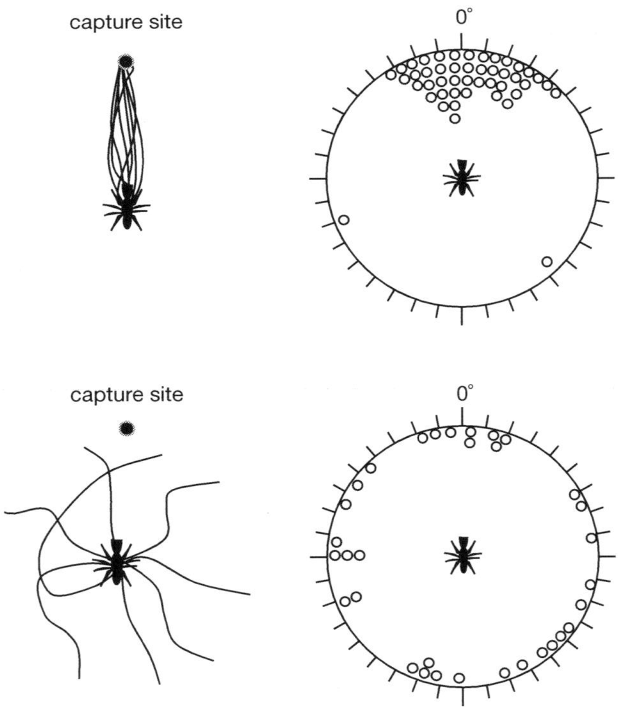

Figure 8.8 (*Above*) A "blind" travelling spider with intact strain gauges exhibits successful odographic (orienting) and odometric (distance determining) behavior with respect to location (0°) of the site of a previous prey. (*Below*) A "blind" spider lacking strain gauges behaves randomly in its effort to return to the site.

to Berkeley's hypothesis. At the same time, this evidence for a purely tactile odometer[17] is paradoxical for his broader thesis. A constancy of tangible distance perception over variations of configuration and motion would seem to be a problem of the very kind that Berkeley was seeking to resolve. Variable strains in the body's tissues are like variable faintness and variable confusion in the retinal image. They are not, in any obvious sense, incorrigible sources of ideas of distance. In his *Principles* published in 1710, Berkeley admitted to the "vulgar error" of supposing that tangible ideas of distance were distinct from visible ideas of distance on the dimension of direct versus indirect. He wrote (1710/1998):

> So that in strict truth the ideas of sight, when we apprehend by them distance and things placed at a distance, do not suggest or mark out things actually existing at a distance, but only admonish us what ideas of touch will be imprinted in our minds at such and such distances of time, and in consequence of such and such actions . . . visible ideas are the language whereby the governing spirit . . . informs us what tangible ideas he is about to imprint upon us, in case we excite this or that motion in our bodies.
>
> (p. 117)

In the *Principles*, the mystery of original meaning and the grounding problem were returned to divine providence, as recommended by Descartes.

Notes

1 The geometric categories can be elaborated (Gibson, 1950). *Extensity* in two dimensions expresses the "spread" of space and corresponds to the plane of the y (vertical) and x (horizontal) axes of geometry. *Location* in two dimensions corresponds to the x and y coordinates of geometry. *Shape* or *form* corresponds to the abstract forms of Greek geometry (circle, triangle, octahedron, etc). *Depth* or *distance*, the third dimension of space, corresponds to the z-axis of geometry.

2 Imagine a person who lives in two-space, a Flatlander, explaining to a person who lives in one-space, a Linelander, that he can distinguish by sight Linelanders who are lines and Linelanders who are points. The Linelander might retort "You speak of an impossibility, you must have seen a vision; for to detect the difference between a Line and a Point by the sense of sight is, as every one knows, in the nature of things, impossible . . ." So wrote Edwin Abbott (1884/1952) in his classic work *Flatland* (see Section 8.2).

3 Malebranche was an advocate of *occasionalism*. This is the doctrine that finite created beings cannot cause things to happen; the only true causal agent is God (Audi, 1999). A paradigmatic argument is that arm movements follow the intention to move because God intervenes, on each and every occasion, to bring about the coincidence of an individual mental act of will and its associated physical action.

4 See also Hinton (1907) and Burger (1965/1994). The richest elaboration of Abbott's tale is Dewdney's (1984) *Planiverse*.

5 This formulation has a long history. It can be found in the works of Alhazen (Sabra, 1989). In 1263, John Pecham wrote (Lindberg, 1970, p. 147): "However, as experience proves, the faculty that apprehends size considers the magnitude of the distance [from the observer] and not only the angle."
6 Consider words such as *watch* (a time piece, a visual act), *bark* (what dogs do, what trees have), and so on.
7 From Hume (1739/2000, 1.3.15.1, p. 116) "the constant conjunction of objects determines their causation" and, similarly, "There must be a constant union betwixt the cause and effect."
8 Again, from Hume (1739/2000, 1.3.15.1, p. 116): "The same cause always produces the same effect, and the same effect never arises but from the same cause."
9 This term is Bunge's (1979). It follows from his definition of the *genetic principle*: "Nothing comes out of nothing; there are neither absolute beginnings nor absolute terminations."
10 In the sense of requiring no improvement, alterations or amendments; perfect as formed.
11 Haptic is derived from a Greek term meaning "able to lay hold of."
12 Jammer (1993, p. 135) observes that, for Berkeley, "tangible space . . . needs no explanation."
13 Sechenov (1903/1960) equated the muscular sense, divisible in the course of the periodic movements of walking and running, with a differentiating analyzer or instrument for measuring space.
14 So-called, in part, because it seeks and catches its prey on solid substrates rather than in a web.
15 Strain exhibited by a material segment is the change in its length relative to its original length. A man-made strain gauge is typically a metal foil or semi-conductor that varies in electrical resistance with the amount of strain.
16 The ablation of slit sensilla of the tibia and fibula did not noticeably impede a spider's ability to coordinate its limbs in locomotion and to capture prey, only its ability to function as a touch odometer. One implication is that different strain gauges function in coordination and distance determination.
17 Touch also functions as a relative speedometer. Judgments of en route speed in a car by seated passengers with blindfolds and earplugs obey the same power function as observed for passengers with unimpeded vision and audition (Semb, 1969).

References

Abbott, E. A. (1952). *Flatland*. New York: Dover (original work published 1884).

Abdolvahab, M., Carello, C., Pinto, C., Turvey, M. T., & Frank, T. (2015). Symmetry and order parameter dynamics of the human odometer. *Biological Cybernetics*, *109*, 63–73.

Atherton, M. (1990). *Berkeley's revolution in vision*. Ithaca, NY: Cornell University Press.

Audi, R. (1999). *The Cambridge dictionary of philosophy*. Cambridge, UK: Cambridge University Press.

Barth, F. G. (2002). *A spider's world: Senses and behavior*. Berlin, Germany: Springer.

Bell, C. (1979). *The hand: Its mechanisms and vital endowments as evincing design*. Brentwood, UK: Pilgrims Press (original work published 1833).

Berkeley, G. (1948). Essay towards a new theory of vision. In A. A. Luce & T. E. Jessop (Eds.), *The works of George Berkeley, Bishop of Cloyne*. London: Thomas Nelson (original work published 1709).

Berkeley, G. (1963). *Works on vision*. C. M. Turbayne (Ed.). Westport, CT: Greenwood Press (original work published 1709).

Berkeley, G. (1998). *A treatise concerning the principles of human knowledge*. J. Dancey (Ed.). Oxford, UK: Oxford University Press (original work published 1710).

Bunge, M. (1979). *Causality and modern science* (3rd ed.). New York: Dover.

Burger, D. (1994). *Sphereland: A fantasy about curved spaces and an expanding universe*. New York: HarperPerrennial (original work published 1965).

Cassirer, E. (1950). *The problem of knowledge*. New Haven, CT: Yale University Press.

Descartes, R. (1985). Optics. In J. Cottingham, R. Stoothoff & D. Murdoch (Trans.), *Philosophical writings of Descartes, Vol. 1* (pp. 152–175). Cambridge, UK: Cambridge University Press (original work published 1637).

Dewdney, A. K. (1989). *The Turing omnibus*. New York: Freeman (reissued as *The new Turing omnibus*, 1993, New York: Holt).

Gibson, J. J. (1950). *The perception of the visual world*. Boston, MA: Houghton Mifflin.

Gibson, J. J. (1966). *The senses considered as perceptual systems*. Boston, MA: Houghton Mifflin.

Haber, R. N., & Levin, C. A. (2001). The independence of size perception and distance perception. *Attention, Perception, & Psychophysics*, 63, 1140–1152.

Hamlyn, D. W. (1967). Contingent and necessary statements. In P. Edwards (Ed.), *The encyclopedia of philosophy, Volume 4* (pp. 198–205). New York: Macmillan.

Haugeland, J. (1985). *Artificial intelligence: The very idea*. Cambridge, MA: MIT Press.

Helmholtz, von H. (1968). Recent progress of the theory of vision. In R. M. Warren & R. P. Warren (Eds.), *Helmholtz on perception: Its physiology and development* (pp. 59–136). New York: Wiley (original work published 1868).

Hinton, C. (1907). *An episode of Flatland*. London: Swann Sonnenschein.

Hume, D. (2000). *A treatise of human nature*. D. F. Norton & M. J. Norton (Eds.), Oxford, UK: Oxford University Press (original work published 1739–40).

James, W. (1983). *The principles of psychology*. Cambridge, UK: Cambridge University Press (original work published 1890).

Jammer, M. (1993). *Concepts of space: The history of theories of space in physics*. New York: Dover (original work published 1954).

Kant, I. (1998). *Critique of pure reason*. (P. Guyer & A. Wood, Trans. and Eds.). Cambridge, UK: Cambridge University Press (original work published 1781/1787).

Kline, M. (1980). *Mathematics: The loss of certainty*. New York: Oxford University Press.

Lindberg, D. C. (1970). *John Pecham and the science of optics: Perspectiva communis*. Madison: University of Wisconsin Press.

Lombardo, T. (1987). *The reciprocity of perceiver and environment: The evolution of James J. Gibson's ecological psychology*. Hillsdale, NJ: Erlbaum.

Lukatela, G., Carello, C., Savic, M., Urosevic, Z., & Turvey, M. T. (1998). When nonwords activate semantics better than words. *Cognition*, 68, B31–B40.

Malebranche, N. (1997a). Elucidation on optics. In T. M. Lennon & P. J. Olscamp (Eds.), *Search after truth: With elucidations of the search after truth* (pp. 687–719). Cambridge, UK: Cambridge University Press (original work published 1678).

Malebranche, N. (1997b). *Search after truth: With elucidations of the search after truth* (T. M. Lennon & P. J. Olscamp, Trans. and Eds.). Cambridge, UK: Cambridge University Press (original work published 1712).

Pastore, N. (1971). *Selective history of theories of visual perception, 1650–1950*. Oxford, UK: Oxford University Press.

Politz, A. (1979). On the origin of space perception. *Philosophy and Phenomenological Research*, *40*, 258–264.

Sabra, A. I. (1989). Form in ibn al-Haytham's theory of vision. *Zeitschrift für Geschichte der Arabisch-Islamischen Wissenschaften*, *5*, 115–140.

Schaefer, M., & Wehner, R. (1993). Loading does not affect measurement of walking distance in desert ants Cataglyphis fortis. *Verh.Dt. Zool. Ges.*, 86, 270.

Schwartz, M. (1999). Haptic perception of the distance walked when blindfolded. *Journal of Experimental Psychology: Human Perception and Performance*, *25*, 852–865.

Sechenov, I. (1960). *The elements of thought*. In G. Gibbons (Ed.), *I. Sechenov: Selected physiological and psychological works*. Moscow, USSR: Foreign Languages Publishing House (original work published 1903).

Semb, G. (1969). Scaling automobile speed. *Perception & Psychophysics*, *5*, 97–101.

Seyfarth, E-A., & Barth, F. G. (1972). Compound slit organs on the spider leg: Mechanoreceptors involved in kinesthetic orientation. *Journal of Comparative Physiology*, *78*, 176–191.

Turvey, M. T. (1977). Contrasting orientations to the theory of visual-information processing. *Psychological Review*, *84*, 67–88.

Turvey, M. T. (2004). Space (and its perception): The first and final frontier. *Ecological Psychology*, *16*, 25–29.

Turvey, M. T., Romaniak-Gross, C., Isenhower, R. W., Arzamarski, R., Harrison, S., & Carello, C. (2009). Human odometry is gait-symmetry specific. *Proceedings of the Royal Society B: Biological Sciences*, *276*, 4309–4314.

Wade, N. J. (1988). On the late invention of the stereoscope. *Perception*, *16*, 785–818.

Walk, R., & Dodge, S. (1962). Visual depth perception of a ten-month-old monocular infant. *Science*, *137*, 529–530.

Wheatstone, C. (1964). Some remarkable phenomena of binocular vision. In W. N. Dember (Ed.), *Visual perception: The nineteenth century* (pp. 114–129). New York: Wiley (original work published 1838).

Wittgenstein, L. (1961). *Tractatus-logico philosophicus*. London: Routledge & Kegan Paul (original work published 1921).

Wittlinger, M., Wehner, R., & Wolf, H. (2006). The ant odometer: Stepping on stilts and stumps. *Science*, *312*, 1965–1967.

Wittlinger, M., Wehner, R., & Wolf, H. (2007). The desert ant odometer: A stride integrator that accounts for stride length and walking speed. *Journal of Experimental Biology*, *210*, 198–207.

Zill, S. N., & Seyfarth, E-A. (1996). Exoskeletal sensors for walking. *Scientific American*, *275* (July), 86–90.

Lecture 9

The Space Enigmas II: Kant, the Nature of Geometry, and the Geometry of Nature

One reason that some ancient Greek thinkers found emanation theory appealing, and eidolon theory less so, was because sending light to an object situated the object *there* (in the environment) and not *here* (in the eye, or in the mind). Alhazen, it will be recalled, repudiated the notion of inside light and established the notion of optical images formed in the eye from reflected outside light. In response to the question of why a visible object was seen *there* and not *here*, he offered a mental process to play the role previously played by emanation. He proposed that a person inferred that a perceived object is *there* because that is the sensible thing to do given the facts. These facts, Alhazen observed, are that the perception occurs only if the eyes are open and only if they are oriented toward the object (Howard, 1996; Sabra, 1989). Eight centuries later, Lotze (1888) would refer to the same facts for the same purpose. Alhazen's and Lotze's resolution of the "*there* not *here*" enigma rests on an implicit metaphysical assumption that gives validity to the noted facts. For any inner visual property to be referable to something external, a prior intuition or conception of space is required—*at the very least.*

The problem introduced here is general and enduring. It is a further example of the paradoxical epistemology imposed by the mechanistic hypothesis of the 17th century and its "man in the inner room" model. Malebranche and Berkeley referred to the problem through the neologism "outness." Its nature was often illuminated through a thought experiment suggested by Molyneux. Imagine a man born blind who in adulthood has his vision restored. What will be his visual experience? Berkeley's answer is simply that the Molyneux Man will see things as *here* not *there*, in the mind or the eye rather than in the environment. "Outness" is not a given for vision. In the absence of correlated tactile experience there is no way to determine by vision alone what is mind-independent, what is out there, what for the man in the inner room has an existence outside the house. While the Molyneux Man is blind to "outness" he can, nonetheless, experience "outness" in the manner in which he had done so prior to the restoration of his sight—by locomotion, reaching, and touching.

Berkeley's solution to *Molyneux's problem*, as history refers to it, became the standard. Stating the matter most generally, within Descartes' scheme, the third grade of sense must extradite or project the sensations of the second grade of sense (e.g., color) so that they appear located in the outer world. A typical 19th-century psychologist (here Ladd, as quoted by James, 1890/1983) might identify the "outness" problem and its solution thus:

> Sensations . . . are psychical states *whose place*—so far as they can be said to have one—*is the mind*. The transference of these sensations from mere mental states to . . . qualities or things projected in space external to the body, is a mental act.
>
> (p. 678)

The most ingenious student of sensory systems in the 20th century (von Bekesy, 1967) expressed the enigma in the following manner:

> The funneling of sensations into a space outside the body is an important feature . . . for it controls practically all our behavior. For example, reflected light from an external object produces an image on the retina. The sensations exist only within our body, yet we localize the image outside the eye, even when we use a single eye and look at an object far away . . . *This external projection has probably been learned early in life*.
>
> (pp. 220–221; italics added)

The anomalous nature of this mental act of external projection is highlighted by the implied *veridical hallucination* (James, 1890/1983, p. 680). Sensations and percepts are really located in the perceiver but they are projected by the mind erroneously, yet accurately, onto the very real environmental objects to which they belong. How could mind be so constructed that it could do such things—prescribing space and, further, prescribing how it should look? For those 18th- and 19th-century scholars puzzling over the extradition of sensations and percepts from inside to outside, the German philosopher Immanuel Kant provided an influential proposal. In *The Critique of Pure Reason*, Kant (1781/1787/1998) claimed:

> By means of outer sense (a property of our mind) we represent objects as outside us, and all as in space . . . Space is not an empirical concept that has been drawn from outer experience. For in order for certain sensations to be related to something outside me (i.e., to something in another place in space from that in which I find myself), thus in order for me to represent them as outside and next to one another, thus not merely as different but as in different places, the representation of space must already be their ground . . . Space is a necessary representation, *a priori*.
>
> (pp. 174–175)

9.1 Kant's Perspective on the Man in the Inner Room

Consider once again the parable of the man in the inner room (see Figure 9.1) and, this time, let his personality be such that while having no doubts about there being a world outside the house[1] he has plenty of doubts about his ability to know what that world is really like. Of particular intrigue to him are the seemingly fundamental and ubiquitous spatial and temporal patterns manifest in the TV images. (These, you will recall, had caused the man in the inner room, from Hume's perspective, to believe that the images seen were of events outside the house, even though he had no means to validate this belief.) The man in the inner room begins to suspect that the synchrony and coherence of the TV images may not be due to the outside world or to the communication channels relaying the signals from the sensors attached to the house. Surprisingly, they seem to be due to some remarkable properties of the inner room itself. On close inspection, he notices that the TV and the room mesh, as if the TV and the room are not two separate things but one thing. He discovers that as the images outside the house are delivered to the TV they are subjected *immediately* to synchronizing circuits built into the walls of the inner room (as Toulmin, 1967, has most insightfully phrased it). These circuits impose spatial and temporal structure on the images. The man in the inner room arrives, thereby, at a startling conclusion. How he experiences space and time is strictly due to the inner room, by how it has been designed.

Prior to his insight, the man in the inner room had been cataloguing certain geometric properties of the images on the screen. General principles of space could be identified. For example, a straight line is the shortest distance between two points and three points determine a plane. One of these principles was particularly complicated but as far as he could tell it was that two straight lines that were parallel at one place would continue to be parallel at each and

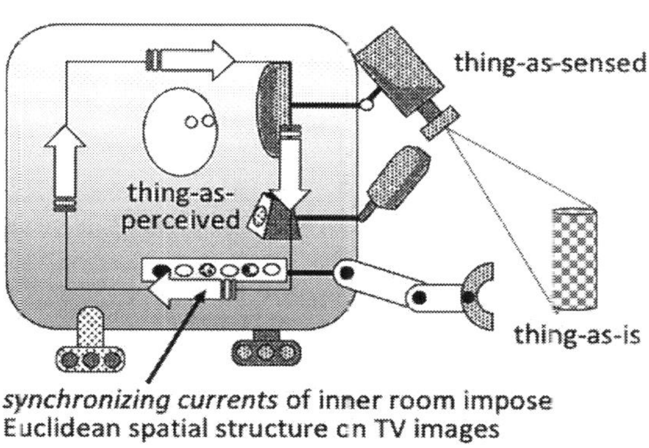

Figure 9.1 The man in the inner room according to Kant.

(From Figure 1, Turvey, 2004, adapted with permission, *Ecological Psychology*.)

every place if they happened to be extended infinitely. The man in the inner room now realizes that these geometric principles that he first thought belonged to the world outside (or, in his more spiritual moments, belonged to God) actually belonged to the inner room. All the TV images of the outer world—past, present and future—must necessarily appear to him in this particular geometric form because of the way the inner room was designed prior to reception of the first signals from the outer world. Space, therefore, is not an object of perception, as the man in the inner room might have been compelled to believe originally, but something very different, namely, a mode of perceiving objects.

With a little contemplation, it becomes patently evident that the proper question to address is not whether there is a necessary fit between the TV images and the outer world, but rather whether there is *a necessary fit of the outer world to the TV images*. For the man in the inner room, this revelation is his personal Copernican Revolution. The world for him becomes a threefold entity consisting of a known world, a sensed world, and the real world. Genuine knowledge of the real world (that outside the house) is impossible because his only access to it is the TV and the TV images are, for him, *phenomena* (appearances or objects of experience shaped by the perceptual modes) rather than *noumena* (the things-in-themselves outside the house).[2] He appreciates, however, that these phenomena, for all intents and purposes, might as well be the real things. They are the things to which he can apply his reasoning. He can use his reasoning or understanding to construct a model of the real world that he cannot possibly know directly from the TV images.[3] This model *is* the known world. In forming this model, the man in the inner room becomes well aware that, for whatever reason, he cannot avoid certain biased ways of thinking. The model reflects, therefore, not only the impositions of space (and time) as rendered by the special properties of the inner room in mesh with the TV, but also the impositions of his own categories of reasoning. The known world, therefore, is very much a product of the inner room and its inhabitant. Stated more fully, the proper form of the proper question identified above is whether there is *a necessary fit of the outer world to the model*.

9.2 Is the Spatial Organization of Visual Experience Necessarily Euclidean?

Contained within the above parable of the man in the inner room is Kant's thesis of space as a *pure form of intuition*.[4] The proof lay with four metaphysical arguments based on the nature of space and one transcendental[5] argument derived from the special character of Euclidean geometry. In the unfolding history of theories of space and space perception, the metaphysical and transcendental arguments live separate lives.

The first metaphysical argument is that space is not derived from sensory experience but, rather, is presupposed by sensory experience. For example, the idea of space does not follow from noticing that some sensed regions of the retinal image are next to each other or that some sensed regions are superposed on others. The spatial predicates "next to" and "on top of" have meaning only if there is already an appreciation of how things can be situated in space. Sensations fall into pre-established spatial patterns. The second argument is that whereas "no space" is unimaginable, "no objects" *can* be imagined, implying that space is a necessary precondition for the possibility of the appearances of objects. Kant's third metaphysical argument focuses on the unique nature of our representation of space. Rather than construing "this space right here" and "that space over there" as representatives of multiple distinct spaces or as component spaces from which a single space is constructed, we understand them as *in* or *encompassed by* a single space. The final metaphysical argument is that space, as we represent it, is not a concept. The defining quality of a concept is that it is a representation *contained in* infinitely many representations. In contrast, our representation of space *contains within itself* infinitely many representations (namely, parts of space) and contains them simultaneously. We represent space, Kant argued, as an infinite magnitude.

Turning now to the transcendental argument, we must first appreciate the form and purpose of such an argument.[6] Its form is deductive in the following sense: The argument proceeds from a premise that asserts the existence of a fundamental phenomenon to a conclusion that asserts the existence of (interesting, substantive) conditions that enable that phenomenon. (Roughly, we could not have cognition C if such-and-such were not the case; we do have C, therefore, such-and-such is necessarily the case.) The argument's purpose is to show the objective validity of conditions prior to and absolutely independent of all experience that make certain experiences possible. A second appreciation that is needed is conditioned by the phenomenon in question—namely, geometry constituted as formal propositions about space. The needed appreciation is this (Kant, 1781/1787/1998): "[M]athematical propositions are always *a priori* judgements and are never empirical, because they carry necessity with them, which cannot be derived from experience" (p. 144). To which should be added (Kant, 1781/1787/1998): "Necessity and strict universality are . . . secure indications of an *a priori* cognition" (p. 137).

As Berkeley and Hume had argued, experience can present us with no more than contingent (possible but not-necessary) truths. Abiding this argument, one must look outside experience for the origin of necessary truths. Kant focuses on two kinds of judgments, both of which can be put into subject–predicate form. An analytic judgment such as "An orange is a fruit" is one in which the predicate merely clarifies the subject (since by definition an orange is a fruit of a particular genus of tree). Because the connection between subject and predicate is that of conceptual identity, an analytic judgment is necessarily true or false without any appeal to experience. Use of the subject and predicate definitions and the principle of contradiction are all that is needed to authenticate an analytic judgment. In contrast are synthetic judgments such as "An orange is a rich source of vitamin C." In this case, the predicate adds something to the subject (the idea of orange does not comprise the idea of vitamin C) and authentication typically requires consulting experience (e.g., running an experiment) to see whether the asserted connection between subject and predicate does indeed hold. Analytic judgments are obviously a priori and synthetic judgments are obviously a posteriori. But Kant raised the original question of whether there could also be *synthetic a priori judgments.* The potential significance of such judgments for knowledge is that, where applicable, they would ensure that the knowledge expressed by predicates that amplified their subjects was necessary rather than contingent. To this purpose, Kant brought the transcendental argument to bear in order to establish that the principles of mathematics and the natural sciences were synthetic a priori judgments and to reveal, thereby, the certainty of the knowledge they contained.

We are now able to identify the transcendental argument for space as a pure form of intuition: Euclidean geometry is a synthetic a priori. Kant (1781/1787/1998) put it into these terms:

> Geometry is a science that determines the properties of space synthetically and yet *a priori*. What then must the representation of space be for such a cognition of it to be possible? It must originally be intuition; for from a mere concept no propositions can be drawn that go beyond the concept . . . But this intuition must be encountered in us *a priori* . . . For geometric propositions are all apodictic, i.e., combined with consciousness of their necessity, e.g., space has only three dimensions; but such propositions cannot be empirical or judgements of experience, nor inferred from them. (p. 176)

As a mathematical and scientific enterprise, geometry is to be understood, therefore, as the exploration of the consequences of the principles and theorems of the mind's pure form of spatial intuition (Kline, 1980). Geometry can be known a priori without reducing to mere tautology precisely because it is at the very basis of perception (Jammer, 1954/1993). All human minds are spatially prefabricated in like manner and all, therefore, organize their visual sensations in accordance with the laws of cognition made explicit in the axioms of Euclidean geometry.

So what does it mean to say that space is pure intuition? It means that space is subjective and ideal *not* objective and real. It means that for the man in the inner room there is no entity, no physical thing called "space" outside the house. It means that space is not a material thing that one perceives but a mode (manner or form) in which one perceives material things. It means that space is described in purely mathematical terms; Euclidean geometry is not a representation of space—it is space.

The meanings of space as pure intuition, although somewhat alarming when stated so explicitly, are as they should be from the perspective of 17th-century science and the everyday measurement of distances and sizes. The meanings are simply the logical consequences of internalizing Newton's *absolute or container view of space*. Material systems such as point masses exist in space—are contained in space—but space itself is not material. To be a physical object satisfying the mechanistic hypothesis (see Lecture 7) is to be something that occupies an amount of space. Obviously, therefore, space cannot be a physical object; it cannot occupy itself. Equally obvious, physical objects can undergo catastrophic change or cease to exist without any consequences for space. Newton's space is abstract (or mathematical) and self-existent (or absolute).[7] On this view of space as a container independent of what it contains, distance or size is indifferent to (a) the kinds of physical things whose separations and magnitudes we desire to measure and (b) the resolution of our measuring instrument.

9.3 A Plurality of Geometry and the Possibility of Geometric Empiricism

Euclidean geometry was the most venerated of all mathematical achievements. It was the first to be established by the deductive method and, for two millennia, both practical application and extensive formal analyses had shown that its theorems matched the physical facts.[8] Scholars presumed that either the world-in-itself is Euclidean or (following Kant) the world as the mind can know it is Euclidean. In this context, it is reasonably easy to enjoin Cassirer's (1950) claim that

> In all the history of mathematics there are few events of such immediate and decisive importance for the shaping and development of knowledge as the discovery of the various forms of non-Euclidean geometry.
>
> (p. 21)

If the certainty of geometry arises from pure reason, and pure reason yields both Euclidean and non-Euclidean geometry—that is, distinctly different, incongruous axiomatic systems—then pure reason would seem to be fallible, contrary and ambiguous. Further, if there are different incongruous systems of geometrical axioms, then there can be different incongruous kinds of space and, perforce, different incongruous kinds of worlds. A central and hitherto unquestioned presupposition of the mechanistic hypothesis (Lectures 5–7), that nature's truths were mathematically enshrined, could no longer inspire confidence. Cassirer (1950) called this state of affairs in the history of ideas a "crisis" and Kline (1980) called it a "debacle."

How did it come about? The spur was the fifth postulate of Euclid, the *parallel axiom*. Mathematicians regarded the wording of this axiom as overly complicated and sought either to simplify it or to demonstrate that it was a consequence of Euclid's other nine axioms. They failed miserably on both counts (Jammer 1954/1993; Kline, 1980). Here's Euclid's irksome wording (Kline, 1980):

> If a straight line falling on two straight lines makes the interior angles on the same side less than two right angles, then the two straight lines if extended will meet on that side of the straight line on which the angles are less than two right angles.
>
> (p. 78)

Looking at Figure 9.2, if angles A and B add up to less than 180°, then lines 1 and 2 will meet if extended in sufficient degree; if, however, the angles sum exactly to 180°, then Line 1 and Line 2 will never meet. For any straight line, therefore, there can be only one line in the plane that is parallel to it. The latter way of expressing the parallel postulate, the one introduced explicitly by John Playfair in 1795, is the one commonly taught (Kline, 1980; see top row, Figure 9.3). In either version, the wording of the parallel postulate is irksome because it asserts the *existence* and *uniqueness* of this parallel line. Simultaneously, it asserts that for all other lines in the plane, there is always some point no matter how far, at which they will eventually intersect. To the mathematicians of the early 19th century (notably, Gauss, Lobatchevsky, and Bolyai), it became evident that Euclidean geometry was unfounded in the absence of an additional axiom about parallelism. This latter realization opened the door on the creation of a new set of axioms obtained by merely adopting a contradictory stance on the 5th postulate (see middle and bottom rows of Figure 9.3). The upshot was a variety of non-Euclidean geometries, each self-consistent, each as equally rigorous as the next, and all apparently able to describe space as thoroughly as Euclidean geometry (Cassirer, 1950; Kline, 1980). Gauss in 1830 took the giant step and proposed that geometry be relegated from the comfortable heights of pure reason to the grind of empirical science (Cassirer, 1950): "[S]pace has a reality outside the mind whose laws we cannot prescribe a priori" (p. 37).

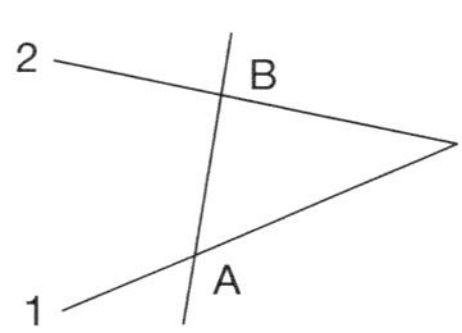

Figure 9.2 Euclid's fifth postulate (see text).

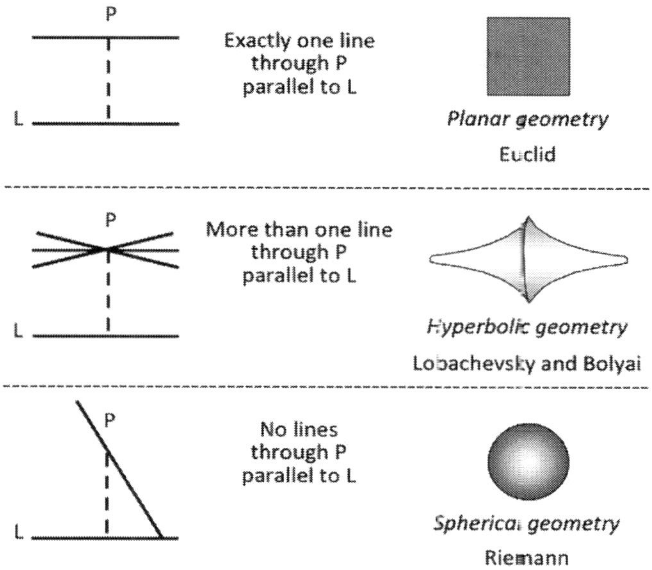

Figure 9.3 Variations on the parallel postulate create different kinds of self-consistent geometry of equal rigor.

(From Figure 2, Turvey, 2004, adapted with permission, *Ecological Psychology*.)

9.3.1 *How can Geometry be Empirical?*

An empirical geometry could take a benign form. Euclid's conceptual basis could be preserved intact with the critical issues limited to the kinds of experiments that would distinguish between Euclidean geometry and non-Euclidean geometry in respect to whether one represented space better than the other. The general development of this form of geometrical empiricism is limited by the fact that Euclidean and non-Euclidean geometry are equally distant from reality since both deal with entities that cannot be experimented upon (Cassirer, 1950). Experiments are conducted on material objects, not concepts such as points, lines and planes. The type of experiment that could be conducted was suggested by Gauss: Measure the angles of a very large triangle defined over distant objects in the environment and determine whether they sum to two right angles; if they do not, then space is non-Euclidean. Gauss surveyed a triangle with sides of 69, 85 and 107km formed by three mountains (Jammer, 1954/1993). His failure to find a deviation from 180° led him to conclude that space at the terrestrial scale was, for all intents and purposes, Euclidean. The result was otherwise inconclusive.

A truly empirical science of geometry would comprise collecting, systematizing and testing observations on the material layout of the environment.

Further, the means by which the observations are made should be expected to become more numerous and refined. At the outset, one can imagine that a sincere geometrical empiricism would have to question Euclid's foundations—his abstract geometric elements of point, straight line and plane—because of their tenuous connection to observable facts. In the latter part of the 19th century, Pasch (1882) sought to show in detail what an empirical geometry must be like and how it might be constructed without abandoning the rigor expected by either geometry or science. In so doing, he argued that although Euclid's elements can be derived from observable facts by idealization (limit processes), this idealization—its necessity and legitimacy—is at issue. Euclid's elements are not grounded in matter. Viewed as a fact of the environment, a *point*, for example, is not something lacking parts but rather a *material body* whose division does not lie within the limits of observation (Pasch, 1882, cited in Cassirer, 1950). Materially, there are segments with length and breadth, not Euclidean lines possessing only length. By continually extending a segment along its length in both directions one derives the Euclidean intuition of a straight line. Restrictions on the axioms of Euclid quickly arise. For example, the proposition that a unique straight line can always be drawn between any two points must be qualified: The two points qua material bodies cannot be at any arbitrary proximity. Restrictions on measurement are also implied. Whereas measures conducted in Euclidean and non-Euclidean geometries based on abstract points and real numbers can be infinitely precise, those conducted in a geometry based on segments and natural numbers can be no more precise than the resolution provided by the shortest segment (Shaw & Cutting, 1980).

Table 9.1 Differences between the Plane of Abstract Geometry (e.g., Euclidean) and the Surface of Ecological Geometry

A plane	*A surface*
is insubstantial	is substantial
is colorless	is colored
is transparent	is opaque or transparent or semi-transparent
can only be visualized	can be seen
is without texture	is textured in both pigmentation and layout (it can be rippled, pebbled, granular, ridged, etc.)
has two sides (it is an infinitely thin sheet in space)	has only one side (it is an interface or boundary between a medium, e.g., air, and a substance, e.g., soil)
forms a line when it intersects another plane	forms an edge or corner at the juncture with another surface (when both surfaces are flat)

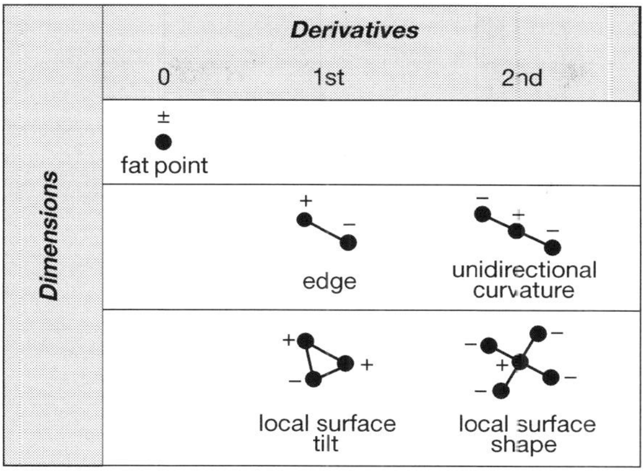

Figure 9.4 Five basic surface structures. Think of + and – as a local elevation relative to a local depression, respectively. Between any + and – pair, a zero crossing will be defined. The order of a surface primitive is given by the number of zero crossings (dimension (derivative).

(From Figure 1, Lappin, 1995, adapted with permission, Elsev er.)

In the 20th century, Pasch's concern with grounding the elements of geometry in the observable facts of the environment was addressed most vigorously by the perceptual psychologist James Gibson (1979/1986). The contrast between the abstract geometrical notion of *plane* and the ecological notion of *surface* suffices as an introduction to Gibson's effort to develop an applied geometry appropriate for the study of perception and behavior. Table 9.1 summarizes the contrasts (cf. Huntington, 1913). It also opens the door on geometric primitives such as spatial derivatives of 0th, 1st, 2nd and 4th order (Koenderink & van Doorn, 1992) that characterize basic local properties of surfaces as schematized in Figure 9.4.

9.3.2 What is the Dimensionality of Space?

From Lecture 8 we will recall the Flatlander's impertinence with regard to his Spacelander teacher. He raised the question of why, in principle, there might not be further lands of more than three dimensions. The question provoked annoyance and exasperation in the Spacelander for he could no more intuit a four-dimensional space than the Flatlander originally could intuit a three-dimensional space. That the Flatlander's question had to be taken seriously was one of the consequences of the "crisis" and "debacle" that arose with the proliferation of geometries incurred by adopting variants of the parallel postulate. For philosophers, mathematicians and physicists in the latter part of the 19th century, the question of whether space has three dimensions or more was now an empirical question on the same footing as the question of whether space was Euclidean or non-Euclidean (Jammer, 1954/1993). An even more iconoclastic question lay ahead: *Is the dimensionality of space an integer?*[9] This latter question comes to prominence in the 20th century with the demonstration that the study of physical phenomena in spaces of non-integer dimension, spaces with so-called *fractal dimensions*, is a logically consistent possibility (Mandelbrot, 1983).[10] We will have reason to confront the notion of fractals in subsequent lectures. A preliminary introduction here lets us see that dimension, surprisingly, is a loose concept (see Lecture 1) and that the determination of the number of dimensions is strictly an empirical matter.

Intuitively, one dimension (coordinate or degree of freedom) is needed to express the size of a piece of string (geometrically a line). Similarly, intuition suggests that two dimensions are needed to express the size of a sheet of paper (geometrically a square), and three dimensions are needed to express the size of a box (geometrically a cube). A line, a square, and a cube typify the forms or patterns studied by standard geometry. Other forms of note are circle, sphere, and cone. Each of these geometric forms is regular (or smooth) and of a single connected piece. For the most part, however, Nature's forms or patterns are irregular (or rough) and fragmented. In a much-celebrated phrase, Mandelbrot (1983) observes that: "Clouds are not spheres, mountains are not cones, coastlines are not circles, and bark is not smooth, nor does lightning travel in a straight line" (p. 1).

What does intuition suggest about the number of dimensions needed to express the size of a cloud or a coastline or the form shown in Figure 9.5 known as the Koch snowflake (a curve of infinite length containing a finite area)? Whereas *dimension* interpreted as number of coordinates works for regular and connected forms, it became evident on the cusp of the 20th century that it does not work for irregular and fragmented forms.[11]

Consider a line of length l cm. To double the size, you need *two* such lines of length l cm placed end to end. Consider now a square with sides of length l. You will need to stick together a total of *four* such squares in order to make a square twice the size, $4l^2$. For a cube with side l, the number of such cubes

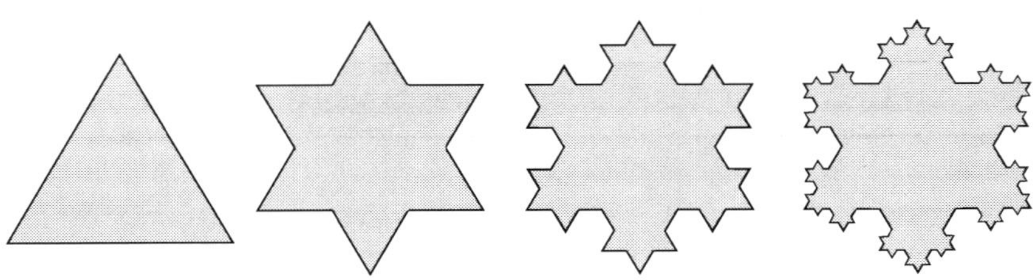

Figure 9.5 The Koch snowflake.

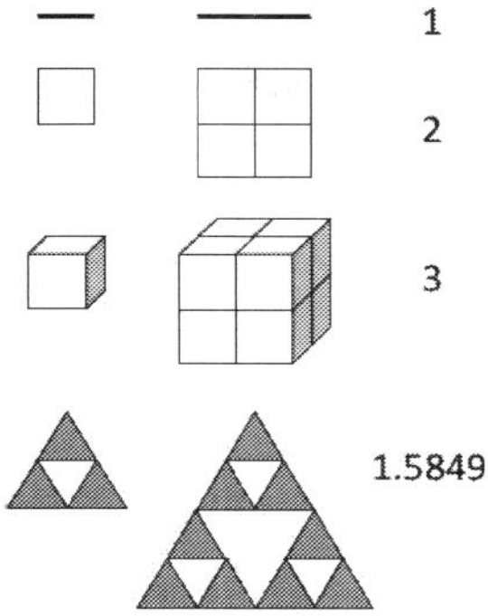

Figure 9.6 (*Top three rows*) A line, a square, and a cube are scaled up by a factor of two. This doubling similarity requires 2 copies of the line, 4 copies of the square and 8 copies of the cube. The dimensionality is calculated according to D = log (number of copies)/log (scaling factor). When the doubling similarity applies to the Sierpinski triangle (*bottom row*), the rule for dimensionality produces a non-integer value.

(From Figure 2 in Turvey, 2004, adapted with permission, *Ecological Psychology*.)

needed to double the size would be *eight*. If you could imagine a hyper-cube of dimension d, then the number c of copies you would need would be 2^d. A simple rule for dimensionality is suggested—namely, d = log$c$/log2. As can be seen in Figure 9.6, this rule gives 1, 2, and 3 as the dimensionality of the line, square and cube, respectively, in agreement with ordinary understanding. Importantly, in respect to the question of the integer nature of the dimensionality of space, this rule implies that if you found a form that required *three* copies to bring about a doubling in size, then it would have a non-integer dimension d = log3/log2 = 1.5849 . . . Such a form is the Sierpinski triangle shown in Figure 9.6. Evidently, rather than being obvious, *dimension* is enigmatic.

The general nature of the rule that expresses the number of copies needed to produce the same d-dimensional object scaled upwards or downwards by a is $c = a^d$ with d = log$c$/log$a$. Let us apply this rule to the Koch snowflake. In constructing the snowflake, one begins by taking a side of an equilateral triangle and dividing it into three equal segments. The middle segment is then removed and replaced by two segments in the form of a peak where these two inner segments are equal in length to the two outer segments. These steps are then repeated forever. Returning to the rule for determining dimension, each new arrangement of one side of the snowflake curve is made up of four copies of the side, c = 4, each of a size one third that of the side's original size, a = 3. So, for the Koch snowflake, d = log4/log3 = 1.2618 . . . Simply, it has a non-integer dimension.

The fractal conception of dimension developed in the preceding paragraphs is non-intuitive and non-Euclidean. Further, it is a conception of dimension that involves more than a consideration of a form's topology (those defining properties of a form that are unchanged when the form is subjected to continuous deformation). Fractal dimension reflects the notion of scale or distance—that is, metrical structure. Whereas topology fails to discriminate—for example, among different island coastlines, in that each is topologically identical to a circle—the metrically infused fractal dimension does so discriminate. If one takes a ruler of fixed length r and moves along a coastline in steps of size r, then the total length of the coastline will be $L(r)$. The use of a shorter ruler, however, would result in a larger estimate because it would permit the detection of sub-bays and sub-peninsulas undetected by the larger ruler. It proves to be the case that as e decreases, $L(r)$ increases steadily without bound—that is, infinitely—according to $L(r) \propto r^{(1-D)}$ where D can be interpreted as the fractal dimension (Mandelbrot, 1967, 1983). Although identical in topology, different coastlines have different values of D.

The lesson learned from measuring objects that are rough and fragmented is at odds with what we had been led to presume from Newton's and Kant's notion of space as absolute. The lengths or sizes or distances of chunks of the natural world are not necessarily fixed quantities but may, in the general case, be contingent on the resolution of the measuring instrument. In the face of this latest enigma, what emerges, as the potentially right degree of freedom to characterize uniquely the spatial magnitudes of a piece of the world, is D. As resolution increases (the "yardstick" becomes smaller), the amount of space increases at the constant rate D that differs from one irregular, fragmented piece of the world to the next.

Perception-action systems are yardsticks. Each organism is a unit measure of its surroundings. Measurements (by scientists) of transects[12] across the surfaces of selected vegetation reveal a fractal dimension of $D = 1.44$ in the mean (Morse, Lawton, Dodson, & Williamson, 1985). The implication is that if arthropods living on a plant's surface perceive the plant in units of body length, then—as shown in Figure 9.7—the expected densities of organisms of different sizes (different r) can be determined from r and D (see also Dibble & Thomaz, 2009; Gunnarsson, 1992; Kalimanis, Sgardelis, & Halley, 2002; Shorrocks, Masters, Ward & Evennett, 1991).

Fractal analysis is typically oriented to the geometry of sets. In respect to the prior example of arthropods and plants the focus was patterns arising from presence/absence data, whether arthropods were present or absent in particular sites. A focus on the *arrangement of quantities*, such as densities or proportions, characterizes multifractal analysis. A waterfall provides a canonical example (Figure 9.8). It can be treated mathematically as an increasingly dense nesting of proportions.

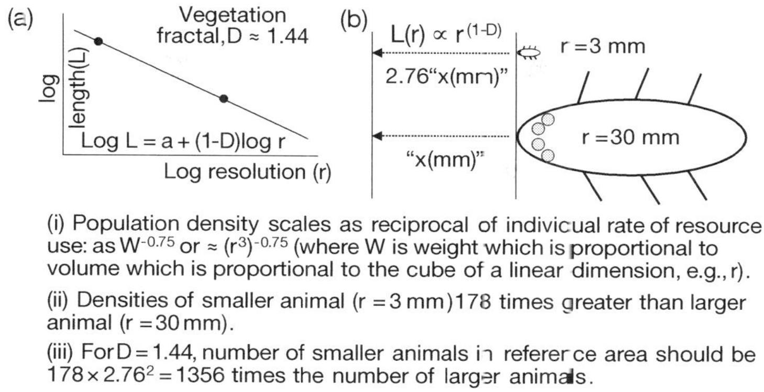

Figure 9.7 Animal density as a function of animal size and the fractal dimension of plants. (a) Length of transect (sample area of vegetation) as a function of resolution of measure in double logarithmic coordinates. Two points on the linear plot identify L for the two animals in (b). Slope yields measure (1-D) where D is fractal dimension. (b) Two animals that differ in size by an order of magnitude. For the smaller animal, the distance between two lines as calculated by the power function for L(r) is 2.76 times greater than for the larger animal. Points (i), (ii), and (iii) spell out the steps used to determine the relative densities of the two animals on the sample of vegetation.

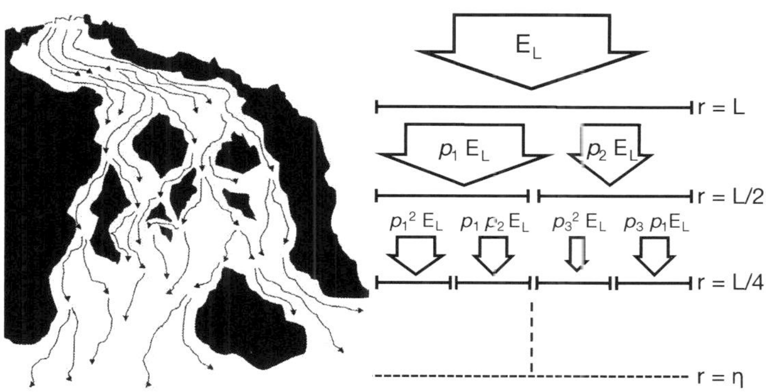

Figure 9.8 The ordinary waterfall (*left*) is a prime example of a natural turbulent cascade. It can be depicted mathematically (*right*) as an indefinite nesting of unequal proportions leading to a so-called multifractal process.

Left: (From Figure 2 of Kelty-Stephen et al., 2013, adapted with permission, *Ecological Psychology*). Right: (From Figure 3, Meneveau & Sreenivasan, adapted with permission. (c) 1987, American Physical Society.)

9.3.3 "Outness" and InformationL

The springboard for this lecture has been the notion and problem of "outness," the "*there* not *here*" enigma, raised by Alhazen, Kant, Lotze and von Békésy, to name but a few. William James treated it with derision ("veridical hallucination"), as noted, but Gibson (1966) offered a counter in terms of the "remarkable fact" that:

> [W]hen a man touches something with a stick he *feels* it at the end of the stick, not in the hand. This is a difficulty for the theory of sensation-based perception; it requires some such postulate as the projecting of sensations outward from the body. But we entertain the hypothesis that information for the mechanical disturbance at the end of the stick is obtained by the hand as a perceptual organ, including information about the length and direction of the stick. The sensations in the hand are irrelevant.
>
> (pp. 100–101)

The point being made can be elaborated. When one taps an object with a hand-held stick, one feels contemporaneously, and one might say independently, the stick in the hand, the end of the stick, and the object at the end of the stick. Each of the preceding is a candidate instance of "outness." Figure 9.9a depicts a participant in an experiment in which there are combinations of three stick lengths of 61, 76, and 91 cm and three object distances of 18, 33, and 48 cm, with stick lengths and object distances as unknowns (Carello, Fitzpatrick, & Turvey, 1992, Experiment 3). The mass moments (mass, static moment, and moment of inertia) of the sticks were manipulated by a 60 g weight attached either 1/4 length from the distal end or 1/4 length from the proximal end. On each trial, the object (a vertical board) and the stick are occluded during the participant's act of tapping or striking with the hand-held stick to perceive, on instruction, either the object's distance or the stick's length. Figures 9.9b and 9.9c summarize the mean data for the group of

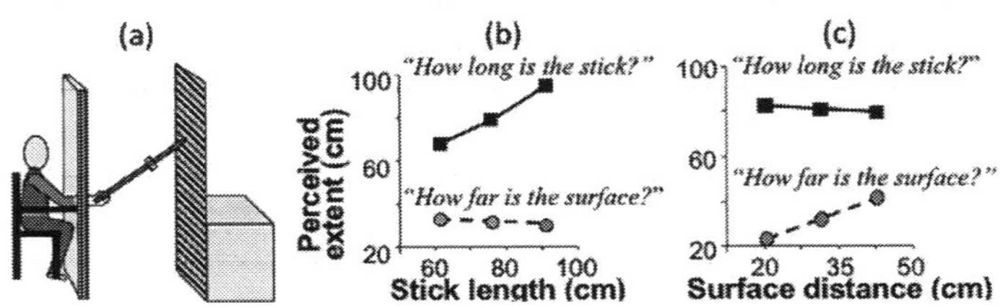

Figure 9.9 (a) Striking a vertically aligned object with the intent to perceive the length of the hand-held stick or the distance of the object as a function of (b) stick length and (c) object distance.

(From Figure 4 of Carello, Fitzpatrick, & Turvey, 1992, adapted with permission, Springer.)

participants. What they show is a close correspondence between perceived and actual stick length, and between perceived and actual object distance. What they also show, in equal importance, is the strict separation of the two perceptual intents.

Repetitive tapping of a surface can be expressed as a dynamical system minimally of the form:

$$\dot{x} = F(x, t; c_i, N) \tag{9.1}$$

with x the stick's displacement at time t, $\dot{x}$ its rate of change, c_i the parameters (the mass moments, center of percussion, and intent), N noise, and F the physics (the relevant laws of motion and change) governing the time evolution of x. During a trial x varies, c_i does not. This time invariance confers on c_i a special quality during the tapping—namely, constraining the specific ways in which the stick's states and, perforce, the states of the participant's body, are coupled to the forces (muscular and contact) imposed upon the stick (Turvey & Carello, 1995). Whereas stick moment of inertia,[13] angle of contact, and center of percussion mattered to the perception of stick length, only stick moment of inertia and angle of contact mattered to the perception of surface distance. The results suggest that the deformations of the muscular and connective tissues of arm and body were specific to stick length under the length intention and specific to surface distance under the distance intention. In terms of the ideas introduced in Lecture 3, we might be disposed to claim that the two kinds of perceiving were specific to two distinct forms of informationL.

9.4 On Space (and Time) Befitting the Facts of Research in Perception

The larger lessons to be learned from this lecture were conveyed by Bentley (1941, p. 478) and echoed by Shaw and Turvey (1981) as follows:

1 Psychology has always concerned itself with facts which do not tolerate description in technical Newtonian space and time.
2 These facts, nevertheless, have their own manifest extensions and durations.
3 Psychology is now at last free to describe them as it finds and observes them.
4 Such observation and description becomes practicable with the frame of a full naturalism for organic and environmental facts.

Notes

1 Kant scorned philosophers who conceived the world as unreal (e.g., Berkeley in *A Treatise Concerning the Principles of Human Knowledge*, 1710/1998) or who questioned the reality of the outside world (e.g., Hume). He regarded such attitudes

as a "scandal of philosophy." For Kant, the world is appearance, not illusion (Jasper, 1962, p. 21).

2 Think of Copernicus (Lecture 5). The daily rotation of the sun around the earth was a *phenomenon*, an appearance, whereas the *noumenon* was the earth's rotation about an internal axis that rotated about the sun.

3 It is an oversimplification to say, but nonetheless useful to do so, that Kant sought to repair the breach between rationalism and empiricism. "Thoughts without concepts are empty, percepts without concepts are blind . . . Understanding can perceive nothing, the senses can think nothing. Knowledge arises from their united action."

4 Intuition is a technical notion in Kant's (1781/1787/1998, p. 172) philosophy: "In whatever way and through whatever means a cognition may relate to objects, that through which it relates immediately to them, and at which all thought as a means is directed as an end, is intuition."

5 Transcendental is also a technical term in Kant's philosophy. It refers to thought that, independently of experience, establishes the possibility and limits of experience and builds an understanding of experience on these foundations (see text below).

6 A 20th-century scholar (Brook, 1994, p. 12) suggests that the transcendental argument "has become a major, perhaps the major, method of cognitive science."

7 The program of Newton, it can be argued (Jammer, 1954/1993), was to demonstrate the existence of true motion and absolute space. His mechanics was a vindication of the theory of absolute space as a logical and ontological necessity (the first law of motion required it). The truth of the matter, however, was that Newton's metaphysical views were irrelevant to his mechanics. What was important was the notion of an inertial system (Jammer, 1954/1993; Smart, 1967).

8 What is Euclidean geometry precisely? It is the study of figures that are unchanged by the group of transformations that leave distances unchanged. The properties of Euclidean geometry (*Euclidean properties*) are those that are preserved over displacements of a rigid figure around the plane. In addition to distance, they include angles, collinearity of points and concurrence of lines.

9 For a representative sample of the forms taken by this question in contemporary physics, consider the titles of the research papers by Zeilinger and Svozil (1985), Jarlskog and Yndurain (1986), and Luo and Schramm (1992).

10 Mandelbrot coined the term *fractal* from the Latin adjective *fractus*. The corresponding verb *frangere* means "to break" with the implication of "creating irregular fragments." Fractal, therefore, connotes both "fragmented" and "irregular."

11 The mathematicians most responsible for this discovery were Cantor, Peano, Lebesgue, and Hausdorff.

12 A transect is a sample area of vegetation in the form of a narrow continuous strip, typically used for the tabulation of data on the properties of vegetation.

13 Defined about the point of rotation in the wrist. As is discernible in Figure 9.9a, the forearm was resting on the chair arm and three-space rotational movements were restricted to the hand and stick.

References

Bentley, A. F. (1941). The factual space and time of behavior. *Journal of Philosophy*, *28*, 477–485.

Berkeley, G. (1998). *A treatise concerning the principles of human knowledge*. J. Dancey (Ed.). Oxford, UK: Oxford University Press (original work published 1710).

Brook, A. (1994). *Kant and the mind.* Cambridge, UK: Cambridge University Press.
Carello, C., Fitzpatrick, P., & Turvey, M. T. (1992). Haptic probing: Perceiving the length of a probe and the distance of a surface probed. *Perception & Psychophysics, 51*, 580–598.
Cassirer, E. (1950). *The problem of knowledge.* New Haven, CT: Yale University Press.
Dibble, E. D., & Thomaz, S. M (2009). Use of fractal dimension to assess habitat complexity and its influence on dominant invertebrates inhabiting tropical and temperate Macrophytes. *Journal of Freshwater Ecology*, 24, 93–102.
Gibson, J. J. (1966). *The senses considered as perceptual systems.* Boston, MA: Houghton Mifflin.
Gibson, J. J. (1986). *The ecological approach to visual perception.* Mahwah, NJ: Erlbaum (original work published 1979).
Gunnarsson, B. (1992). Fractal dimension of plants and body size distribution in spiders. *Functional Ecology*, 6, 636–641.
Howard, I. (1996). Alhazen's neglected discoveries of visual phenomena. *Perception, 25*, 1203–1217.
Huntington, E. V. (1913). A set of postulates for abstract geometry, expressed in terms of the simple relation of inclusion. *Mathematische Annalen, 73*, 522–559.
James, W. (1983). *The principles of psychology.* Cambridge, UK: Cambridge University Press (original work published 1890).
Jammer, M. (1993). *Concepts of space: The history of theories of space in physics.* New York: Dover (original work published 1954).
Jarlskog, C., & Yndurain, F. J. (1986). Is the number of spatial dimensions an integer? *Europhysics Letters, 1*, 51–53.
Jasper, K. (1962). *Kant.* New York: Harcourt, Brace & World.
Kalimanis, A.S., Sgardelis, S. P., & Halley, J. M. (2002). Accuracy of fractal dimensions for small samples of ecological distributions. *Landscape Ecology, 17*, 281–297.
Kant, I. (1998). *Critique of pure reason.* (P. Guyer & A. Wood, Trans. and Eds.). Cambridge, UK: Cambridge University Press (original work published 1781/1787).
Kelty-Stephen, D. G., Palatinus, K., Saltzman, E., & Dixon, J. A. (2013). A tutorial on multifractality, cascades, and interactivity for empirical time series in ecological science. *Ecological Psychology, 25* (1), 1–62.
Kline, M. (1980). *Mathematics: The loss of certainty.* New York: Oxford University Press.
Koenderink, J. J., & van Doorn, A. J. (1992). Second-order optic flow. *Journal of the Optical Society of America A*, 9, 530–538.
Lappin, J. (1995). Visible information about structure from motion. In Epstein & Rogers (Eds.), *Perception of space and motion* (pp. 165–199). New York: Academic Press.
Lotze, H. (1888). *Logic* (2nd ed., B. Bosanquet, Trans. and Ed.). Oxford, UK: Clarendon Press.
Luo, X., & Schramm, D. N. (1992). Fractals and cosmological large-scale structures. *Science, 256*, 513–515.
Mandelbrot, B. B. (1967). How long is the coast of Britain? Statistical self-similarity and fractional dimension. *Science, 155*, 636–638.
Mandelbrot, B. B. (1983). *The fractal geometry of nature* San Francisco, CA: Freeman.
Meneveau, C., & Sreenivasan, K. R. (1987). Simple multifractal cascade model for fully developed turbulence. *Physics Review Letters, 59* (13), 1424–1427.

Morse, D. R., Lawton, J. H., Dodson, M. M., & Williamson, M. H. (1985). Fractal dimension of vegetation and the distribution of arthropod body lengths. *Nature*, *314*, 731–733.

Pasch, M. (1882). *Vorlesungen uber Neuere Geometrie*. Leipzig, Germany: Teubner.

Sabra, A. I. (1989). Form in ibn al-Haytham's theory of vision. *Zeitschrift für Geschichte der Arabisch-Islamischen Wissenschaften*, *5*, 115–140.

Shaw, R. E., & Cutting, J. (1980). Biological constraints on linguistic form: Clues from an ecological theory of event perception. In U. Bellugi & M. Studdert-Kennedy (Eds.), *Signed and spoken language: Biological constraints on linguistic form* (pp. 57–84). Weinheim, Germany: Verlag Chemie.

Shaw, R. E., & Turvey, M. T. (1981). Coalitions as models for ecosystems: A realist perspective on perceptual organization. In M. Kubovy & J. Pomerantz (Eds.), *Perceptual organization* (pp. 343–415). Hillsdale, NJ: Erlbaum.

Shorrocks, B., Masters, J., Ward, I., & Evennett, P. J. (1991). The fractal dimension of lichens and the distribution of arthropod body lengths. *Functional Ecology*, *5*, 457–460.

Smart, J. J. C. (1967). Space. In P. Edwards (Ed.), *The encyclopedia of philosophy, Vol. 7* (pp. 506–511). New York: Macmillan.

Toulmin, S. (1967). Neuroscience and human understanding. In G. C. Quarton, T. Melnechuk & F. O. Schmitt (Eds.), *The neurosciences: A study program* (pp. 822–832). New York: Rockefeller University Press.

Turvey, M. T. (2004). Space (and its perception): The first and final frontier. *Ecological Psychology*, *16*, 25–29.

Turvey, M. T., & Carello, C. (1995). Dynamic touch. In W. Epstein & S. Rogers (Eds.), *Handbook of perception and cognition, Vol. V. Perception of space and motion* (pp. 401–490). San Diego, CA: Academic Press.

von Bekesy, G. (1967). *Sensory inhibition*. Princeton, NJ: Princeton University Press.

Zeilinger, A., & Svozil, K. (1985). Measuring the dimension of space-time. *Physical Review Letters*, *54*, 2553–2555.

Lecture 10

The Space Enigmas III: Local Signs and Geometrical Empiricism

From a contemporary point of view, Kant's (1781/1787/1998) argument was that space (and time) should be studied in terms of mind/brain rather than vice versa. In the 19th century, the weakening of the strong rationalist stance on geometry gave Kant's argument a new twist. The investigation of space as a property of mind (or an embodiment of brain) should proceed not through metaphysical and transcendental arguments, but through the methods and facts of physiology and psychology. The new twist was accompanied by an emphatic promotion of the class of arguments defended by Berkeley (1709/1948). Mind might be predisposed to perceiving objects in the world as spatially extended, but the geometric character of this extension originated entirely in experience. The primary scholar in developing this geometrical empiricism was Herman von Helmholtz—a true intellectual giant in each of the disciplines of mathematics, physics, philosophy, physiology, and perceptual psychology. Cassirer (1950, p. 41) observed that Helmholtz investigated the problem of space in the terms of each of the aforementioned disciplines; it was the focal point of his career.

We will develop Helmholtz's thinking on the concept of space and the nature of its perception in this lecture and the next. The starting point is the claim of Rudolph Hermann Lotze (1852, 1886) that the right theory of space perception cannot begin with the very thing it is a theory about, namely, position and extension. To the contrary, the position and extension of objects—and, pursuant to them, the geometry of points, lines and planes—must be derived through experience from non-spatial beginnings.[1] James (1890/1983) referred to the theory of local sign as "the theory which denies that there can be in sensation any element of actual locality, of inherent spatial order" (p. 798).

In the beginning, there are only intensities. Consider the skin. At each point there is a unique magnitude or intensity of receptor activity due to the unique arrangement of tissue properties at each point. Locally, the skin varies in how it deforms under a specific pressure and in the particular constellation of cutaneous receptors that would be stimulated by the deformation. Because these differences in intensity (more precisely, intensity pattern) are correlated with differences in location, intensity is a *local sign*. Following Kant, Lotze presumed that the mind imposed spatial order but, in his view, could only do so if given local signs. The situation is like that of a postal worker with a handful of envelopes that are missing the names of the areas to which the envelopes are to be sent (Pastore, 1971). Although the worker is fully capable of sorting the mail, of placing envelopes into their appropriate mailbags, he or she cannot sort her handful of envelopes because they are not tagged as to their mailbags—they lack local signs.

We can develop an interpretation of Lotze's theory of space through the notion of space as a *differentiable manifold* which lacks familiar geometric properties such as parallelism, curvature, geodesic (shortest path), length and angle, but which can become endowed with such properties given the right circumstances. This development is in keeping with Riemann's (1854/1953) and Helmholtz's (1868/1977a, 1868/1977b) analytic (as opposed to axiomatic) approach to geometry that begins with the mathematical properties of a manifold of points determined by a set of coordinates.[2] Additionally, this development is in keeping with Riemann's assertion that the structure of a physical space depends on the physical phenomena for which it serves as background. Space as a structureless manifold is endowed with structure by material processes (Weyl, 1920/1952).[3]

10.1 The Concept of a Manifold

In the spirit of Lotze, Riemann, and Helmholtz, therefore, we may conceptualize an arbitrarily chosen patch of skin as a two-dimensional point manifold.[4] By this, we mean the following. First, that each point is uniquely specified by two real numbers (see Figure 10.1). Second, that between any two distinct points there are other points so that the patch is smooth (or continuous) rather than granular (or discrete). We actually think of the patch as composed of a large number of small, virtually planar pieces that are sewn together. Although we

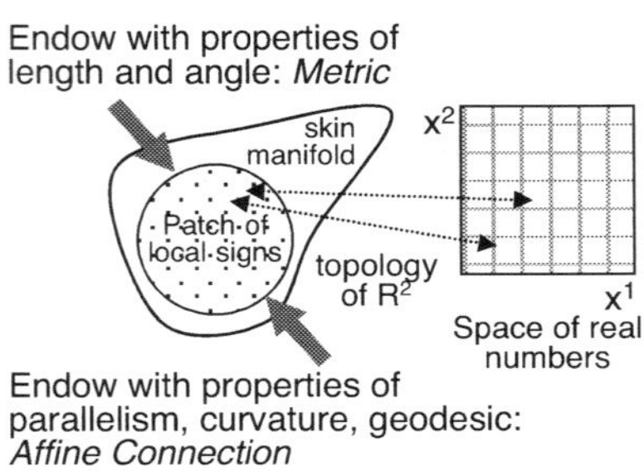

Figure 10.1 Lotze's theory of developing spatiality from intensity interpreted through geometric notions originating with Riemann and Helmholtz.

(From Figure 2 in Turvey, 2004, adapted with permission, *Ecological Psychology*.)

can presume that the small pieces of skin are all sewn together the same way we should note that, in the general case, if there were different ways of sewing the pieces together they would determine different global properties of the patch.[5] The aforementioned smoothness is a property of sewing all the pieces together without any sharp corners or folds. In general, the characteristic of an n-dimensional point manifold is that each of the points composing it may be specified by the assignment of n quantities (coordinates) that are continuous differentiable functions within the manifold.[6]

The smoothness feature of a manifold is actually a very technical notion. Its ascription presumes that the manifold shares the topological properties[7] of real numbers (see Figure 10.1). The latter properties are expressed in terms of unions of open intervals referred to as *open sets*. An open interval (a, b) consists of all the points (real numbers) x such that $a < x < b$ with the end points a and b excluded. Consequently, any point x in (a, b) can be surrounded by another open interval $(x - e, x + e)$, all of whose points are also in (a, b) (Lawrie, 1990).

It is of great importance that the assignment of numbers to points need not involve the geometry of the three-dimensional space in which the skin is embedded. As highlighted, in Lotze's scheme the assignment is done strictly through the anatomically based local signs. However, in order to grasp firmly what is at issue in deriving spatiality from intensity, we will need to consider a conventional mathematical strategy for assigning local signs (coordinates) without leaving the surface. The strategy is due to Gauss (1827/1965). In Figure 10.2, two families of curves have been drawn on a patch of skin in the manner that curves of longitude and the curves of latitude are imposed upon a desktop globe of the world. Call the two families of curves u curves and v curves. Beginning with any curve, we can consecutively label the u curves $u = 1$, $u = 2$, $u = 3$, and so on, and the v curves, $v = 1$, $v = 2$, $v = 3$, and so on. The patch of skin can be covered with these curves, with any curve of one family (a) intersecting none of the curves of the same family and (b) intersecting each of the curves of the other family at a single point. The coordinates of any point are then simply the labels of the u curve and the v curve that intersect at the point.[8] Armed with these coordinates, a geometry of the skin manifold (Figure 10.1) can be developed that deals with measures made entirely on, and belonging solely to, the skin manifold, independently of how it is embedded in the world's x, y, z coordinates (see Figure 10.2).[9]

To repeat, the coordinates (u, v) of the points of the skin manifold are merely labels or identification marks, that is, they are local signs. They do not themselves supply any notion of a distance between two points. Determining the distance along a curve drawn on the skin manifold requires a rule—for example, *Distance* (*D*) = (*function of coordinates*) But any such rule imposes an additional structure, a metric, which does not inhere in the manifold. In the problem that Lotze has defined for himself, this rule would have to arise experientially. It would have to arise from actions upon or involving the skin

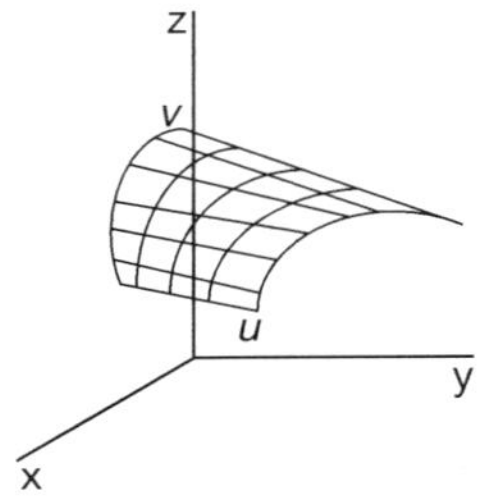

Figure 10.2 Extrinsic (x, y, z) and intrinsic (u, v) coordinates of a patch of skin.

manifold. Lotze presumed that movements of the skin across environmental surfaces or vice versa were the primary means of endowing the manifold with typical spatial properties.[10] The aforementioned *metric*, that provides a meaningful notion of length and a definition of angle between two vectors, would have to be obtained through movement, as would the *affine connection*. The latter is a rule for determining whether a vector at one point in the manifold is parallel to a vector at another point (Lawrie, 1990). Given this rule, the curvature of the skin manifold and geodesics[11] on the skin manifold can also be defined. We ought to note, however, that a special kind of affine connection is deducible from a metric. It is referred to as a *metric connection*. Although duly noted, it is nonetheless valuable to appreciate the distinction between geometric notions that rely only on an affine connection and those that require a metric.

The concepts incorporated in the rules are of significance to several topics that follow in later lectures as well as being essential to our present discussion. We need to make contact, therefore, with their nature and use.

10.2 The Metrical Groundform

It will be helpful to use x_1 and x_2 in place of u and v. Consider two adjacent points P and Q on the surface of Figure 10.2. Let the coordinates of P be (x_1, x_2) and the coordinates of Q be $(x_1 + dx_1, x_2 + dx_2)$, where dx_1 and dx_2 are infinitesimal. Then the distance ds between P and Q is also infinitesimal. Applying Pythagoras's theorem to the surface (a theorem originally introduced in extrinsic coordinates for finite magnitudes) we can write the distance ds as a quadratic function of dx_1 and dx_2. That is,

$$ds^2 = g_{11}dx_1^2 + 2g_{12}dx_1dx_2 + g_{22}dx_2^2. \tag{10.1}$$

This equation defines the *line element* of a surface. Figure 10.3 will let us develop (in the manner of Singh, 1959/2010) an appreciation for the function of the g-coefficients. Consider a part of the mesh covering the surface that is

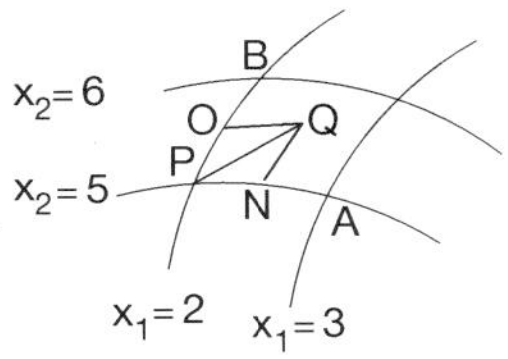

Figure 10.3 A part of the mesh depicted in Figure 10.2.
(From Figure 56 in Singh, 1959, with permission from Dover Publications.)

bounded by x_1 curves 2 and 3 and x_2 curves 5 and 6. Q is a point in the mesh at a distance ds from P, the corner of the mesh with coordinates $x_1 = 2$ and $x_2 = 5$. QN and QO are lines parallel to the mesh lines PB and PA, respectively. We need to identify the coordinates that label points O and N. The ratio of PN to PA varies from 0 to 1 as N travels along PA. This ratio is the increase in the x_1 coordinate of N as N displaces from P. Call this ratio dx_1. Then the x_1 coordinate of N is $2 + dx_1$. By similar reasoning, dx_2 is the ratio $PO:PB$ and the x_2 coordinate of O is $5 + dx_2$. Because dx_1 and dx_2 are ratios, they do not give us the lengths of PN and PO. To get them we need to discover the scales on which PA and PB are drawn. That is, we need to make measures, and for this purpose we can imagine using a very small rigid measuring rod to quantify infinitely small regions of the surface without leaving the surface. Suppose that this yardstick reveals that PA is of length g_{11}. Then, given $PN/PA = dx_1$, the scale number g_{11} converts the ratio dx_1 into the actual distance PN ($g_{11}dx_1 = PN$). Similarly, the measurement of PB provides the scale number g_{22} that converts dx_2 into the actual distance PO. A third scale number is one that converts dx_2 into the length of the projection of QN on PA (a quantity needed in order to apply the well-known form of Pythagoras's theorem in terms of the hypotenuse of a triangle). This latter scale number enters into a product with g_{11} to produce g_{12}.

As long as the mesh is constant, the scale numbers or g-coefficients are constant. If the mesh is changed globally or locally (e.g., made finer or coarser), a different set of scale numbers may be needed, and typically are needed, to determine the distance ds between any P and Q. To appreciate the g-coefficients further, consider the line element of a plane and the line element of a sphere. In the case of the plane, coordinates can be chosen for which

$$ds^2 = dx_1{}^2 + dx_2{}^2,$$

that is, $g_{11} = 1$, $g_{12} = 1$, $g_{22} = 1$. For the sphere, with x_1 as latitude, x_2 as longitude, and r the sphere's radius, the line element is computed according to

$$ds^2 = r^2dx_1{}^2 + r^2\cos^2 x_1dx_2{}^2.$$

Here, the values of the coefficients are $g_{11} = r^2$, $g_{12} = 0$, $g_{22} = r^2 \cos^2 x_1$. In this geometry based on the differentials of infinitesimal magnitudes, the g-coefficients may vary not only with the coordinates but also with the global form of the surface.

Equation 10.1 is referred to as the *metrical groundform* or simply the metric of a surface. It is the "open sesame" (Singh, 1959/2010) of a surface's intrinsic geometry; all the intrinsic properties are determinable if the values of g at every point are known. Defining g_{21} by $g_{21} = g_{12}$, leads to the following useful expression of the metrical groundform:

$$ds^2 = (dx_1, dx_2)\begin{pmatrix} g_{11} & g_{12} \\ g_{21} & g_{22} \end{pmatrix}\begin{pmatrix} dx_1 \\ dx_2 \end{pmatrix} \tag{10.2}$$

Let us call the symmetric 2 × 2 matrix, the *metric matrix* (Synge, 1970). Essentially, this matrix g_{ij} is an *operator:* It operates on the coordinates or local signs of two infinitely close points of the manifold to produce the distance between them.

10.3 Geodesics and Curvature

Let us see how the metrical groundform yields up a surface's internal structure. That geodesics might be defined intrinsically is hinted at by the fact that one could just as well pull a string tight between two points on the surface of a football as one could between two points on a plane. Just as the length of the taut string on the plane gives the shortest distance, so does the length of the taut string on the football. A curve on a surface is composed of many line elements bridging the distance between the two pairs of coordinates. Adding the multiple line elements together is denoted by $\int ds$. To determine the geodesic, one basically perturbs the curve (the taut string) and looks for that length which undergoes a change δ that is much less than the perturbation. Thus,

$$\delta \int ds = 0$$

defines a geodesic as a curve of stationary length. Whether the emphasis is on the idea of a minimal or stationary length, it is nonetheless clear that this surface measure is obtained from the line element and, therefore, the metrical groundform. More challenging is the task of understanding how the metrical groundform enables the determination of surface curvature. Obviously, a comparison between (1) a non-planar surface A, and (2) a planar surface B, ought to provide some impression of just how non-planar or curved is A. The comparison could be conducted in terms of simple Euclidean forms drawn on A and B such as circles and triangles. For example, a triangle drawn on a plane always has angles that sum to 180°, the sum of two right angles. What of a triangle drawn on a sphere? Suppose one were to draw a straight line from the earth's north pole to the equator followed by a right-angled turn and the drawing of a further straight line of the same length followed, finally, by a repeat of the latter maneuver to return to the north pole. The outcome will be a triangle with three right angles, that is, 270° for the sum rather than 180°. On a sphere the sum of a triangle's angles is always in excess of 180°, with the degree of excess proportional to the triangle's area (the smaller the area, the smaller the excess). On a pseudosphere (see middle line of Figure 9.3), the sum of the angles of a triangle with geodesic sides is always *less* than 180°. Again, however, the magnitude of the deviation (here, negative excess) is proportional to the area of the triangle. The area of a triangle is equal to half the product of base and height. It is a metrical quantity and as such is indifferent to the mesh or coordinate system covering the surface. An examination of many small triangles on a non-planar surface reveals that the ratio of excess to area is similarly an invariant, independent of the shapes of the triangles and of the coordinate systems. This invariance over coordinate systems means, of course, invariance over a surface's metrical groundforms (recalling that the metric matrix will vary as the mesh varies). Take this invariant excess-to-area ratio to be the definition of curvature and recall that the line element or metrical groundform contains all the geometry of a surface. Then, it must be the case that there is an operator—let's call it C—that acts on the metrical groundform of each and every surface, whatever the values of the metric groundform's scaling factors, to produce a measure of the local surface curvature. Gauss made this discovery and referred to it as *theorema egregium* (i.e., outstanding theorem). It was the central result of his "Discourse on curved surfaces" published in 1827. In words, the operator C prescribes that the metrical groundform be differentiated twice with respect to the coordinates and that the metrical groundform and its first and second derivatives then be combined in a certain way (Synge, 1970).

We can represent the *theorema egregium* in terms of the intuitive notion of an operator box (Synge, 1970). Such a box is pierced on two sides by one or more rods, and contains an internal mechanism that connects the rods on the two sides in a specific way. A given rod's length indexes the value of a given variable. Figure 10.4 shows a metric operator box and a curvature operator box. Moving over the surface depicted in Figures 10.2 and 10.3 is tantamount to manipulating the rods of the metric box labeled x_1 and x_2. This manipulation, via the inner mechanism of the metric box, brings about variations in the rods labeled g_{11}, g_{12} and g_{22}. These *g* rods operate, by the inner mechanism of the curvature box, on the rod labeled *Cgx*. One reads the length of this latter rod as the curvature magnitude obtained by first applying the metrical operator *g* to the coordinates or local signs to obtain the line element and then applying the curvature operator C to the line element. Whereas the particulars of the metric box's inner mechanism vary with the nature of the surface, those of the curvature box are the same for *all* surfaces.

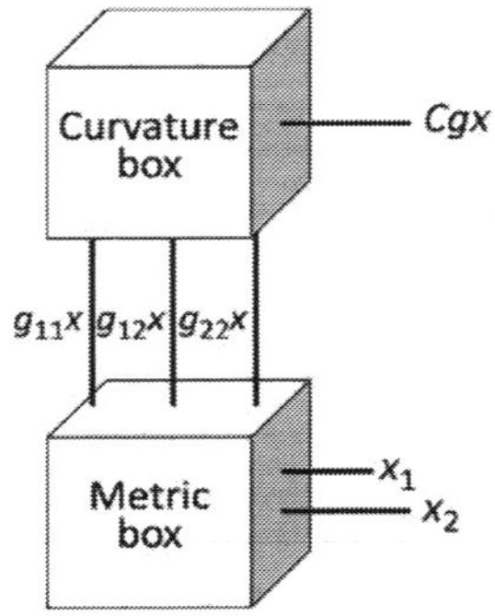

Figure 10.4 The determination of intrinsic curvature expressed in terms of operator boxes.

(From Figure 10.2 in Synge, 1970, adapted with permission, Elsevier.)

10.4 Movement, Metric Geometry and Affine Geometry

Lotze provided little detail of how movements might endow the skin manifold with geometric structure. He limited himself to describing how a stimulus moving across the skin would excite a succession of local signs providing the experience of adjacency or co-linearity or, simply, *line* (the rudimentary form of spatial extent). The experience of *between-ness* might arise in a similar fashion. For example, discerning that local sign *b* is between local signs *a* and *c* could follow from the fact that a continuous back and forth movement would lead to the ordered sensations *a–b–c* and *c–b–a* (Boring, 1942). In both cases—of sensing line and sensing between-ness—the suggested movement is merely one of parallel translation. In neither case does the sensed property rely on an act of measurement. A property of a planar surface that is not characterized by a measure of distance or angle, and which is realized through (or, more precisely, invariant over) parallel translations and anisotropic contractions or expansions, is an *affine* property. Such a property belongs to affine geometry—simply, Euclidean or metric geometry minus the machinery for measuring distances and angles.[12] In terms of the intuitive notion of operator boxes, no metric box is needed to register the co-linearity and the between-ness of the skin's local signs. If Lotze had developed explicit proposals for how the skin manifold acquires metrical properties in addition to affine properties, then he would have had to consider a further kind of movement—that implied by the principle of congruence. On this principle, all geometric measurements are ultimately based.

It will be recalled from the discussion of Figure 10.3 that determining the g-coefficients requires a rigid measuring rod that can brought into coincidence with the mesh lines. This act of measurement assumes that the measuring rod can be moved freely on the mesh to any place and in any orientation and that neither it nor the mesh change size or shape during these motions. Congruence or equality, as Helmholtz (1868/1977a, 1879/1968) took pains to argue, presumes *completely free mobility* and *fixity* (the quality or state of being fixed and stable). Implicit in the axioms of geometry, he argued, is the empirical issue of the mechanical behavior of fixed bodies. In Helmholtz's (1868/1977a) words:

> [T]he axioms of geometry are certainly not propositions belonging to the pure theory of space alone . . . they speak of magnitudes. One can only talk of magnitudes if one knows and intends some procedure, whereby one can compare these magnitudes, split them into parts and measure them. Thus all spatial measurement, and therefore in general all magnitude concepts applied to space, presuppose the possibility of the motion of spatial structure whose form and magnitude one may take to be unchanging despite the motion.
>
> (p. 24)

This assertion brings motion into the forefront of the formal development of geometry (Cassirer, 1950) and gives biological movement[13] added significance as Helmholtz emphasized (Helmholtz, 1868/1977a):

> When we measure, we are only doing, with the best and most reliable auxiliary means known to us, the same thing as that we otherwise ordinarily ascertain through observation by visual estimation and touch, or through pacing something off. In the latter cases, our own body with its organs is the measuring instrument which we carry around in space. At different moments our hands or our legs are dividers, or our eyes turning in all directions is the theodolite with which we measure arcs or phase angles in the visual field.
>
> (p. 19)

"Completely free mobility" needs elaborating. It means that a fixed body qua measuring rod can be moved continuously to any point of the manifold such that mutual congruence of any one region with any other can be discerned (Helmholtz, 1868/1977b, p. 43). "Completely free mobility" means a complete metric. Conversely, "incompletely free mobility," mobility that is subject to restrictions, means an incomplete metric. Affine geometry, when expressed solely in terms of its own axioms, contains none that deal with congruence (Gans, 1969). One might say that affine geometry is a geometry of restricted mobility. An interesting consequence is that distances in affine geometry can be compared in value only when they are on the same line or parallel lines. With "restricted mobility" the evaluation of mutual congruence is possible for only some, not all, regions of the manifold.

In his study of *retinal* local signs, Helmholtz was able to provide insights into the movements that endow the manifold with a metric as well as an affine connection (Koenderink, 1990), insights that did not follow from theorizing on the local signs of the skin. He was also able to identify in what principled ways the metric of the retinal manifold is limited by virtue of the laws governing the movements of the eyes.

10.5 Retinal Local Signs, Donders's Law and Listing's Law

In the case of the skin, a given intensity of mechanical contact creates different intensive patterns at different locations. In the case of the retina, a given photic intensity creates the *same* intensive pattern at different locations. Retinal local signs must be of extra-retinal origin. Lotze (1852, 1886) attributed retinal local signs to eye movements. Any given retinal point could be assigned an intensive value on the basis of the movement that brought the image from the given point to the center of the retina. It was assumed that such associations were likely given the tendency of the eye to fixate objects detected peripherally. It was also assumed that eye movements exhibited a simplicity and constancy that would ensure that the formed associations between retinal points and movement intensity would be reliable. For the determination of retinal local signs, eye movements had to be lawful, not fortuitous (Boring, 1942). Helmholtz (1886/2000) was among the first to appreciate the lawfulness of eye movements and their implications for visual space perception.[14] The law of immediate relevance to Lotze's account of the genesis of local signs is Donders's law. This law states that the attitude of the eye in the head is specified uniquely by the direction of gaze (its angles of elevation and azimuth). Irrespective of its positions and movements prior to arriving at a particular gaze direction, the eye always assumes, at that gaze direction, the same unique three-dimensional orientation. Consequently, any fixation relative to the eye's *primary position* (roughly, the natural position in looking horizontally straight ahead)[15] would always be characterized by the same unique pattern of contractions and elongations of the ocular muscles and, therefore, by the same special feeling of innervation.

Donders's law has additional virtue. For any fixed head orientation, the image of any object that holds a constant position in the field of vision will always cover the same retinal points whenever fixated regardless of the eye movements occurring since the last fixation. This latter feature means that the retina can move back and forth between, say, two parallel lines to determine if the points on the retina that coincide with the end points of one line coincide similarly with the end points of the other line. Here, the retina functions as an analogue of a pair of compasses whose points are placed on the ends of two lines in succession to determine whether they are of equal length (Helmholtz, 1886/2000). The analogy breaks down, however, for non-parallel lines and it does so for reasons of the lawfulness of ocular movements.

It is important to appreciate that Donders's law is not trivial. Each eye has a pair of muscles (horizontal recti) that rotate it leftward and rightward and four muscles (superior and inferior recti and obliques) that rotate the eye up-clockwise (CW), down-CW, up-counterclockwise (CCW), and down-CCW, respectively. Potentially, the eye musculature could rotate the eye about the line of sight without affecting gaze direction, meaning that, for any one direction, there is a multitude of possible eye orientations.

In respect to the larger issue of how the retinal manifold is endowed with geometry, Helmholtz saw the relevance of a further law identified by Listing and related to the fact that the eye does not achieve all possible three-space orientations. The law is that the only achievable eye orientations are those that can be attained by starting from one specific "primary" reference orientation and then rotating about an axis that lies within the plane orthogonal to the primary orientation's gaze direction (line of sight/visual axis). This plane is called Listing's plane (Crawford & Vilis, 1995; Figure 10.5).

Listing's law only applies to axes in Listing's plane for which the saccadic eye movement is toward or away from primary position—the circumstances depicted in Figure 10.5. For any other circumstance (e.g., that shown in the left panel of Figure 10.6), the velocity axis of the saccade must tilt *out of* Listing's plane (right panel of Figure 10.6). The untilted axis points the eye

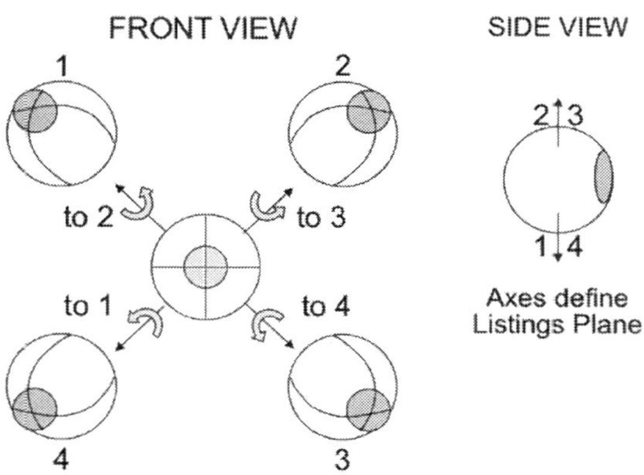

Figure 10.5 Definition of Listing's Law. Saccades reach eccentric eye positions 1, 2, 3 or 4, from the central primary position by rotating the eye about axes (indicated by the arrows) that lie in the plane of the page (viewed edge-on in the side view). The axes relative to primary position are used to describe 3D eye positions. In the depicted case, the final position vectors are parallel to the actual axes of rotation (velocities) of the preceding saccades.

(From Figure 1, Crawford & Vilis, 1995, adapted with permission, *Journal of Motor Behavior*.)

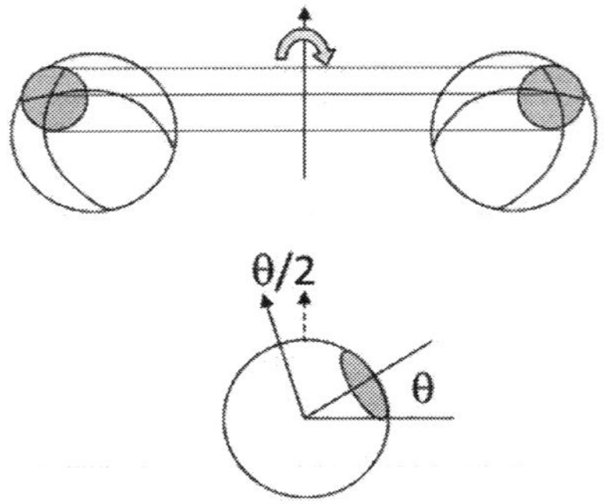

Figure 10.6 The half-angle rule when saccades are not toward or away from primary position. See text for details.

(From Figure 1, Crawford & Vilis, 1995, adapted with permission, *Journal of Motor Behavior*.)

in the correct direction but its 3D position is not in Listing's plane. The tilted axis gives the correct gaze direction and 3D orientation.

10.6 Space and its Geometries: Review and Preview

We conclude with a summary of the issues of space and attendant geometries (cf. Turvey, 2004), both those that have been noted so far and those that we should expect to encounter in forthcoming lectures.

1 Space is Euclidean, describable in terms of points, lines, etc. (e.g., Alhazen, Descartes, Malebranche).
2 Space as related to success of visually guided action, not abstract geometry (e.g., Berkeley).
3 Visible properties are not mathematical entities but signs for types of contact with the environment (e.g., Berkeley).
4 Space-for-agent, not space-as-is (e.g., Kant, Gibson, von Uexküll).
5 Geometry of space as a posteriori, not a priori (e.g., Lotze, Helmholtz, Riemann).
6 Spatial properties relative to transformations of space, degree of free mobility (e.g., Helmholtz, Klein).
7 Space as local and intrinsic, not global and extrinsic (e.g., Gauss, Einstein).
8 Space dependent on its constituents, not absolute and container-like (e.g., Riemann, Clifford, Einstein).
9 Geometric elements as referring to material facts, not idealizations (e.g., Pasch).
10 Spatial forms as irregular, fragmented not regular, connected (e.g., Mandelbrot).

11 Environment as a space of possibilities for action (not a static structure of objects and relations) (e.g., Gibson).

Notes

1 Lotze's formulation of this issue was anticipated in important respects by Steinbuch in 1811 (Rose, 1999).
2 Riemann's "profound suggestion" (Gray, 1989, p. 145) was that *the notion of position is basic to geometry* and that relations of position are expressible in terms of distance and direction. His contention was that all of classical geometry could be re-established on these basic notions and new geometries could be constructed to meet the needs of physics.
3 An apposite analogy is the physical structure of the magnetic or electrostatic field that depends on the distribution of magnetic poles or electric charges (Jammer, 1954/1993; Lecture 13).
4 According to Mach (1906, p. 9), "The space of the skin is the analogue of a two-dimensional, finite, unbounded and closed Riemannian space."
5 Sewn together one way might produce a sphere sewn together a different way might produce a donut shaped object, a torus. Although globally different, locally both objects would appear to be Euclidean planes.
6 When discussing the retinal local signs (see below), Helmholtz (1866/2000, p. 536) thought that it was not unlikely that "the resemblance between the local signs of adjacent points is greater than it is between those of points that are farther apart, and therefore that the nature of a local sign is a continuous function of the coordinates of the retinal point."
7 In two dimensions, topology is sometimes referred to as rubber sheet geometry. This is because topology is the study of properties of forms that are unchanged by stretching or twisting the plane on which they are drawn. The word topology derives from the Greek for "study of position."
8 These latter values are referred to as "Gaussian coordinates." As described below, Gauss proved in 1827 that the curvature of a surface at any point, defined extrinsically through principal curves, could be defined intrinsically in terms of "Gaussian coordinates."
9 We may wish to note that an intrinsic view of a surface would be the only one available to the Flatlanders we met in Lecture 8. A Spacelander, in contrast, would take an extrinsic perspective on the surface, either from above or from below.
10 In the context of describing the skin as a Riemann manifold, Mach (1906, p. 9) suggested that "Through the sensations induced by the movements of the various members of the body (notably, the arms, the hands, and the fingers) something analogous to a third dimension is superposed."
11 Intuitively, the notion of a geodesic is that if one were to walk along a straight line, each step taken must be parallel to the last.
12 The axioms of affine geometry are concerned with only two kinds of geometric objects, *points* and *lines*, and with only two kinds of relations, *between* (an order relation) and *on* (an incidence relation) (Gans, 1969).
13 Alhazen (see Lecture 4) was among the first to argue that dimensions of the body (foot size, arm length, eye height) might provide yardsticks for the implementation of congruence (see Sabra, 1989, p. 136).
14 Helmholtz did not follow Lotze in assuming that intensive patterns due to eye movements determined local signs. His assumption was that nerve-fiber differences

would suffice to explain differences in sensed retinal location (Boring, 1942). Helmholtz was generally ambiguous about whether local signs were acquired or innate.

15 Helmholtz (1886/2000, p. 44) defined the primary position of the line of fixation as that from which turning the eye to look straight up or down, or straight left or right, involved no rolling of the eye.

References

Berkeley, G. (1948). Essay towards a new theory of vision. In A. A. Luce & T. E. Jessop (Eds.), *The works of George Berkeley, Bishop of Cloyne*. London: Thomas Nelson (original work published 1709).

Boring, E. G. (1942). *Sensation and perception in the history of experimental psychology*. New York: Appleton-Century-Crofts.

Cassirer, E. (1950). *The problem of knowledge*. New Haven, CT: Yale University Press.

Crawford, J. D., & Vilis, T. (1995). How do motor systems deal with the problems of controlling three-dimensional rotations? *Journal of Motor Behavior*, *27*, 89–99.

Gans, D. (1969). *Transformations and geometries*. New York: Appleton-Century-Crofts.

Gauss, C. F. (1965). *General investigations of curved surfaces* (A. Hiltebeitel & J. Morehead, Trans.). Hewlett, NY: Raven Press (original work published 1827).

Gray, J. (1989). *Ideas of space: Euclidean, non-euclidean and relativistic*. Oxford, UK: Oxford University Press.

Helmholtz, von H. (1968). The facts of perception. In R. M. Warren & R. P. Warren (Eds.), *Helmholtz on perception: its physiology and development* (pp. 207–231). New York: Wiley (original work published 1879).

Helmholtz, von H. (1977a). On the origin and significance of the axioms of geometry. In R. S. Cohen & Y. Elkana (Eds.), *Herman von Helmholtz: Epistemological writings*. Boston, MA: Reidel (original work published 1868).

Helmholtz, von H. (1977b). On the facts underlying geometry. In R. S. Cohen & Y. Elkana (Eds.), *Herman von Helmholtz: Epistemological writings*. Boston, MA: Reidel (original work published 1868).

Helmholtz, von H. (2000). *Treatise on physiological optics, Vol. III* (J. P. C. Southall, Trans.). Bristol, UK: Thoemmes (original work published 1866).

James, W. (1983). *The principles of psychology*. Cambridge, UK: Cambridge University Press (original work published 1890).

Jammer, M. (1993). *Concepts of space: The history of theories of space in physics*. New York: Dover (original work published 1954).

Kant, I. (1998). *Critique of pure reason* (P. Guyer & A. Wood, Trans. and Ed.). Cambridge, UK: Cambridge University Press (original work published 1781/1787).

Koenderink, J. J. (1990). The brain a geometry engine. *Psychological Research*, 52, 122–127.

Lawrie, I. D. (1990). *A unified grand tour of theoretical physics*. Bristol, UK: Adam Hilger.

Lotze, H. (1852). Medicinische Psychologie, oder Physiologie der Seele. Leipzig, Germany: Weidmann'sche Buchhandlung.

Lotze, H. (1886). *Outlines of psychology* (G. Ladd, Trans.). Boston, MA: Ginn.

Mach, E. (1906). *Space and geometry*. LaSalle, IL: Open Court.

Pastore, N. (1971). *Selective history of theories of visual perception, 1650–1950*. Oxford, UK: Oxford University Press.

Riemann, B. (1953). Über die hypothesen, welche der geometrie zu grunde liegen. In H. Weber (Ed.), *Collected works of B. Riemann* (pp. 272–286). New York: Dover (original work published 1854).
Rose, D. (1999). The historical roots of the theories of local signs and labelled lines. *Perception, 28*, 675–685.
Sabra, A. I. (1989). Form in ibn al-Haytham's theory of vision. *Zeitschrift für Geschichte der Arabisch-Islamischen Wissenschaften*, 5, 115–140.
Singh, J. (2010). *Great ideas of modern mathematics*. New York: Dover (original work published 1959).
Synge, J. L. (1970). *Talking about relativity*. Amsterdam Netherlands: North-Holland.
Turvey, M. T. (2004). Space (and its perception): The first and final frontier. *Ecological Psychology, 16*, 25–29.
Weyl, H. (1952). *Space–time–matter*. New York Dover (original work published 1920).

Lecture 11

Doctrines of Sensations and Unconscious Inferences

Here we venture further into the circle of ideas that define Helmholtz's geometrical empiricism and give shape to his influential variant of the Cartesian Program. By way of preview, we can take note of how he chose to summarize his understanding of perception (Helmholtz, 1866/2000, Volume III):

> The general rule determining the ideas of vision . . . is that such objects are always imagined as being present in the field of vision as would have to be there in order to produce the same impression on the nervous mechanism, the eyes being used under ordinary normal conditions.
>
> (p. 2)

> The fundamental thesis of the empirical theory is: The sensations of the senses are tokens for our consciousness, it being left to our intelligence to learn how to comprehend their meaning.
>
> (p. 533)

> The psychic activities that lead us to infer that there in front of us at a certain place there is a certain object of a certain character, are generally not conscious activities, but unconscious ones. In their result, they are equivalent to a conclusion, to the extent that the observed action on our senses enables us to form an idea as to the possible cause of this action; although as a matter of fact, it is invariably the nervous stimulations that are perceived directly, that is, the actions, but never the external objects themselves.
>
> (p. 4)

In terms of the model of the man in the inner room—the Cartesian model—the first quotation defines the problem of perception as that of determining what conditions outside the house would normally give rise to the current mosaic of colors on the TV screen. Descartes had formulated the problem of perception as determining the primary qualities that were the outer physical causes of the current secondary qualities (see Lecture 6). In terms of the model, the second quotation recalls Berkeley's insistence that the TV images are merely signs that the man in the inner room comes to understand through the process of learning. These signs bear only a contingent, not necessary, relation to the things that they signify (see Figure 8.3). In terms of the model, the third quotation reiterates two principal Cartesian themes (see Lecture 6). First, perception involves an intellectual reasoning-like process with sensations as the premises. Second, awareness is directly of states of the sensory nerves and only indirectly of states of the world.

We learned in Lecture 6 that the 2nd grade of sense in Descartes' trialism, commonly referred to as sensation, is at the interface of matter and mind. For Descartes, sensation is a physical–mental hybrid.[1] The development of the technical notion of sensation in the 19th century and the role ascribed to it within the theory of how we know the world by sight reflect this peculiar status. Whereas investigations by physiologists and physiological psychologists focused primarily upon sensation's physical side, investigations by philosophers and philosophical psychologists focused primarily upon sensation's mental side. The *doctrine of sensations* that would become the bedrock of Helmholtz's perceptual theory is a hybrid of these distinct, yet conceptually linked, lines of inquiry.

Scientists of the 19th century took very seriously the following questions framed by the founding fathers of the mechanistic hypothesis (see Lecture 5). In the founders' language, the questions were: 'How does the first grade of sense work, that is, how are external physical motions transformed into internal physical motions of the sense organs, nerves, and brain?" "How do the physical motions of the sense organs, nerves, and brain produce the second grade of sense?" The discovery of receptors in the eye, skin, and ear provided an answer to the first question (let's call it the *doctrine of elemental receptors*). The discovery that a given kind of sensation depends strictly on the nerve excited not on how it was excited provided an answer to the second question (known historically as the *doctrine of specific nerve energies or qualities*). Our primary and immediate goal is to develop these two answers into the doctrine of sensations and, from that, Helmholtz's refinement of the Cartesian Program. One ancillary goal in this development will be that of recognizing the epistemological consequences of these two answers.

11.1 Doctrine of Elemental Receptors

The first answer gave rise to a new and more general version of the argument that the simulacrum (Lecture 4) under-specifies the environment. The properties of the environment perceived visually exceed in both number and kinds those given in the simulacrum. This argument, it will be recalled, became firmly established through the study of the retinal image and gave impetus to the indirect view of visual perception characterized in Figure 3.2. The properties that are not copied in the retinal image must be derived from or added to those that are copied in the retinal image. With the discovery of receptors, the argument could now be extended beyond vision to the other senses that lack anything analogous to the retinal image (Figure 11.1). The properties that receptors do not encode must be deduced or constructed from the properties that they do encode.

Following the form of the first question above, the science of the 19th century identified receptors as special nervous mechanisms, microscopic in size, which convert the external physical motions into internal physical motions. Consider sound. The external physical motion is a travelling wave that can be compactly described in terms of amplitude (the sound's intensity) and the rate at which the wave pattern repeats per second (the sound's frequency). Auditory receptors encode these descriptors. That is, they *transduce* these two aspects of the external physical motions of air particles into the internal physical motions—the electrical currents—of the auditory nerves.[2] The mental counterpart to the physical variable intensity is called "loudness" and the mental counterpart to the physical variable frequency is called "pitch." They compose the second grade of sense in the case of hearing. The thrid grade of sense in the case of hearing comprises infinitely many more kinds of mental counterparts—not in respect to acoustic energy, of course, but in respect to the infinitude of sound producing environmental events. As simple examples, the sounds produced by rubbing, scraping, rolling and brushing are readily distinguished (Gibson, 1966) and dogs, birds, doors and drums are quickly identified (Schubert, 1975). Patently, the achievements of the third grade of auditory sense go beyond the registrations of the receptors of the ear (the first grade of auditory sense) and the sensations they give rise to (the second grade of auditory sense).

A key strategic component of the doctrine of elemental receptors is conveyed by our auditory example. Receptors were discovered that transduced various forms of mechanical energy, chemical energy, and radiated energy, notably that in the photic and thermal frequency bands. In each case the advocated strategy was, as above, to take the descriptors of these energy forms

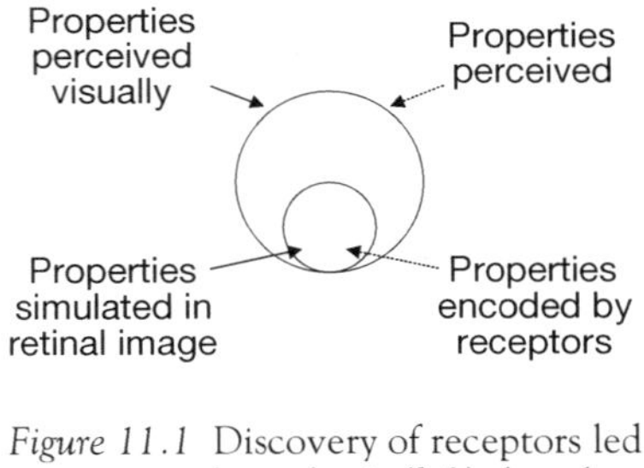

Figure 11.1 Discovery of receptors led to a generalization of the traditional hypothesis (*left*) that the properties given in stimulation are far fewer in number and kinds than the properties perceived.

provided by physics and chemistry as the properties predicated of the corresponding receptors. However, while the strategy could be implemented for audition and vision it could not be implemented for smell and taste and was implemented only approximately for touch. The problem was that the physical or chemical descriptors befitting the impressions of these senses were simply not known; the needed physical and chemical principles had not been discovered and might not even exist (Boring, 1942). Nonetheless, the guiding assumption remained firmly in place. For each sense, there would be only a few types of receptors and what they encoded would be the variables known to physics. The upshot, from the point of view of 19th-century epistemology was a substantial mismatch in type and number between the descriptors encoded by receptors (strictly, descriptors of energy) and the descriptors of environmental objects and events as perceived by an observer. Theorizing, therefore, had to be constrained by this apparent fact: A description of the environment that was not typically framed in terms of the ordinary variables of physical energy had to be derived from a description that *was* framed in such terms.

Because the number of variables that describe the relevant energy form restricts the receptor variety within a sense, the resultant set of receptor types takes on the status of "elements" or "atoms." Echoing Locke (Lecture 7), receptor responses as the physiological interpretation of simple ideas could be envisaged as composing all complex ideas through a kind of associative fusion. For example, if the sensory qualities of sweet, saline, bitter and sour referred elliptically to the elemental receptor responses of taste, as Vintschgau suggested in 1880 (Boring, 1942), then allowing just 10 distinct response levels for each receptor would yield 10,000 distinct four-element patterns. In principle, a very small number of elemental receptor types together with a mechanism capable of associating their responses could produce a multitude of complex (compound) ideas. That the number of receptor types would always be small was countered, however, by Helmholtz's analysis of the auditory sense. Much to the dismay of some of his peers who presumed an underlying parsimony of elements (Boring, 1942), he advanced a successful theory of audition on the grounds that receptor types existed for each audible frequency. That is, the auditory receptor types numbered in the thousands.

In Helmholtz's view of things, the receptors, regardless of the number of kinds, obeyed a *law of isolated conduction* (Figure 11.2). The nerve fiber from each receptor extended to the brain in isolation so as to conduct to the brain precisely the impression it receives (Helmholtz, 1868/1968). With other things being equal, therefore, there would be a fixed or constant relation between excitation on the retina and excitation in the brain. Isolated retinal excitations would be isolated brain excitations. For these isolated receptor responses to go together (as in producing, for example, the taste of chocolate from particular values of the excitation levels of the sweet, saline, bitter and sour "receptors") it would be necessary for associative connections to be formed among them

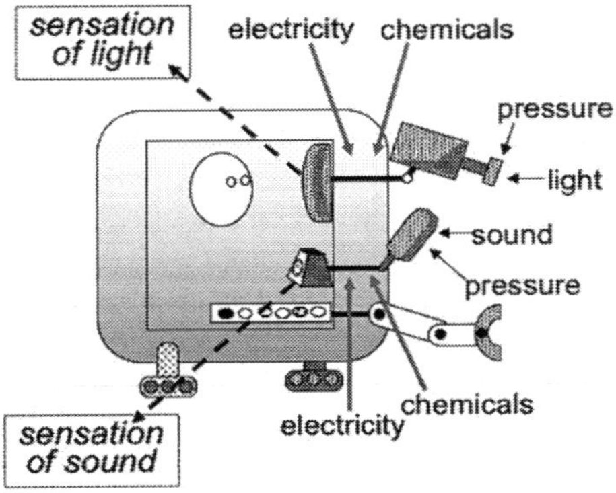

Figure 11.2 Doctrine of specific nerve energies. Whether excited by light, pressure, chemicals or electricity, the first grade of visual sense gives rise to the same kind of second grade of visual sense—namely, a sensation of light. Similarly, whether excited by sound, pressure, etc., the first grade of auditory sense gives rise to the same kind of second grade of auditory sense, namely, a sensation of sound.

(From Figure 1 in Turvey, 2004, adapted with permission, *Ecological Psychology*.)

in the brain. Returning to the man-in-the-inner-room model, the law of isolated conduction means that the image on the TV screen, like that at the camera eye, is a mosaic of independent pixels. Consequently, any departure from the *constancy hypothesis*, that is, any interdependency or organization evident among the pixels of the TV image, was evidence of an extra-sensory process. Helmholtz assumed it was associative learning.

11.2 The Doctrine of Specific Nerve Energies

The answer to the second question of the founders of the mechanical hypothesis is characterized in Figure 11.3. It was formulated by Johannes Müller in 1826 (Boring, 1942) and discussed in detail by Helmholtz (1868/1968, 1866/2000).[3] No matter how a given sensory nerve is excited, the resultant sensation is the same; and when the same kind of excitation is applied to different sensory nerves, the resultant sensation is different. In respect to the origin of sensation, it is the nerve rather than the stimulus exciting the nerve that matters. It should be underscored, however, that this doctrine of specific nerve energies is a far-from-complete answer to the question of the mechanical genesis of the 2nd grade of sense. It does not explain how a sensation comes to have the quality that it has (Humphrey, 1992/1999). What is lacking is an account of how the qualitative character of the sensation of blue, for example, follows systematically from the neural activity in the optic nerve and visual cortex. Modern philosophers refer to the *explanatory gap* (e.g., Levine, 1983)—the

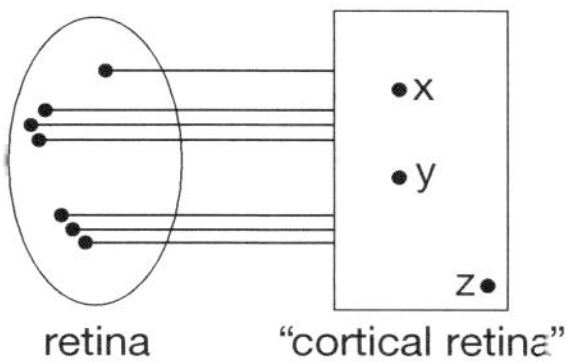

Figure 11.3 The law of isolated conduction (the constancy hypothesis).

inability to explain the *qualitative* distinctiveness of a sensation in terms of the quantifiable physical properties of nerves.

11.2.1 Relational Properties and Kantian Metaphysics

Helmholtz interpreted the doctrine of specific nerve energies as a way to return to Kant's metaphysics, but this time through physiology and psychology rather than mathematics and mathematical physics (Cassirer, 1950). Looked at from the perspective of the doctrine, Helmholtz (1868/1968) saw Kant's theory of a priori forms of intuition in a positive light. It was, he said "a very fortunate and clear expression of the state of affairs" (p. 238).

The doctrine of specific nerve fibers, Helmholtz (1866/2000, Volume III) argued, was in a certain sense "the empirical fulfillment of Kant's theoretical concept of the nature of human reason" (p. 20)

Kant's plea for principled constraints on what can be known seemed to be answered by the discovery of specific nerve energies. The senses mediate our contact with the world, but as physical devices they have physical modes of operation such that how the world appears to us is not how the world is. Helmholtz wished to make very clear that there is no scientific anomaly here (1866/2000, pp. 20–22; 1868/1968, pp. 101–102). At issue is the understanding of what is meant by a property that an object is said to have. From the practical perspective of experimental science, the property of any one thing A, he argues, is the *effect* that it exerts on another thing *B*. The properties said to characterize A are not, in fact, possessed by A. Rather, they are possessed by A in relation to *B*. Often, when remarking on A's properties, *B* is implicitly understood and not explicitly mentioned. This is particularly the case in respect to secondary qualities—for example, where A is light, *B* is the visual sensory system, and *color* is the property of A. As observed in Lecture 5, a relational or mutual property of A may or may not depend causally on *B*. Helmholtz's concern is with the causal cases (e.g., force on a body, solubility of lead in nitric acid, color of light) and the observation that those causal cases involving the senses are not inherently different on formal grounds from those involving inanimate objects. To pose questions such as "Is vermilion really red or an illusion of the visual sense?" is nonsensical. "Red" is the mutual or relational property given in the juxtaposition of light and normally formed eyes. The color-as-illusion move supposes that there are properties of light that belong to light absolutely, independent of all other things—a supposition that Helmholtz (1868/1968, p. 102) regards as "a contradiction in itself."

11.2.2 Elaborating the Doctrine: Nerve Fibers and Signs

Müller's original doctrine was restricted to nerve trunks (e.g., optic, auditory) and modes of sensation. Helmholtz's extension included the nerve fibers within a nerve trunk and, thereby, the qualities of sensation within a mode. Thus, within the optic nerve, Helmholtz posited three visual specific energies, one for each of the primary colors as implied by the color theory proposed by Thomas Young in 1811 (Boring, 1942). (It was this extension of the doctrine to the fibers of the optic nerve that we exploited earlier in our discussion of deriving multiple compound ideas from a few receptor responses.) The general principle was that, given a sensation, there must be a part of the anatomy to which it is specific.[4] Indeed, the Müller–Helmholtz doctrine was presented as a potential Rosetta stone for comprehending key perception capabilities of the nervous system: Units of function correspond to units of anatomy or compounds of units of anatomy.

The doctrine of specific nerve fiber energies was the 19th century's upgrade of Descartes' 17th-century doctrine of corporeal ideas (Lecture 6; Reed, 1982). As Descartes had proposed, and as expressed in the man-in-the-inner-room model, we have direct awareness only of the states of the body, specifically the sensory nerves. The third quotation at the beginning of this lecture indicates that Helmholtz was of the same opinion.[5] Descartes proposed further that because the states of the nerves are "mechanical motions" they were more properly conceived as symbols, signs, or tokens rather than as images or copies. On this latter point, Helmholtz (1866/2000, Volume III) was also in firm agreement, summarizing his own arguments on sensations thusly: "[S]ensations have been described as being simply *symbols* for the relations in the external world. They have been denied every kind of similarity or equivalence to the things they denote" (p. 18).

There is a pragmatic flavor to Helmholtz's perspective on sensations as signs or symbols that recalls the position taken by Berkeley in the *New Theory* (see Lecture 8). They become, through learning, the means by which movements and actions are regulated (Helmholtz, 1866/2000, Volume III): "Having learned correctly how to read those symbols, we are enabled by their help to adjust our actions so as to bring about the desired result" (p. 19).

In pressing this point, Helmholtz adheres to the criterion of workability identified in Lecture 7 (Section 3). The question of whether sensations and their derivatives correspond to real things, whether they are true or false, is nonsensical. Sensations and the ideas they compose have no truth apart from their practical use.

11.2.3 Do Perception and the Qualities of Sense Serve Different and Independent Purposes? Reid's Alternative Possibility

The Müller–Helmholtz doctrine that the same sensation follows from very different causes, most of them unrelated to the properties of external visible objects, would seem to worsen the paradox and epistemological puzzles discussed in Lecture 7 (Section 6). The first grade of sense cannot be a source of epistemologically sound (that is, unquestionable) premises for the subsequent judgmental processes of the third grade of sense. Helmholtz (1868/1968) put it sternly: "[W]e must never forget . . . that there is no exclusive relation between the sensation of light and light itself" (p. 86).

In brusque terms, the Müller–Helmholtz doctrine is at odds with the empiricist stance on the senses. Whereas it suggested that the senses are mere conveyers of sensory qualities, empiricism of the 17th and 18th century assigned the senses a much loftier role: sources of knowledge about the world. We can turn to the 18th-century philosopher Thomas Reid for potential resolution. Reid drew the distinction between sensation and perception[6] in these terms:

> [S]ensation . . . appears to be something which can have no existence but in a sentient mind, no distinction from the act of the mind by which it is felt. Perception . . . hath always an object distinct from the act by which it is perceived; an object which may exist whether it be perceived or not.
> (Reid, 1764/1997, p. 168)

The conception and belief which nature produces by means of the senses, we call perception. The feeling which goes along with the perception, we call sensation. The perception and its corresponding sensation are produced at the same time. In our experience we never find them disjoined (Reid, 1785/1969, p. 16).

The senses, he argued, do double duty. They make us feel and they make us perceive. They serve different purposes. Sensation answers the question, "What is happening in here, to me?" and perception answers the question, "What is happening out there, to the world?" (Humphrey, 1992/1999). According to the philosophy and physiology that spawned the man-in-the-inner-room model, perceiving is predicated on what is felt—that is, the answer to the question about "out there" must be derived from the answer to the question about "in here." Thomas Reid (1764/1997) considered nature's options in this matter and recognized that there was an alternative possibility. The two answers could have been independent: "The perceptions we have, might have been immediately connected with the impressions upon our organs, without any intervention of sensations" (p. 176).

Although he did not subscribe to this option of sensationless perception in his larger scheme, he did allow perception and sensation as co-occurring, different, and non-overlapping experiences (Figure 11.4). In smelling a rose, the experience of being stimulated by a most agreeable smell accompanies the experience that the object I am sniffing, a rose, possesses a pleasant scent (Reid, 1785/1969, p. 17; see Humphrey, 1992/1999). A parallelism of sensation and perception, indexing different meanings of stimulation, is implied by the second of the above quotations from Reid. Despite this momentary flirtation with parallelism, Reid adhered closely to the classical serial notion that he regarded as acutely problematic. He interpreted the empiricists' understanding that sensations bear no resemblance to external objects to mean that drawing inferences about external objects from sensations is impossible. There are no discoverable connections, he argued, between sensations and the properties of objects that would justify the use of inference. For Reid (1764/1997, p. 174), therefore, turning sensations into perceptions can involve no intellectual act (no reasoning, no calculating and no inferring). He would argue for a providential naturalism: Sensation's immediate metamorphosis into perception is by way of the (God-given) natural constitution of the senses.

Reid's alternative possibility warrants more attention for it bears upon the issue of indirect versus direct perception of Lecture 3. Gibson (1966) hypothesized two centuries later that realizing the alternative, and dissolving the opposition between the Müller–Helmholtz doctrine and the empiricist's view of the senses, might depend on the viability of two key distinctions. One distinction is between the *energy of stimulation* and the *order in stimulation* (roughly, the sequential order of changes in energy and the adjacent order of relations of energy). The other distinction is between the *sensitivity of a passive receptor* and the *sensitivity of an active perceptual organ* (roughly, a collective of very many receptors that is mobile, like the eye or the hand). In Gibson's (1966) formulation of Reid's alternative possibility, sensation is evoked by "stimulus energy"—the description of stimulation at the level of passive

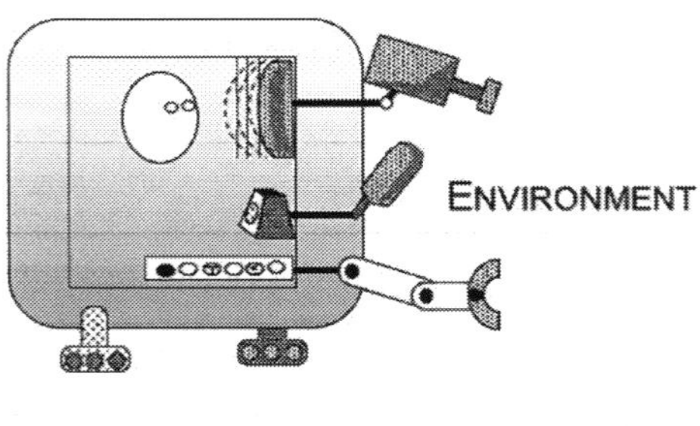

Figure 11.4 A crude attempt to capture Thomas Reid's conjecture within the man-in-the-inner-room model. The man has simultaneously and independently the third grade of sense of the world (communicated by the curves) and the second grade of sense of the states of the transmitters (communicated by the vertical lines).

(From Figure 1 in Turvey, 2004, adapted with permission, *Ecological Psychology*.)

receptors—and perception is evoked by "stimulus order"—the description of stimulation at the level of active perceptual organs. In these terms, sensation is not the basis of perception, and sensation may co-occur with perception or it may not. Further, whereas the cause of a single receptor's excitatory state may not get past the receptor, the cause of an active perceptual organ's excitatory state may get past the organ (Gibson, 1966)—that is, the Müller–Helmholtz doctrine need not be an insurmountable epistemological problem.

The idea of an active perceptual organ is not alien to Helmholtz's thinking. First, as we saw in Lecture 10, he recognized that, in both geometry and perception, constraints on mobility had non-trivial consequences for measurement. Second, he was of the opinion that without free mobility of the sensory organs perceptual judgments would be forever uncertain (Helmholtz, 1866/2000, Volume III):

> It is only by voluntarily bringing our organs of sense in various relations to the object that we learn to be sure as to our judgments of the causes of our sensations . . . If the objects had simply been passed in review before our eyes by some foreign force without being able to do anything about them, probably we should never have found our way about amid such an optical phantasmagoria.
>
> (pp. 30–31)

In extending these ideas, Helmholtz observed that when objects are explored visually or manually, it becomes evident that some sense-impressions vary with our voluntary movements while others vary independently of them. These changes in the sense-impressions that we are unable to alter by free mobility, that are invariant over our willed exploratory movements, depend on the nature of the object. The implication is that the idea of an active perceptual system capable of detecting different orders of stimulation may also not be alien to Helmholtz's thinking.

11.3 The Doctrines of Sensations and Unconscious Inference

It became standard practice in the 19th century to link the philosophers' notion of sensation to the output of receptors in either one of two ways. Sensations could be mental experiences, elemental and conscious, that result from receptor responses. Alternatively, and more simply, sensations could be identified with the receptor responses. In this alternative, the elemental character of sensations is retained free of reference to conscious states. In either case, the philosophical concept of sensation was amplified by the doctrines of elemental receptors and specific nerve energies. Here is the resultant inventory of properties. Sensations are:

1 punctate (discrete, pointillistic);
2 momentary (transient, ephemeral);
3 integrable (association-able, combinable);
4 immutable (uneducable, non-pliable);
5 irreducible;
6 anatomically specific;
7 mental correlates of energy variables;
8 signs (meaningless, non-significant);
9 private;
10 necessary occasions of perception.

Collectively, these properties constitute the doctrine of sensations. Properties 1–5 define the elemental nature of sensations. Property 6 identifies the physical basis of sensations in the anatomy. Properties 7–10 express the mental aspect of sensations.

Sensations are adjudged to be *punctate* for a variety of reasons, historical and technical. We can consider a small sample. Alhazen had suggested that sensations begin with the "sensory point-forms" defined, approximately, by the Euclidean points on the eye that coincide with Euclidean ray lines from the distal object (Sabra, 1989; see Lecture 4, Figure 4.1). Berkeley (1709/1948) had identified a smallest discernible expanse of color that he referred to as the "minimum visible." Any percept of visual extent was composed of these color-sensation atoms. Sensation as *punctate* was tied to sensation as *irreducible* in conformity with Euclid's definition of a point as "that which has no parts." Notions such as those of Alhazen and Berkeley set the stage for, and were reinforced by, the microscope-aided discovery of receptors—anatomical points potentially coordinate with geometric points and sensation points. The law of isolated conduction and its close ally, the constancy hypothesis, ensured that this punctate-ness of receptor responses was maintained from the periphery to central anatomical sites. For the central mechanisms that implement the third grade of sense, a major challenge, therefore, would be composing a unified percept of spatial extent from discrete sensations. How, otherwise, would many point sensations of green be seen as that "green patch over there"? Sensations must be *integrable*. A mechanism that integrates point sensations with their different local signs is implied.

Prior to the development of 19th century physiology, the *momentary* property of sensations was suggested by experience: Sensations are tied to instants. As the eyes flit over an object, the sensations of a prior view are replaced immediately (it seems) by the sensations of a current view. This vague intuition of sensations as momentary was made concrete by the discovery that the response of an electrically stimulated receptor is transient. With a persisting stimulus, a response generated at stimulus onset declines within a fraction of a second to its pre-stimulus level. A stimulus moving across a receptor surface (retina, skin) would generate a sequence of momentary responses at adjacent receptor locations. Given the law of isolated conduction, a major challenge for central mechanisms would be composing a unified percept of motion from momentary sensations. A mechanism that integrates over instants of excitation is implied.[7] If the case in question were a receptor translated across an environmental surface, then the challenge would be composing a unified percept of spatial extent from a sequence of momentary sensations. The latter case makes clear that the process of integration must bring each momentary sensation forward into the present so that perception in the present is possible (Gibson, 1979/1986, p. 221). Most importantly, it makes clear that *integration ensures satisfaction of the principle of local causality or local action* (Lecture 4). Because of integration a past sensation becomes part of a simultaneous whole that is causal *now*. Without integration, a sensation no longer present would have to be causal *now*, in violation of the principle.

The interpretation of sensations as irreducible points and irreducible instants forecloses on the possibility that the first and second grades of sense are changeable by learning. If a sensation has no internal structure, then it has no room for change—it is *immutable*. For it to change in its entirety, to become some other sensation, its *anatomical specificity* would have to undergo a radical change: Its anatomical base, its receptor type and specific nerve, would have to become receptive to different energy variables. The immutable feature of sensations, therefore, restricts learning-to-perceive to the third grade of sense. Either one learns to reason differently about the sensations (the rationalist's interpretation) or one learns to connect them in ways dictated by experienced contingencies (the empiricist's interpretation). In Helmholtz's variant of the Cartesian Program, both kinds of learning were assumed.

In Figure 11.5 are diagramed the main features of Helmholtz's proposal on the nature of perception (Hochberg, 1974). The doctrine of sensations allowed Helmholtz to address immediately the challenge of the infinitude of differences among objects and scenes. It provided a particulate system very familiar to the modern-day chemist, elementary particle physicist, geneticist and linguist. Given a finite number of atom-like particulars and a finite means of combining them, an infinite number of differences are possible. The focus in Figure 11.5 is on the means by which the infinitely many object sizes are perceptible. A distal object S_1 is represented on the TV screen in the inner room as the sensations s_a*, s_b* and s_c*. These sensations (color points or pixels) have been produced by the responses $R(s_1)$ of the specific nerve fibers to the proximal retinal stimuli, s_a, s_b, and s_c. They are the *private* and *necessary occasions for perception*. Because of eye movements and reaching movements made in relation to adjacent proximal stimuli in the past, the visual sensations s_a*, s_b* and s_c* are richly connected in memory with kinesthetic sensations. Together, the visual sensations and their associated memories yield a unified percept of the object's extensity as projected on the retina—the retinal-size percept S_1*.

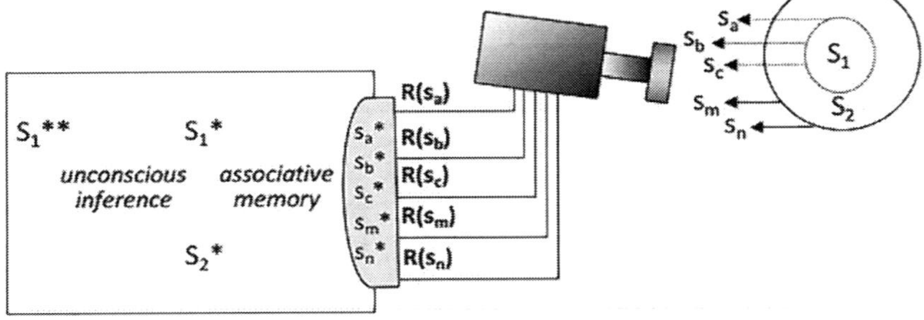

Figure 11.5 A truncated version of the man in the inner room expresses Helmholtz's variant of the Cartesian Program. See text for details.

The distal object S_1 in Figure 11.5 is surrounded by many other distal stimuli. In the figure those distal stimuli most relevant to the problem at hand are identified by S_2. These are distal stimuli that have to do with the object's distance. The sequence of processes beginning with the corresponding proximal stimuli (s_m and s_n), proceeding via the specific nerve energies to sensations (s_m*, s_n*) and kinesthetic memories (established through movements such as walking, reaching, accommodating and converging), yields the apparent-distance percept, S_2*.

Helmholtz's proposal for how these preliminary size and distance percepts are achieved follows closely the empiricism of Berkeley (Lecture 8). Helmholtz, however, departed from Berkeley in presuming a necessary linkage between size and distance. Consonant with Descartes and Malebranche he proposed that an inference from the perceived retinal size S_1* about the actual object size S_1 could be made by taking S_2* into account. The basis of the inference is the necessary Euclidean truth that in order for a distal object to produce an extent on the retina of a particular size I (more correctly, subtend a particular visual angle θ), object size must increase with object distance, $S_1 = I \times S_2$ or $S_1/S_2 = I$. Given that the processes in the inner room can only be conducted in strictly mental (not physical) terms, the inferred size S_1** is the product of $S_1^* \times S_2^*$. The implementation of this calculation, Helmholtz suggested, occurs outside of consciousness. When generalized, this is Helmholtz's *doctrine of unconscious inference*—the doctrine that we encountered in the third quotation of the present lecture. In the general case, unconscious inferences produce spatial percepts from non-spatial sensations. These unconscious inferences are irresistible and irreversible. In illusions, such as the Ponzo illusion of Figure 8.3, the perceiver makes the normal inference in abnormal conditions resulting in a false conclusion, the illusory appearance. This occurs even when it is the case that the perceiver knows that the conditions are abnormal and that the conclusion is false. The unconscious inference is immune to conscious reasoning.

11.4 The Invisibility of Light and its Implications

According to the doctrine of sensations, an animal in an illuminated environment is directly in contact with the illumination (light) and indirectly in contact with that which is illuminated (the surrounding environment). It is understood that retinal receptors are excited by light and give rise to sensations of light. And it is further understood that these sensations of light are the necessary occasions for the visual perception of the environment that the light illuminates. This fundamental tenet of the doctrine can be tested.

What is required for the test is an experimental arrangement in which light can be encountered as such by itself, that is, light when it is not illuminating[8] any surfaces (Zajonc, 1993; Figure 11.6). The arrangement involves a carefully constructed box (black rightward part of Figure 11.6) into which light is beamed by a powerful projector (white leftward part of Figure 11.6). The construction ensures that none of this light that fills the box is reflected light. There is illumination in the absence of things illuminated. In this situation, what the person experiences when looking into the box, and therefore at the light, is darkness (Zajonc, 1993). A handle attached to the box permits one to introduce an object (a wand) into the box's interior—and to retract it, providing thereby a necessary contrast. The introduction of the object results in a visual experience. The object is seen, strongly lit on one side. With the object's retraction, the experience of absolute darkness is restored. The experience is that of an astronaut in space walk with the spacecraft, earth, and moon out of view. Although the sun's light is present everywhere, it falls on nothing, and nothing is seen. The astronaut experiences absolute darkness (Zajonc, 1993, p. 3). Reflecting surfaces are necessary for the phenomenon we call vision.

The light-in-a-box demonstration and the astronaut's experience invite a question that must, at this point, be seen as a question long waiting to be

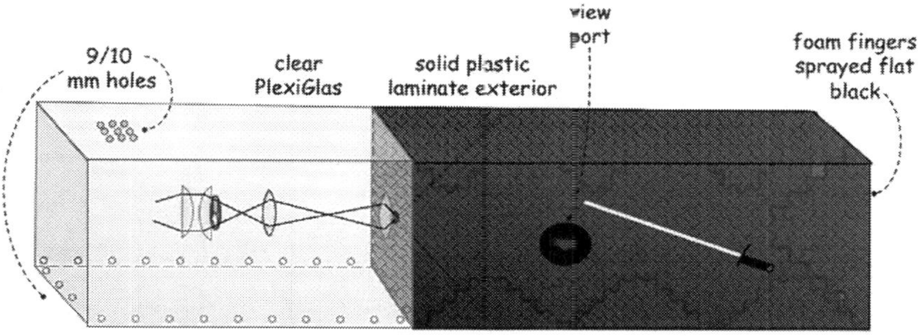

Figure 11.6 Demonstrating the invisibility of light. See text for details. The image interceptor rod can be entered into the box by a small entry port such as that adjacent to the depicted view port.

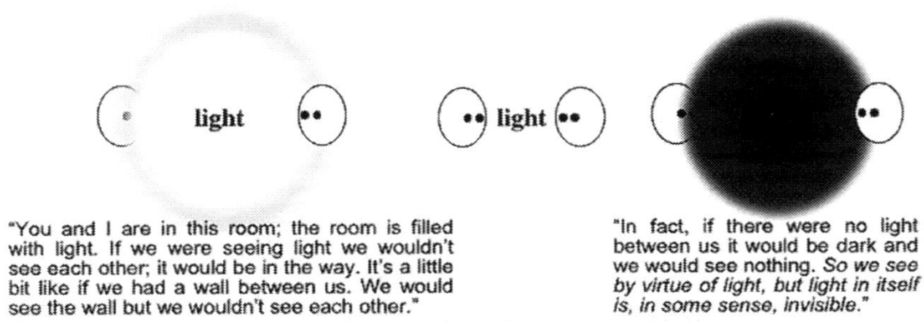

Figure 11.7 Do we ever see light as such? (Quotations, A. Zajonc, personal communication.)

asked: *What would be the case if light were visible?* In a transparent medium, all separations between an observer and surrounding environmental surfaces would be densely filled with light. If light was visible, then the observer would see light, not surrounding surfaces. The observer's surroundings would be occluded as if by a wall that has no beginning or end (Figure 11.7). The fact of light's invisibility and its implications were previewed by Gibson (1979/1986):[9]

> The only way we see illumination, I believe, is by the way of that which is illuminated, the surface on which the beam falls, the cloud, or the particles that are lighted. We do not see the light that is in the air, or that fills the air. If all this is correct, it becomes quite reasonable to assert that all we ever see is the environment or facts about the environment, never photons or waves or radiant energy.
>
> If light in the exact sense of the term is never seen as such, it follows that seeing the environment cannot be *based on* seeing light as such. The stimulation of the receptors in the retina cannot be seen, paradoxical as this may sound. The supposed sensations resulting from this stimulation are not the data for perception.
>
> (p. 55)[10]

A distinction is needed between the physics of light—illumination, which is not seen—and the ecology of light—the illuminated environment, which is seen. Three ecological factors affecting the structure of light ambient to a point of observation can be identified: (a) different *facing* of different surfaces, large or small (*layout-structuring*), (b) different *whiteness* of reflecting surfaces, large or small (*pigment-structuring*),[11] and (c) different illuminatedness (differential shadowing) of different parts of a surface (*illuminatedness-structuring*) (Gibson, 1966, p. 214). In each case, the possibility can be entertained that the ambient light structure is specific to the source of its structure (Gibson, 1966, 1979/1986), that is for each ecological factor there is informationL (Lecture 3). Intuitively, obtaining informationL for any one source co-occurs with obtaining informationL for the other two.

11.5 The Seeing of Things as Black, Gray or White

It may come as a surprise to know that the most prominent aspect of everyday visual experience—the lightness or perceived reflectance of the surroundings—is yet to be explained. In the bluntest of terms, science has yet to explain why some surfaces appear black and others appear white (Gilchrist, 2006). The challenge is more than you might have expected: "The seeing of things as black, gray, or white is not at all a simple matter . . . seems likely that they are features of the world on the same level as geometrical space and the fact of sunlight" (Gibson, 1966, p. 215).

In conventional physical terms, the reflectance R is the proportion of incident light E (the intensity of illumination or radiant energy) that a surface reflects L (the luminance or physical amount of light at the viewpoint). That is, R = L/E. As Gilchrist (2006) emphasizes, an explanation of lightness is thwarted by the fact that R varies by a factor of no more than 30 whereas E can vary by a factor of 100 million—that is, there is no correlation between R and E. Black paper in high E (e.g., bright sunlight) and white paper in low E (e.g., shadow) can yield the same R but still be seen as black and white, respectively.

In accord with our subheading, we will limit our introduction to the enigma that is lightness to neutral or achromatic (colorless) surfaces, those that reflect the same percentage of light at all wavelengths.[12] Blackness or black is the quality or state of the achromatic color of least lightness (bearing the least resemblance to white). Whiteness or white is the quality or state of the achromatic color of greatest lightness (bearing the least resemblance to black). Grayness or gray is a neutral achromatic color midway between black and white.

Gelb introduced science to the enigma that is lightness in 1929 (see Gilchrist, 2006). A viewed black surface that appears light under illumination (by a lamp) will appear dark when a similarly black surface adjacent to it is also illuminated (by a lamp) so as to appear light. A stepwise variant of Gelb's original experiment, introduced by Cataliotti and Gilchrist (1995), is schematized and summarized in Figure 11.8. In this staircase Gelb effect, a black surface in a spotlight appears white and becomes darker as four lighter shades of gray are added within the spotlight.[13] Each new square is seen as white until the next square is added[14] (an effect that is relatively indifferent to the viewer's distance from the array of surfaces). The amount of darkening depends only on the amount by which each new square increased the maximum luminance of the group of squares. It does not depend on spatial proximity to the black square. The implication is that lightness value is tied to the highest luminance.

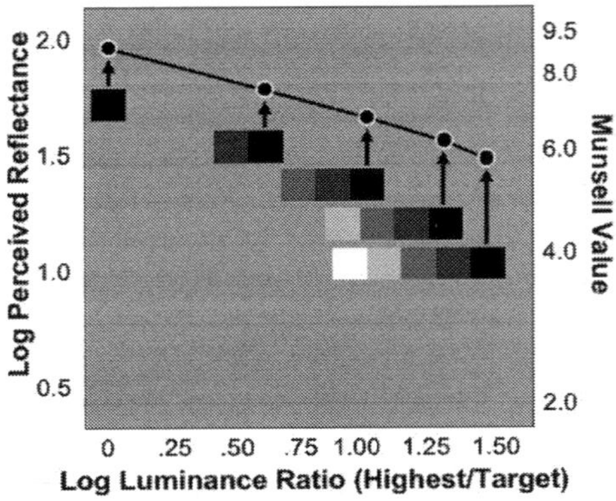

Figure 11.8 Perceived lightness of a black square in a spotlight as squares of higher lightness are added (see text for details).

(Adapted from Figure 11.5 in A. Gilchrist, 2006, *Seeing black and white*. By permission of Oxford University Press, USA.)

There is an additional feature, however: The assignment of lightness values to the squares is compressed; they are far smaller than actual values. The perceivers in Cataliotti and Gilchrist's experiment erred in the sense that perceived R did not abide R = L/E. As depicted in Figure 11.9, one can hypothesize that the error arises from the fact that two distinct reference

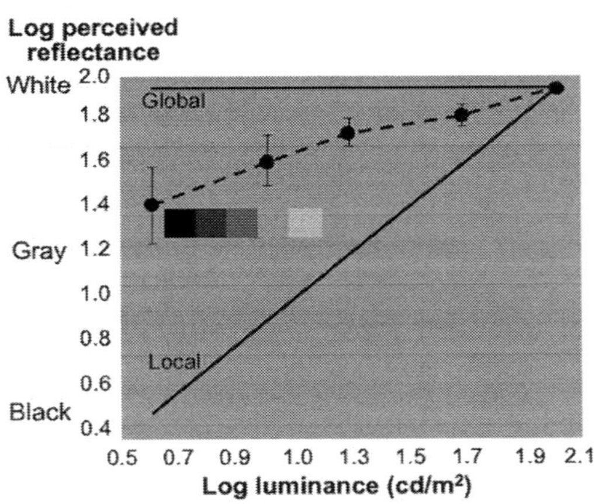

Figure 11.9 Gelb's co-determination phenomenon as an example of impredicativity in visual perception. x-axis is luminance values; y-axis is predicted lightness values.

(From Figure 7, Gilchrist et al., *Psychological Review, 106*, 795–834, 1999, APA, adapted with permission.)

frames are involved, one local (the adjacent squares) and one global (the visible parts of the laboratory). Perceived R is compromised by their conjunction.

The wrongness of perceived R is asserted on grounds of not satisfying the conventional physical definition of R. Such errors in respect to R in experiments of the preceding kind are seemingly common and systematic suggesting that the manner in which they pattern has the potential to reveal the means by which R is determined, say, computationally (Gilchrist, 2006, p. 267). The need to invoke two reference frames suggests, however, that the error at play is not on the side of the human observer but on the side of scientific definition: At the ecological scale, R is an impredicative concept. Reflectance of any given surface is a property definable only in terms of the whole arrangement of surfaces to which it belongs (Lecture 3), as the following quotation contends.

> [F]rom an ecological point of view, the color of a surface is relative to the colors of adjacent surfaces; it is not an absolute color. Its reflectance ratio is specified only in relation to other reflectance ratios of the layout. . . . The colors are not seen separately, as stimuli, but together, as an arrangement.
>
> (Gibson, 1979, p. 91)

Kardos seems to have anticipated such a view 44 years earlier in his conception of co-determination. On this conception, lightness perception of each square in Figure 11.8 is determined by the lightness of its neighboring squares and of the environment (e.g., the laboratory) that encompasses them (see Gilchrist, 2006, p. 309). Related observations go a step further: In displays of a target patch embedded in a context, accounting for the perception of target lightness requires that the target itself be included in the lightness description of the target's visual context (Allred, Radonjić, Gilchrist & Brainard, 2012). Impredicativity is implied.

Notes

1 Bertrand Russell (1921/1997, p. 144) concurred: "Sensations are what is common to the mental and physical worlds; they may be defined at the intersection of mind and matter."

2 The concept of electricity as motion was in place at the start of the 19th century (Segré, 1984). The phenomena of electrostatics were well documented by 1770 and Coulomb had proposed the "inverse square law" in 1788. Galvani published his discovery of electrically induced muscular contractions in dissected frogs in 1791 and by 1801 Volta inspired by Galvani's discovery was able to produce a continuous electric current by combining different kinds of conductors.

3 Hobbes (1651/1968, Book 1, Chapter 1) anticipated their efforts to explain sensory qualities in terms of physical motions that could be produced by diverse causes.

4 Müller suggested that this specificity lies either in the body of the nerve or in the location in the brain where the nerve ends (Boring, 1942). As implied by Figure 11.2, the evidence indicated that sensation arose from stimulation beyond the receptors, so the locus of anatomical specificity could not be in the periphery. Helmholtz (1868/1968, pp. 83–85) was inclined to the terminus view. He drew an analogy with the telegraph system. The same copper wires conveying the same kind of electrical motion produce different results as a function of the apparatus to which they are connected at the terminal station (e.g., ringing a bell, moving a railway signal, setting a recording device to work).

5 Not surprisingly, Müller (1843, p. 707) held the same position: "The immediate objects of the perception of our senses are merely particular states induced in the nerves and felt as sensations."

6 It is this distinction for which Thomas Reid is best known in the history of philosophy and psychology (Boring, 1950; Pastore, 1971).

7 The doctrine of sensations, with its irreducible points and instants, impressed upon the general investigation of knowing about the world by sight an enduring notion: visual perception necessarily entails integration over space and time. Although the historical tendency is to interpret the terms points and instants to mean "without size" or "infinitesimally small," such interpretations are not necessary (Huntington, 1913; Koenderink, 1990). For the practical purposes of analyses, a point and an instant refer, respectively, to a spatial entity and a durable event with an internal structure, internal *df*, that the scientist chooses simply to ignore. Later theories that abide the notion of integration over space and time do so with points and instants that are defined in this more general, operational sense. For example, a point can be a retinal image and an instant can be the duration of the iconic memory of a retinal fixation (Neisser, 1967).

8 Illuminance is the total luminous flux (intensity of light) incident on a surface per unit area. It is a measure of how much the incident light illuminates the surface in lux or lumens per square meter (candelera $\times$ steradian $\times$ $1/m^2$). Gibson (1979/1986, p. 307) defines illumination in these terms: the steady state of reverberating radiant energy such that light is *ambient* at all points in the medium.

9 One of Gibson's so-called "purple perils" written in May 1971 asked: "Do we ever see light?"

10 We will recognize Gibson's quotation as the conjecture of Thomas Reid (Figure 11.4 and note 6, above).

11 Pigment is a substance that gives color to something else. For example, chlorophyll and melanin are substances that produce a characteristic color in the tissues of plants and animals, respectively.

12 Gilchrist (2006, p. 9) suggests that all the important perceptual problems are to be found in the achromatic domain including the fundamental problem of perceptual constancy.

13 Some details are needed. The illumination of the laboratory was adjusted so that a black test-square in the projector beam was adjudged to be completely identical to a true white test-square located just outside the projector beam. Lightness judgments were in respect to selecting a match from a separately illuminated Munsell chart of 16 samples. To accommodate the five squares the projector beam formed a rectangle aligned horizontally.

14 The five data sets in Figure 11.8 were obtained from five different groups of 10 participants.

References

Allred, S. R., Radonjić, A., Gilchrist, A. L., & Brainard, D. H. (2012). Lightness perception in high dynamic range images: Local and remote luminance effects. *Journal of Vision, 12*, 7,1–16.

Berkeley, G. (1948). Essay towards a new theory of vision. In A. A. Luce & T. E. Jessop (Eds.), *The works of George Berkeley, Bishop of Cloyne*. London: Thomas Nelson (original work published 1709).

Boring, E. G. (1942). *Sensation and perception in the history of experimental psychology*. New York: Appleton-Century-Crofts.

Boring, E. G. (1950). *A history of experimental psychology*. New York: Appleton-Century-Crofts.

Cassirer, E. (1950). *The problem of knowledge*. New Haven, CT: Yale University Press.

Cataliotti, J., & Gilchrist, A. L. (1995). Local and global processes in lightness perception. *Perception & Psychophysics, 57*, 125–135.

Coulomb, C. A. (1788). Premier mémoire sur l'électricité et le magnétisme. Construction & usage d'une balance électrique, fondée sur la propriété qu'ont les Fils de métal, d'avoir une force de réaction de Torsion proportionnelle à l'angle de Torsion. *Mémoires de l'Académie Royale des Sciences. Paris*, 569–657.

Galvani, L. (1791). *De Viribus Electricitatis in Motu Musculari Commentarius*. Bologna, Italy: Institute of Sciences at Bologna.

Gibson, J. J. (1966). *The senses considered as perceptual systems*. Boston, MA: Houghton Mifflin.

Gibson, J. J. (1971). The information available in pictures. *Leonardo, 4*, 27–35.

Gibson, J. J. (1986). *The ecological approach to visual perception*. Mahwah, NJ: Erlbaum (original work published 1979).

Gilchrist, A. (2006). *Seeing black and white*. Oxford, UK: Oxford University Press.

Helmholtz, von H. (2000). *Treatise on physiological optics, Vol. III* (J. P. C. Southall, Trans.). Bristol, UK: Thoemmes (original work published 1866).

Helmholtz, von H. (1968). Recent progress of the theory of vision. In R. M. Warren & R. P. Warren (Eds.), *Helmholtz on perception: its physiology and development* (pp. 59–136). New York: Wiley (original work published 1868).

Hobbes, T. (1968). *Leviathan*. London: Penguin Books (original work published 1651).

Hochberg, J. (1974). Higher-order stimuli and inter-response coupling in the perception of the visual world. In R. B. MacLeod & H. L. Pick (Eds.), *Perception: Essays in honor of James J. Gibson* (pp.17–39). Ithaca, NY: Cornell University Press.

Humphrey, N. (1999). *A history of the mind: Evolution and the birth of consciousness*. New York: Springer-Verlag (original work published 1992).

Huntington, E. V. (1913). A set of postulates for abstract geometry, expressed in terms of the simple relation of inclusion. *Mathematische Annalen, 73*, 522–559.

Koenderink, J. J. (1990). The brain a geometry engine. *Psychological Research, 52*, 122–127.

Levine, J. (1983). Materialism and qualia: The explanatory gap. *Pacific Philosophical Quarterly, 64*, 354–361.

Müller, J. (1843). *Elements of physiology* (2nd ed., W. Baly, Trans.). London: Taylor & Walton.

Neisser, U. (1967). *Cognitive psychology*. New York: Appleton-Century-Crofts.

Pastore, N. (1971). *Selective history of theories of visual perception, 1650–1950*. Oxford, UK: Oxford University Press.

Reed, E. S. (1982). Descartes's corporeal ideas hypothesis and the origin of scientific psychology. *Review of Metaphysics*, 35, 731–752.

Reid, T. (1969). *Essays on the intellectual powers of man*. Cambridge, MA: MIT Press (original work published 1785).

Reid, T. (1997). *An inquiry into the human mind on the principles of common sense*. D. Brookes (Ed.). University Park: Pennsylvania State University Press (original work published 1764).

Russell, B. (1997). *The analysis of mind*. London: Routledge (original work published 1921).

Sabra, A. I. (1989). Form in ibn al-Haytham's theory of vision. *Zeitschrift für Geschichte der Arabisch-Islamischen Wissenschaften*, 5, 115–140.

Schubert, E. D. (1975). The role of auditory perception in language processing. In D. D. Duane & M. B. Rawson (Eds.), *Reading, perception and language* (pp. 97–130). Baltimore, MD: York Press.

Segré, E. (1984). *From falling bodies to radio waves: Classical physicists and their discoveries*. New York: Freeman.

Turvey, M. T. (2004). Space (and its perception): The first and final frontier. *Ecological Psychology*, 16, 25–29.

Volta, A. (1801). De l'électricité dite galvanique. *Annales de chimie*, 40, 225–256.

Zajonc, A. (1993). *Catching the light*. New York: Bantam Books.

Lecture 12

The Space Enigmas IV: On Learning Space Perception

Helmholtz's theory of visual space perception from the point of view of empiricism can be summarized as follows.[1] The perceived properties of space are, in all cases, the results of an unconscious inference to the best explanation. *Given current sensations, one sees the spatial properties that would routinely cause them.* The current sensations themselves are never intrinsically spatial because if they were, they would not be so readily overcome as the illusions of space show them to be. Because both illusory and real space perceptions are traceable to experience, then all hypothesized intuitions of space must be traceable solely to experience. For Helmholtz, the sole mechanism responsible for these space perception capabilities is learning by association—that is, unconscious inferences are learned and the learning is associative. Can this be so?

12.1 The Paradox of Unconscious Inference

The immediate problems for Helmholtz's doctrine of unconscious inference to which we must attend are already familiar: the problem of non-repayable loans of intelligence and the problem of original meaning (Lecture 6, Section 5). Returning to the man-in-the-inner-room model, how does the man know the principles employed in the unconscious inferences (such as $S_1/S_2 = I$, the ratio of object size to object distance is the retinal image size)? How are the inferences to the spatial properties of the world outside the house justified? The knowledge necessary for unconscious inference is that of the connection between the second grade of sense (sensations) and the external spatial reality. Unconscious inference, however, is proposed as an explanation of how the outside spatial reality is known. Here's the paradox: *The third grade of sense must be endowed with knowledge of the connection between sensations and spatial reality prior to knowing about that reality through unconscious inference.* In commenting on Helmholtz's theory, James (1890/1983) asked:

> How can we by induction or analogy infer what we do not already generically know?
>
> (p. 909)

Contrary to the tenor of strict empiricism, the doctrine of unconscious inference seems to presume some knowledge that is a priori. Helmholtz does grant that unconscious inference presupposes the law of causality. It must be assumed that sensations are caused, and if prior experiences are to be beneficial, it must be assumed that the same cause always has the same effect. The law of causality, he claims, is a law of our thinking that precedes all experience and cannot be deduced from experience (Helmholtz, 1886/2000; 1868/1968).

In terms of the problem of original meaning, we have already taken note of Helmholtz's appeal to touch (Lecture 8). He spoke of tactile experiences as if they were the original materials of our percepts of space. He did so infrequently, however, leaving the issue of original meaning very much unresolved.[2] In consequence, Helmholtz's many efforts to explain percepts of space through processes whereby one sensation reproduces via association another sensation were basically silent on what, in fact, is reproduced, leaving William James (1890/1983) to claim that: "Helmholtz's *Optics* and the 'empirisistic theory' therein professed must not be understood as attempts at answering the *general* question of how space-consciousness enters the mind. They simply deny that it enters with the first optical sensations" (p. 909).

12.2 Unconscious Inference and Peirce's Abduction

At various points in these Lectures we will need to elaborate further on the preceding since much of the contemporary science of perception-action is, to put it bluntly, Helmholtzian in spirit. Here we take an essential first step beyond Section 12.1 and relate the Helmholtzian form of inference to the more familiar forms of deduction and induction. Following Charles Peirce (see Hanson, 1969; Harris and Hoover, 1983), the Helmholtzian form of inference will be termed *abduction*.

In the case of deduction, a conclusion necessarily follows from the premises. It explicates that something *must be*. In the cases of induction and abduction, the conclusion does not follow necessarily from the premises. Induction shows that something *actually is* operative. Abduction merely suggests that something *may be*.[3] The latter two kinds of inference differ as follows. Induction is an inference from sample to whole, from specific knowledge to a general rule or law. Abduction is an inference from observation to explaining hypothesis, from effect to cause.

We can give a concrete example of each using football (soccer).

Deduction

Hypothesis: All field players on the Arsenal team wear red and white shirts.
Fact: Field player X is on the Arsenal team.
Observation/conclusion: Field player X wears a red and white shirt.

Induction

Fact: Field player X is on the Arsenal team.
Observation/conclusion: Field player X wears a red and white shirt.
Hypothesis: All field players on the Arsenal team wear red and white shirts.

Abduction

Observation/conclusion: Field player X wears a red and white shirt
Hypothesis: All field players on the Arsenal team wear red and white shirts.
Fact: Field player X is on the Arsenal team.

Abduction can be expressed through a Bayesian[4] formulation of the following kind:

$$Probability\ (H/O) \quad = \quad \frac{Probability\ (O/H)\ \times\ Probability\ (H)}{Probability\ (O)} \qquad (12.1)$$

In the formulation as applied to Helmholtz's construal of perception, observation O is *current sensations* and hypothesis *H* is, for example, *an environmental object at distance d meters* (e.g., Figure 11.5). To implement abduction for a single case presumes knowledge of each of the three right-side probabilities specific to that abduction. For abduction in the large—indefinitely many environmental objects of indefinitely many shapes, sizes, orientations, and colors at indefinitely many depths moving in indefinitely many ways—the formulation must be so amplified as to accommodate Malebranche's bold challenge (Lecture 8, Section 8.1): infinite perceptions at an instant.[5]

12.3 Experience: Obvious and Non-obvious

When an empiricist trumpets the significance of experience (Lecture 7) to the successful perceiving of space, what precisely is meant by the term *experience*? Most typically, the empiricist has in mind experiences of a particular kind—those that can be related to the achievements of space perception in an obvious, transparent way. What kind of experiences would one assume to be causal antecedents to three-dimensional visual perception? As we can now appreciate, the implicit Helmholtzian answer would be "binocular visual experiences with objects in depth."

Traditionally, a candidate experiential precursor to a spatial perceptual ability is an experience that can be linked to the ability by a plausible, rational argument (cf. Johnston, 1997). Oppositely, an experience that bears no obvious, transparent, easily rationalized, relation to the spatial perceptual ability is presumed to be an unlikely precursor to the perceptual ability on prima facie grounds (cf. Johnston, 1997). Where rational precursors have not been identified, or have been deemed impossible, then the spatial ability in question is likely to be regarded as an unlearned ability, one that is genetically determined (see Section 12.3.1). It will become important to appreciate, however, that the lack of identifiable experiences that relate to the perceptual spatial ability in a straightforward manner does not mean that experience is irrelevant to the emergence of that ability. Unlearned or "instinctive" abilities—those not traceable to frank learning or practice—can be experientially based (Gottlieb, 1992, 1997).

Consider the following non-obvious influences on highly stereotypic perception–action abilities. Chicks handle mealworms in a species-typical fashion. If they are prevented from seeing their toes during the first two days after hatching, they do not pick up mealworms and do not eat them in the standard ways. Rather, they simply stare at them (Wallman, 1979). Squirrel monkeys fed during rearing with live insects develop the species-specific avoidance behavior toward snakes. If they are instead fed fruit or chow, the fear of snakes fails to emerge (Masataka, 1994). Honey bee larvae incubated at a lower temperature than normal do not differ as adults in within-hive behavior, but do differ in the post-foraging return-to-hive dance that communicates a food source. Compared to bees incubated at the normal temperature, their waggle dance is significantly reduced in likelihood of occurring, number of circuits, and duration of the waggle phase (Tautz, Maier, Groh, Rossler & Brockman, 2003). It seems that there is an experiential context, a possibly dense network of experiences (as introduced in Lecture 3 in the form of Figure 3.4 top), which entails the emergence of stereotypic mealworm eating, stereotypic snake avoidance, and stereotypic bee communication. The stereotypic behaviors fail to emerge when aspects of the context—however subtle, however disingenuous—are omitted.[6]

A causal context C will bring about an effect *E* if C contains all the necessary causes and at least one sufficient cause. An efficient cause labeled *sufficient* is one that precedes and initiates a state change. An efficient cause labeled *necessary* is one whose absence from an otherwise sufficient C disallows the expected state change. Generally, a C sufficient for producing *E* provides many necessary causes that are so indirectly related to *E* that they go unnoticed and unnamed (Killeen & Nash, 2003). Moreover, they are—by virtue of their normalcy, their commonness—taken for granted. The sufficient causes for triggering stereotypic mealworm eating and stereotypic snake avoidance were present in the two cases above. What were absent, apparently, were the necessary causes of previously looking at one's toes and previously eating live insects, respectively. In terms of the causal support versus causal sequence analogy of Lecture 3 (Section 3.4), C is more like the legs of a table than the links in a chain.

The non-obvious experiences supporting the emergence of a species-specific behavior span the prenatal, perinatal (near to birth) and postnatal periods. The significance of perinatal experiences has been revealed in studies on the responses of mallard ducklings to the maternal assembly and alarm calls

(Gottlieb, 1997; Miller, 1997). Mallard ducklings begin to vocalize 2–3 days before hatching. If the self-produced sounds are eliminated by temporarily closing off the embryo's vocal chords,[7] then the probability that the hatched duckling will respond selectively to the mother's postnatal call to assemble (for departure from the nest) will be significantly reduced. For a duckling with operative vocal chords, the absence of perinatal sounds arising from within the nearby eggs of sibling embryos can also reduce the probability of subsequent selective responding to the mother's assembly call. Importantly for matters of interpretation, the specifics of the self- and sibling-vocalizations are crucial to the effects (Gottlieb, 1997). It is these missing specifics of perinatal hearing, not simply the absence of opportunities for auditory stimulation, that result in the reduced likelihood of selectively responding after birth to the maternal assembly call of one's species and not to that of another species.

The intricacy of this developmental causal network resulting in perceptual attunement to the assembly call deserves highlighting. First, the duckling must experience the vocalizations as an embryo. The experience is ineffective after hatching. Second, the embryo must experience embryonic vocalizations. The postnatal vocalizations of ducklings lack the structure that tunes the embryo to the maternal call.

A similar conclusion has been reached for the freezing behavior that occurs in ducklings as a response to the maternal alarm call—a response that, like the response to the assembly call, occurs when the call is heard for the very first time (Miller, 1988, 1997). The investigation of the perinatal and postnatal influences on the freezing response reveals, additionally and importantly, what can only be termed "unreasonable" relations between the non-obvious auditory and social experiences. Consider a duckling deprived of both self-produced sounds and the sounds emanating from its siblings' eggs during the perinatal period. If this duckling is kept in social isolation after hatching and during the alarm call, it will not, in all probability, exhibit the freezing response. However, a duckling subjected to the same perinatal sound deprivations but placed after hatching into, and tested with, a social group of similarly deprived and now hatched ducklings, will freeze with a high probability. Further, a devocal duckling that hears sibling-produced sounds during the perinatal period and is then reared and tested in social isolation, will freeze to the alarm call with a high probability (Miller, 1997). The phenomena depicted in Figure 12.1 round out the illogical relations. In sum, aural and social non-obvious experiences can trade off, apparently, in providing different routes to this species-specific perception-action ability.[8] And non-obvious environmental activities can influence the development of unlearned perception–action abilities in ways that are as specific and essential as genetic activities (West-Eberhard, 2003).

This brief overview of prenatal roots of so-called instinctive behavior makes room for furthering our understanding of the loose concept of experience. To begin with, the concept refers to a relation in the sense that what

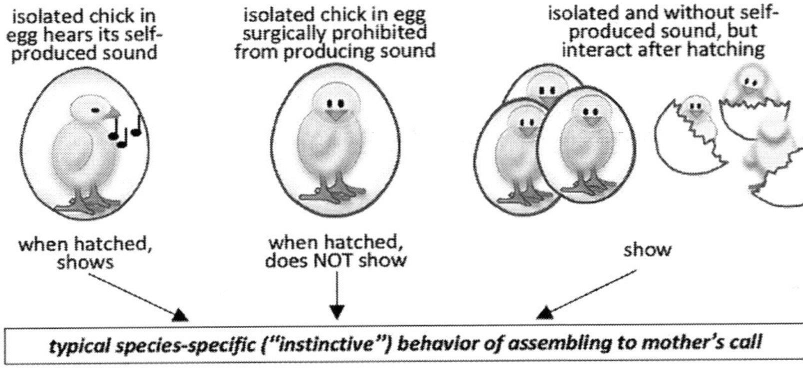

Figure 12.1 Non-obvious experiences and multiple experiential paths.

makes development happen is the relation of (minimally) two events (Gottlieb, 1997). To fix this idea, we can use a variant of Helmholtz's way of expressing relational properties introduced in Lecture 11 (Section 11.2.1). Let A be *embryonic vocalization*, let *B* be *perinatal embryo*, and let *development* be of the *response to the assembly call*. Then it is the case that, although one is tempted to ascribe the cause of development to A, the cause is not in fact A but, rather, the *A–B* relation. Second, the concept refers to a variety of functions of which the following three are the most prominent (Gottlieb, 1997). An experience can *induce* a change in a developmental state of affairs, it can *facilitate* an induced change (bringing it about sooner rather than later), and it can *maintain* an induced change.

12.3.1 Central Dogma and Probabilistic Epigenesis

Helmholtz's stance (and Berkeley's) in regard to space perception is that its development is strictly exogenous (externally constrained). In the absence of confirming evidence for obvious exogenous experiences, the contemporary student of perception is likely to be drawn to the opposite position: that space perception develops through strictly endogenous (internal) processes. An unambiguous position would be that these processes are those identified by the central dogma of molecular biology (Crick, 1970, 1982). The dogma asserts that influences flow in only one direction, from the DNA of a set of master genes to the DNA of genes, to the transcription of messenger RNA, to the formation of (or translation into) proteins. As Gottlieb (2000, 2007) underscores, the dogma suggests that the genome (the totality of DNA molecules transmitted from generation to generation) is insulated from influences above the genetic level and that genetic activity constructs the organism and endows it with its species-specific and species-general competencies.

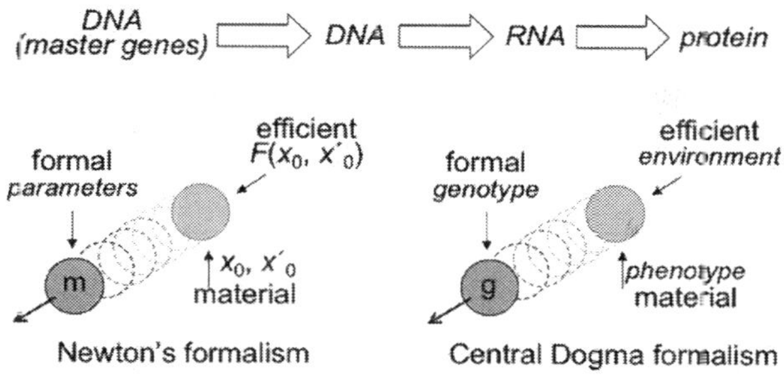

Figure 12.2 Central Dogma's formalism as an analogue of Newton's formalism.

On this commonly held view, genome and environment constitute a dichotomy or dualism (Lecture 2; see West-Eberhard, 2003). Figure 12.2 portrays the central dogma and its relation to the paradigm of system description inherited from Newton (discussed in Lecture 2) in which causal categories are reflected in logically independent aspects of system description.

The investigations of non-obvious influences on development discussed above and the ideas that motivated them (Kuo, 1967; Lehrman, 1953, 1970; Schneirla, 1960) provide an alternative to the central dogma and its implications. *Probabilistic epigenesis* is defined as follows (Gottlieb, 1997):

> Individual development is characterized by an increase of complexity of organization—that is, the emergence of new structural and functional properties and competencies—at all levels of analysis (molecular, subcellular, cellular, organismic) as a consequence of horizontal and vertical coactions among its parts, including organism–environment coactions. (p. 90)

Figure 12.3 is a simple diagram that conveys the essential form of probabilistic epigenesis as defined. To draw the contrast with the central

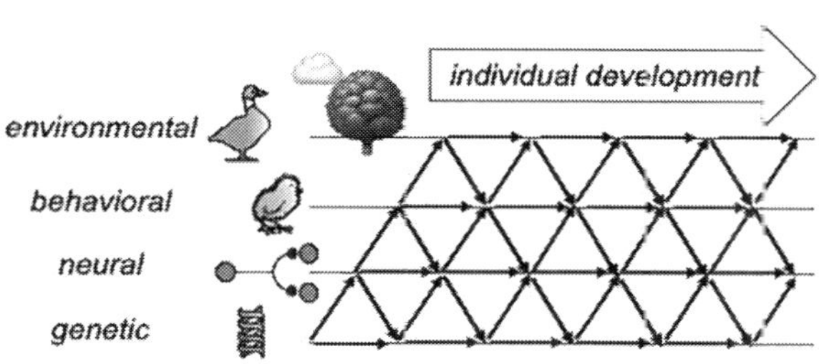

Figure 12.3 Self-organizing developmental system: co-active, co-equal, and co-evolving parts.

(From Figure 14-3 in Gottlieb, 1992, adapted with permission.)

dogma, Figure 12.3 shows that genetic activity affects neural, behavioral, and environmental activities and is affected, in turn, by each of them (indirectly or directly).[9] The evidence for influences exerted on genetic activity by normal environmental and behavioral activity is considerable (Gottlieb, 1998; Lewkowicz, 2011).[10]

Hopefully, one can infer from Figure 12.3 that probabilistic epigenesis is an explanation of development that satisfies the minimal model $m(s) = \langle C(s), E(s), S(s)\rangle$ identified in Lecture 1. It is an explanation in the style of *systemism*: Every part is connected, minimally, with some other part or parts (Mahner & Bunge, 1997). Further, one should be able to infer that it is an explanation that rejects genome-environment dualism. Contrary to the central dogma, probabilistic epigenesis holds that these binary opposites do not make identifiably separate contributions to the development of phenotypic behavior and anatomy (Gottlieb, 1998, 2000; Ho, 1984).

There is a further way in which probabilistic epigenesis can be characterized as different from the central dogma. The central dogma is clearly a view of phenotypic development as *program driven*. It is a claim that current and future developmental states are dependent on prior (stored) states, those of the genome. These prior prescripts are assumed to be sophisticated in their where and when directives, and thorough in their detail. In contrast, probabilistic epigenesis is a view of phenotypic development as *execution driven* (Kugler, 1986; Kugler & Turvey, 1987, 1988; Turvey & Fitzpatrick, 1993). Only crude initial conditions are required for the start-up and fulfillment of phenogenesis. Once initiated, the characteristic developmental processes unfold, dependent upon and driven by the current organization of causal relations expressed over the system's full complement of levels. In its detail and precision, phenogenesis exceeds (by far) the detail and precision of its initial conditions.

The inquiries into non-obvious experience reviewed above suggest a potentially bothersome question to which an answer might now be forthcoming. The question is, how can phenotypic behavior (or structure) be so contingent on apparently minor experiences and yet be completely robust? The answer might have the following form. The detail and precision of any execution-driven system's resultant organization is a function of *the intrinsic stability of the dynamic configuration itself* (the nexus of causal relations) and of the system's self-sensitivity to this dynamic configuration (Kugler & Turvey, 1987). A full appreciation of this latter point will have to await subsequent deliberations on the physics of self-organization. For the present, it is valuable to have the intuition of conceptual proximity between phenotype development and generic ordering principles. Indeed, two important distinctions between the views on development depicted in Figures 12.2 and 12.3 do spadework for future discussions of complexity. First, whereas the different causal categories can be ascribed to distinct components in the view based on the central dogma, such ascription is difficult and perhaps impossible in probabilistic

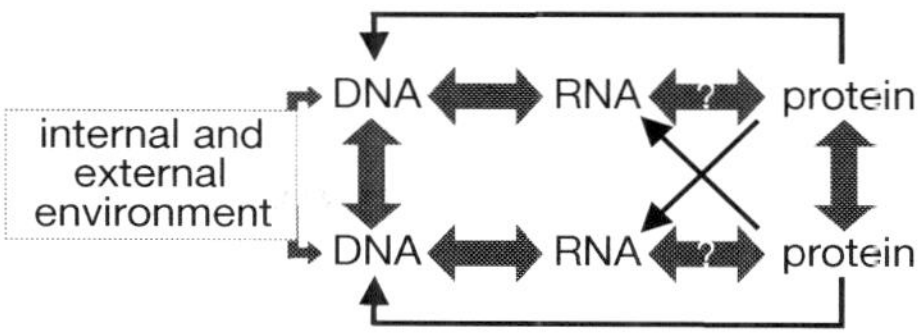

Figure 12.4 In the central dogma, genetic activity is dictated solely by genes (DNA → DNA), whereas in probabilistic epigenesis, internal and external environmental events activate genetic expression through proteins (protein → DNA), hormones, and other influences. Question mark on influence from protein back to RNA indicates what remains a theoretical possibility in probabilistic epigenesis but is prohibited in the central dogma (as are protein ⟷ protein influences).

(From Figure 4 in Gottlieb, 2000, adapted with permission, Sage Publishing.)

epigenesis. In the causal network of Figure 12.3, the causal categories seem intertwined or entangled (Lecture 4). Second, whereas the emphasis in the view based on the central dogma is on what the components do (component-dominant dynamics), the emphasis in probabilistic epigenesis is on what the interactions among the components do (interaction-dominant dynamics). Figures 12.2 and 12.4 provide a useful comparison of the two views in terms of the linkages among DNA, RNA, and proteins.

12.3.2 What Natural Selection Selects

One lesson of the preceding observations and arguments is that phenotypic form and function arise if and only if the necessary and sufficient causes implicit in the activities of Figure 12.3 are present at the right times and in the right places. The other lesson is that the varied factors identified in Figure 12.3 are of comparable causal and formative significance. The upshot of these lessons for comprehending the notion of heredity and the evolution-development relation are far from trivial.

In the simplest of terms, *heredity is the passing on of all developmental conditions* (Oyama, 2000). Under this definition, there is no dichotomy of hereditary versus acquired. Genes are involved in all traits, in all differences, and all traits, all differences, are heritable. All perceptual and behavioral variations that can be subjected to natural selection or selective breeding will change in the selected direction across generations. The variations will do so in consequence of these selective operations only to the degree that the pre-, peri-, and post-natal developmental conditions are kept constant across generations (Gottlieb, 1992; see his Table 12–1). Once the constancy of developmental conditions is interrupted, even a behavior bred over 39 generations will not endure (Hood, 2005).

12.3.3 Obvious and Non-obvious Experiences are not Fundamentally Different

The image of development projected by Figure 12.3 is that of a dense network of causal relations. It is an image of development as replete with necessary and sufficient experiences—as massively entailed. What the figure does not project is the image of these experiences occurring at multiple, nested time-scales. There are experiences of all temporal sizes. An experience's temporal extent may be measured in milliseconds, minutes, days, months, years, or tens of years (depending on the species). What the figure also fails to project is the status of an experience as obvious or non-obvious. Of these two failings, that relating to temporal size is probably unfortunate, that relating to obviousness is probably not. A reasonable bet, given the growing understanding of self-organizing complex systems, is that what may be construed as major experiences—those that are patently obvious and of well-defined extent—do not play a special role.[11] Rather, in respect to their influence on development, on perception and action, they follow the same laws as minor experiences (those that are patently indiscernible and of ill-defined extent). If so, the implication is that it is not a specific theory of the effect of major experiences that is needed but a general theory encompassing all experiences—the logically major and minor, the obvious and non-obvious, the prolonged and instantaneous, the recurring and the once only.

12.4 Learnability of the Size–Distance Invariance Hypothesis

We conclude this lecture by examining the thesis that if an object (*o*) aligned vertically at a perceived distance (*d*) projects a retinal angle/proximal size (*s*), then *o*'s perceived size (*S*) is given by $S = sd$. This equality is representative of the rules or algorithms that Helmholtz promoted and a common textbook example of the proposed inferential nature or assumptive context of visual perception (see Epstein, 1967). Following Turvey and Shaw (1979), we will regard the size–distance invariance rule as a concept that has to be acquired in the (outwardly) empiricist tradition of Helmholtz. Figure 12.5a shows minimal grounds for inferring the concept $S = s_1d_1 = s_2d_2$, that is, actual size is invariant over the product of retinal angle/proximal size and perceived distance. Given a change in the observer-to-*o* distance of any reasonable magnitude, retinal angle/proximal size changes from s_1 to s_2, and perceived distance changes from d_1 to d_2. But to acquire the concept, there has to be conviction that any change in *s* from t_1 to t_2 (where *t* is time) was solely due to a change in *d*. It could have been due to a change in the type of *o* (*constancy of identity* problem), the size of *o* (*constancy of actual size* problem), the orientation of *o* (*constancy of orientation* problem, see Figure 12.5b), the shape of *o* (*constancy of shape* problem, see Figure 12.5c), or the eyes/head orientation

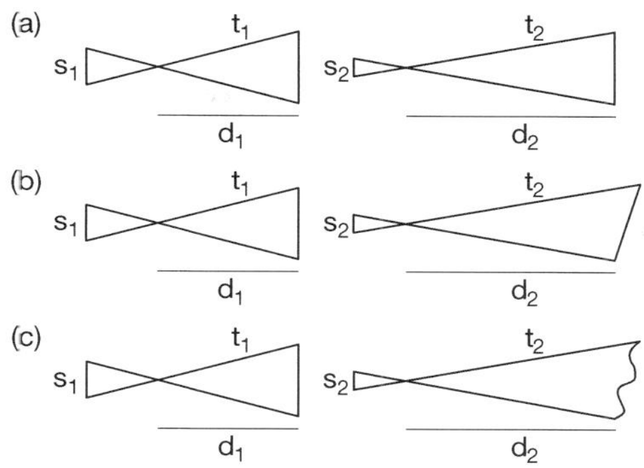

Figure 12.5 The challenges of acquiring the size–distance invariance rule as a concept in the (outwardly) empiricist tradition of Helmholtz. See text for details.

(From Figures 9.1–3 in Turvey & Shaw, 1979, adapted with permission.)

of the perceiver (*constancy of eyes/head orientation* problem). The point here is that if there is a set A of algorithms to mediate the set C of perceptual constancies, then determining the consistency of any one algorithm a_i (to mediate the constancy c_i) requires that the set A be at the perceiver's disposal.[12] The foregoing requirement seems contrary to the tradition of empiricism.

12.5 Agreement from Afar

Surprisingly, a major voice in the contemporary rationalist perspective—namely, Fodor (1983)—can be dismissive of the logical order that grounds Helmholtz's unconscious inference:

> [F]eedback [13] is effective only to the extent that *prior* to the analysis of the stimulus, the perceiver knows quite a lot about what the stimulus is going to be like. Whereas the *point* of perception, is surely, that it lets us find out how the world is, even when the world is some way that we *don't* expect it to be . . .
>
> So: The perceptual analysis of unanticipated stimulus layouts (in language and elsewhere) is possible only to the extent that the output of the transducers is insensitive to the beliefs/expectations that the transducers supply. This is to say that the perception of novelty depends on bottom-to-top perceptual mechanisms.
>
> (pp. 67–68)

They are quotations befitting an ecological realist.

Notes

1 This summary is modeled after William James's (1890/1983, p. 908).
2 A commentator on Helmholtz suggested in jest (see James, 1890/1983, p. 909) that the various senses bear the same relation to space perception as a "troop of jolly drinkers" bear to the landlord's bill. No one has any money but each hopes that one of the others will pay.
3 This overview of deduction, induction, and abduction is from Pierce's *Collected Papers*, Volume 5, cited by Hanson (1969, p. 85).
4 Referring to Bayes's theorem that relates current belief (or evidence) to prior belief (or evidence). It is derivable from the basic axioms of probability theory, specifically conditional probability.
5 Integral to abduction of any scale are questions of which *H* to apply on any given occasion and which *H*s to ignore. These issues are discussed, contemporarily, relative to the so-called frame problem, particularly in robotics. In planning an action, there are determinations of which causes to apply and which to ignore, which environmental aspects will change, and which will not (see papers in Ford & Pylyshyn, 1996).
6 It is similarly the case that stereotypic development of the somatosensory nervous system fails to occur when aspects of the context, as subtle and disingenuous as twitching when sleeping, are omitted (Khazipov, Sirota, Leinekugel, Holmes et al., 2004; Petersson, Waldenstrom, Fahraeus & Schouenborg, 2003).
7 See Chapter 2 in Gottlieb (1997) for the embryonic devocalization procedure.
8 A refinement of the notions of sufficient and necessary causes, along probabilistic lines, is in order. One lesson from the examples just given is that one sufficient cause for a given *E* may differ from another in the constellation of necessary causes required for its efficacy. Another lesson is that the role of an experience as "sufficient" or "necessary" may be only part-time (Killeen & Nash, 2003). Let experience or functional activity *X* be probabilistic and graded (rather than simply either present or absent). Then, if the probability of *E* given *X* is greater than the base line probability of *E*—that is, $P(E \mid X) > P(E)$—then *X* is a part-time sufficient cause. If the probability of *E* in the absence of *X* is less than the base line probability of *E*—that is—$P(E \mid absent\ X) < P(E)$, then *X* is a part-time necessary cause.
9 As proffered by Noble (2006, 2008): In biological systems, there is no program of the kind promoted by Jacob and Monod (1961) and there is no privileged level of causality as proclaimed by Dawkins (1976/2006). Related arguments are to be found in Coen (1999).
10 Here are some examples (Gottlieb, 2000). Visual stimulation increases RNA complexity in visual cortex of cats. Conspecific song increases forebrain messenger RNA in canaries and zebra finches. Tactile stimulation enhances the expression of genes and increases their protein production for the formation of somatosensory neurons in rats. Practicing balancing changes the RNA of vestibular nerve cells in rats.
11 The Guttenberg–Richter law of the distribution of earthquake magnitudes is the basis for the "reasonable bet" (cf. Bak, 1996). It suggests that large earthquakes are not singular. In a plot of frequency of occurrence against size in double logarithmic coordinates, large earthquakes and small earthquakes (including aftershocks) tend to fall on the same line (Bak, Christensen, Danon, & Scanlon, 2002). As Bak (1996, p. 14) asks: "How can the dynamics of all the elements of a system as complicated as the crust of the earth . . . conspire, as if by magic, to produce a law with such extreme simplicity?"

12 In subsequent lectures, we will refer to the problem intimated here as the problem of intractable non-specificity.
13 Alias, top–down influence.

References

Bak, P. (1996). *How nature works*. New York: Springer Verlag.

Bak, P., Christensen, K., Danon L., & Scanlon, Y. (2002). Unified scaling law for earthquakes. *Physics Review Letters*, 88, 178501.

Coen, E. (1999). *The art of genes*. Oxford, UK: Oxford University Press.

Crick, F. (1970). Central dogma of molecular biology. *Nature*, *227*, 561–563.

Crick, F. (1982). DNA today. *Perspectives in Biology and Medicine*, *25*, 512–517.

Dawkins, R. (2006). *The selfish gene*. NewYork: Oxford University Press (original work published 1976).

Epstein, W. (1967). *Varieties of perceptual learning*. New York: McGraw-Hill.

Fodor, J. A. (1983). *Modularity of mind*. Cambridge, MA: MIT Press.

Ford, K. M., & Pylyshyn, Z. W. (1996). (Eds). *The robot's dilemma revisited*. Norwood, NJ: Ablex.

Gottlieb, G. (1992). *Individual development and evolution: The genesis of novel behavior*. New York: Oxford University Press.

Gottlieb, G. (1997). *Synthesizing nature and nurture: Prenatal roots of instinctive behavior*. Mahwah, NJ: Erlbaum.

Gottlieb, G. (1998). Normally occurring environmental and behavioral influences on gene activity: From central dogma to probabilistic epigenesis. *Psychological Review*, *105*, 792–802.

Gottlieb, G. (2000). Environmental and behavioral influences on gene activity. *Current Directions in Psychological Science*, 9, 93–97.

Gottlieb, G. (2007). Probabilistic epigenesis. *Developmental Science*, *10*, 1–11.

Hanson R. N. (1969). *Patterns of discovery*. Cambridge, UK: Cambridge University Press.

Harris, J. F., & Hoover, K. (1983). Abduction and the new riddle of induction. In E. Freeman (Ed.), *The relevance of Charles Peirce* (pp. 132–144). La Salle, IL: Monist Library of Philosophy.

Helmholtz, von H. (2000). *Treatise on physiological optics*, *Vol. III* (J. P. C. Southall, Trans.). Bristol, UK: Thoemmes (original work published 1866).

Helmholtz, von H. (1968). Recent progress of the theory of vision. In R. M. Warren & R. P. Warren (Eds.), *Helmholtz on perception: Its physiology and development* (pp. 59–136). New York: Wiley (original work published 1868).

Ho, M-W. (1984). Environment and heredity in development and evolution. In M.-W Ho & P. T. Saunders (Eds.), *Beyond neo-Darwinism: An introduction to the new evolutionary paradigm* (pp. 267–289). San Diego, CA: Academic Press.

Hood, K. (2005). Development as a dependent variable: Robert B. Cairns on the psychobiology of aggression. In D. M. Stoff & E. J. Susman (Eds.), *Developmental psychobiology of aggression* (pp. 225–251). New York: Cambridge University Press.

Jacob, F., & Monod, J. (1961). Genetic regulatory mechanisms in the synthesis of proteins. *Journal of Molecular Biology*, 3, 318–356.

James, W. (1983). *The principles of psychology*. Cambridge, UK: Cambridge University Press (original work published 1890).

Johnston, T. D. (1997). Comment on Miller. In C. Dent-Read & P. Zukow-Goldring (Eds.), *Evolving explanations of development* (pp. 509–513). Washington, DC: American Psychological Association.

Khazipov, R., Sirota, A., Leinekugel, X., Holmes, G. et al. (2004). Early motor activity drives spindle bursts in the developing somatosensory cortex. *Nature*, *432*, 758–761.

Killeen, P., & Nash, M. R. (2003). The four causes of hypnosis. *International Journal of Clinical and Experimental Hypnosis*, *51*, 195–231.

Kugler, P. N. (1986). A morphological perspective on the origin and evolution of movement patterns. In M. G. Wade & H. T. A Whiting (Eds.), *Motor development in children: Aspects of coordination and control* (pp. 459–525). Dordrecht, Netherlands: Martinus Niijhoff.

Kugler, P. N., & Turvey, M. T. (1987). *Information, natural law and the self-assembly of rhythmic movement*. Hillsdale, NJ: Erlbaum.

Kugler, P. N., & Turvey, M. T. (1988). Self-organization, flow fields, and information. *Human Movement Science*, *7*, 97–129.

Kuo, Z.-Y. (1967). *The dynamics of behavior development: An epigenetic view*. New York: Random House.

Lehrman, D. S. (1953). A critique of Konrad Lorenz's theory of instinctive behavior. *Quarterly Review of Biology*, *28*, 337–363.

Lehrman, D. S. (1970). Semantic and conceptual issues in the nature-nurture problem. In L. R. Aronson, E. Tobach, D. S. Lehrman, & J. S. Rosenblatt (Eds.), *Development and evolution of behavior* (pp. 17–50). San Francisco, CA: Freeman.

Lewkowicz, D. J. (2011). The biological implausibility of the nature-nurture dichotomy and what it means for the study of infancy. Infancy, *16*, 331–367.

Mahner, M., & Bunge, M. (1997). *Foundations of biophilosophy*. New York: Springer.

Masataka, N. (1994). Effects of experience with live insects on the development of fear of snakes in squirrel monkeys, *Saimiri sciureus*. *Animal Behavior*, *46*, 741–746.

Miller, D. (1988). Development of instinctive behavior: An epigenetic and ecological approach. In E. M. Blass (Ed.), *Handbook of behavioral neurobiology, Vol. 9: Developmental psychobiology and behavioral ecology* (pp. 415–444). New York: Plenum Press.

Miller, D. (1997). The effects of nonobvious forms of experience on the development of instinctive behavior. In C. Dent-Read & P. Zukow-Goldring (Ed.), *Evolving explanations of development* (pp. 457–507). Washington, DC: American Psychological Association.

Noble, D. (2006). *The music of life: Biology beyond the genome*. Oxford, UK: Oxford University Press.

Noble, D. (2008). Genes and causation. *Philosophical Transactions of the Royal Society* A, *366*, 3001–3015.

Oyama, S. (2000). *A system's view of the biological-cultural divide*. Durham, NC: Duke University Press.

Petersson, P., Waldenstrom, A., Fahraeus, C., & Schouenborg, J. (2003). Spontaneous muscle twitches during sleep guide spinal self-organization. *Nature*, *424*, 72–75.

Schneirla, T. C. (1960). Instinctive behavior, maturation, experience and development. In B. Kaplan, & S. Wapner (Eds.), *Perspectives in psychological theory: Essays in honor of Heinz Werner* (pp. 303–334). New York: International University Press.

Tautz, J., Maier, S., Groh, C., Rossler, W., & Brockmann, A. (2003). Behavioral performance of honey bees is influenced by the temperature experienced during their pupal development. *Proceedings of the National Academy of Sciences, 100*, 7343–7347.

Turvey, M. T., & Fitzpatrick, P. (1993). Commentary: Development of perception-action systems and general principles of pattern formation. *Child Development, 64*, 1175–1190.

Turvey, M. T., & Shaw, R. E. (1979). The primacy of perceiving: An ecological reformulation of perception for understanding memory. In L.-G. Nilssen (Ed.), *Perspectives on memory research: In honor of Uppsala University's 500th anniversary* (pp. 167–222). Hillsdale, NJ: Erlbaum.

Wallman, J. (1979). A minimal visual restriction experiment: Preventing chicks from seeing their feet affects later responses to mealworms. *Developmental Psychobiology, 12*, 391–397.

West-Eberhard, M. J. (2003). *Developmental plasticity and evolution*. Oxford, UK: Oxford University Press.

Lecture 13

Gestaltism I: Atomism, Anatomism, and Mechanistic Order

In the country of its origin (Germany) and in the country of its adoption (America), Gestalt psychology was a reaction against two "–isms": *atomism* and *anatomism*. The school of perceptual psychology derived from Helmholtz and known as Structuralism or Introspectionism and the school of learning psychology known as Behaviorism differed markedly in goals and methods. From the perspective of Gestalt psychology, however, the well-advertised differences between the two schools were superficial. The two opposing points of view shared in common deep-seated assumptions about the most fundamental notion: the source of order. Percepts are organized (rather than disorganized) and behaviors are orderly (rather than disorderly); at issue is how should this order be explained.

Recall the depiction of Helmholtz's variant of the Cartesian Program (Figure 11.5). A key feature of that depiction is the labeled lines—the specific nerve fiber energies. They obey the so-called law of isolated conduction. Given that the fibers do not interact and are subject to no other external influences, each sends to the brain precisely the impression that the receptor of each receives. The nerve fibers behave as linear causal chains (Lecture 3): Isolated retinal excitations, as efficient causes, produce isolated sensations. As we appreciated in Lecture 11, the elemental or atomistic nature of the produced sensations is at the core of the doctrine of sensations. A further lesson of Lecture 11 was that association is the means by which these "atoms" of experience attach, so as to become the "molecules," "polymers" and so on, of experience.

Developments in histology in the latter half of the 19th century boosted the atomism of perceptual theory and provided a way in which associations could be comprehended anatomically (Boring, 1950). The discovery that each nerve cell and its fibers formed an independent unit became the basis of the neuron doctrine.[1] The discovery that there were an almost infinite number of such independent units in the brain fit with the common intuition that the number of separate simple and complex ideas possessed by one mind was uncountable. Further, the discovery that this infinity of distinct cell structures was richly interconnected fit with the major hypothesis that ideas were associated in multiple ways with other ideas. The discoveries of histology provided the necessary spadework for encoding the philosophical/psychological thesis of associationism into the topography[2] of the central nervous system. The association of ideas championed by Locke, Berkeley, Hume and Helmholtz could become—in the hands of a theorist who was so disposed—an anatomical concept.

The constancy hypothesis, so long a major departure point for the theorizing of empiricists (Pastore, 1971), was for 19th-century physiological psychologist the logical consequence of the law of isolated conduction. Given the law, one had to argue that the initial distribution of punctate excitations on the cortical sheet (area 17) to which the retina projects had to be topologically identical to the distribution of excitations on the retina. The topography of retina-to-cortex labeled lines (consider the $R(s_i)$ lines in Figure 11.4) dictated the initial distribution of cortical excitations—that is, the "cortical retinal image" (e.g., Köhler & Wallach, 1944) is strictly a consequence of the anatomy. Two reasons could be given for those many cases in which the percept's properties are not explainable by the retinal distribution and its cortical isomorphism. One reason was unconscious inference (as with the Ponzo Illusion of Figure 8.3). The other reason was the induction of extra cortical units into the distribution of excited cortical units. The discoveries of histology enabled the conjecture that repeated experiences facilitated the anatomical connections among cortical cells. If cells *a*, *b* and *c* were in the initial cortical distribution, the final distribution might include cells *d*, *e*, *f* and *g*, inducted into the final distribution by virtue of their active anatomical connections with *a*, *b* and *c*. By this reasoning, the final distribution of cortical excitations governing the percept, like the initial distribution, is a consequence of the topography of the nervous system.

We are now in a position to identify *anatomism*. As applied to perception, it is *the tendency to attribute the order in perception to the order in (or topography of) the anatomy*. Anatomism is the natural extension of the doctrine of specific nerve energies. For structuralism, not only was sensation specific to the anatomy, but so was the spatial order of percepts. For behaviorism, the order that had to be accounted for was that manifest by movements. A particular anatomical arrangement was presumed to underlie each simple reflex as the grantor of its spatial and temporal order, and reflexes, both unconditioned and conditioned, were presumed to be the anatomically specific atoms of behavior. With these movement atoms situated at different locations, or embodied in different networks of anatomical components, the production of complex behavior such as locomotion required that the movement atoms be connected. Again, the histological discoveries of endless connectivity allowed an anatomical interpretation of association. Elemental movements, like simple ideas, could be chained together via neural links.

For Gestalt psychologists to inveigh against *atomism* and *anatomism* was to inveigh against the machine theory of the nervous system introduced by

Descartes (Lectures 5 and 6) and reinforced by Newton's mechanics (Lectures 2 and 3). We cannot truly come to terms with Gestalt psychology in the absence of a more detailed understanding than that developed thus far of the related concepts of *machine*, *mechanism*, and *mechanistic order*.

13.1 Machine as Superposed Mechanical Units

Structurally, a machine is made up of independent parts where each part is a "simple machine" with a shape, a size, and a designated role. Think of an old-fashioned clock (as displayed in Figure 13.1) or a modern automobile. The parts are fabricated separately, for example, by casting, such that one part is cast using one mold, one part is cast using another mold, and so on. When assembled, the independent parts are made to interact through the principle of nearby action (Lecture 3) where the particular manifestation of the principle depends on how the parts are arranged. The forms of nearby action permitted by the topography of the juxtaposed parts affect the state (Lecture 2) of a part as a unit, but do not alter the part structurally and do not, therefore, change the part's designated role (its essential nature). The specific chain of part-to-part interactions determines the characteristic behavior of the machine.

Because of the generic structural principles, it is possible to understand any given machine by a process of dissection or fractionation. Imagine taking apart a clock (see Figure 13.2) or an automobile. The aforementioned process

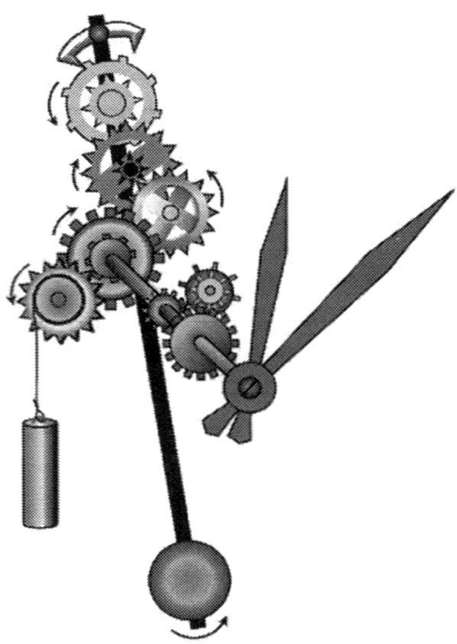

Figure 13.1 The machine metaphor can be nicely expressed by means of an old-fashioned pendulum clock.

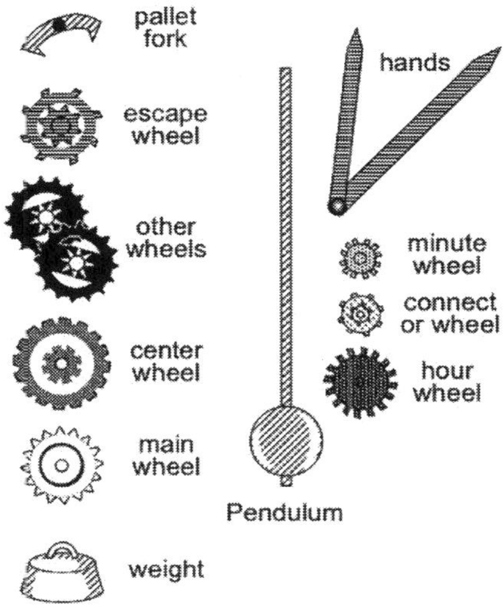

Figure 13.2 The parts of an old-fashioned pendulum clock provide an immediate appreciation of the concept of mechanical units and, by analogy, anatomical units.

results in the independent parts or "simple machines" that constitute the clock or automobile. They are the machine's natural analytic units. By means of them one can understand, in principle, how the machine was constructed and how it works. This is because, as an aggregate, the properties of the isolated parts qua the machine's natural analytic units entail the properties of the machine. Each independent part causes an effect, and the summing or superposing of these independent causes and effects yields the overall effect—the machine's characteristic behavior.

Together, the disassembling (analysis) and assembling (synthesis) of a machine manifest what might be called a *principle of superposition*. A machine can be decomposed into independent parts; each part can be studied and understood individually; the parts can be reassembled to understand the machine. Figure 13.2 identifies the parts into which the machine depicted in Figure 13.1 can be analyzed and from which it can be synthesized. Self-evidently, superposition means that the machine (the whole entity) cannot be more than the sum of its parts or, synonymously, the machine cannot exhibit a property that is not contained in its parts. By the same token, superposition also means that there is no impredicativity (Lecture 3): The parts define the whole and there is no definition of any part in terms of the whole. The vexing chicken–egg situation of "characterizing the parts requires understanding the whole but understanding the whole requires a characterization of the parts" does not arise. Superposition is in keeping with

Russell's (1903) predicative view. Simply, to understand a system, look only to its subsystems.

13.2 The Machine Metaphor

Descartes presented us with the thesis that the world is a machine. He argued that the physical world and everything in it must be explained in the way that we explain machines, through the sizes, shapes, and motions of their independent parts. His thesis did not distinguish between inanimate and animate physics. Descartes' observations of machines that sometimes appeared lifelike—that is, as automata—suggested to him that living things were analogous to automata. The *machine metaphor* was his legacy to physics and biology (for example, *Principles of Philosophy*, IV, Section 203; see Cottingham, Stoothoff & Murdoch, 1985, Volume 1).

> [I] do not recognize any difference between artefacts and natural bodies except that the operations of artefacts are for the most part performed by mechanisms which are large enough to be easily perceivable by the senses
>
> (p. 288)

On the functions exhibited by living things, he remarked (*Treatise on man*, Section 202; see Cottingham et al., 1985, Volume I):

> I should like you to consider that these functions follow from the mere arrangement of the machine's organs every bit as naturally as the movements of a clock or the other automaton follow from the arrangement of its counter weights and wheels.
>
> (p. 108)

This latter quotation is a clarion call—one that has been heard down the centuries—to conceptualize the body's organs, its anatomical units, as mechanical units. What is intended by this conception can be made clear by considering the mechanical units in Figure 13.2. First, the function of each unit is implicated strictly by the unit's form and material composition—that is, a unit's function is defined predicatively in terms of the unit and not impredicatively in terms of the larger system, the clock, of which the unit forms a part. Second, each unit is absolute in the various senses of "stands alone," "not dependent on anything else," and "self sufficient." The existence of a mechanical unit is independent of whether the machine is operative. Thus, the mechanical units in Figure 13.2 continue to exist when the clock has stopped running. They also continue to exist in isolation from the clock, as the comparison of Figure 13.2 with Figure 13.1 makes apparent.

The machine metaphor and its central notion of mechanical unit constitute the cornerstone of the modern methodological principle of reductionism.

Abiding the metaphor, fractionation of a machine into independent parts (into simple machines) can be extrapolated to the world at large. For any material system, including the universe, there is always a set of parts into which it can be decomposed without losing information about the system. For any material system, including the universe, reduction to parts is a necessary and sufficient strategy to account for the system and its properties.

13.3 On Billiard Balls and Being Particulate

An object akin to a billiard ball has often been used to convey the image of a particle and, on extension, a mechanical unit. Think of a billiard ball's properties. It is spatially localized, having a well-defined size and occupying a particular region. It is stable in that it is not likely to fragment of its own accord. It possesses a definite mass and color. It has a name. It is separable from other billiard balls. It is capable of interacting with other billiard balls. It has properties that can sensibly be added to the like properties of other billiard balls (e.g., mass) and properties that cannot (e.g., color). We can anticipate from the foregoing the features that are essential to something being *particulate*. It is (a) localized and separate, (b) stable and objective with a distinct name, and (c) individual and additive (Krieger, 1992).

The member of the preceding inventory that is most challenging is "localized." The immediate interpretation in terms of ordinary geometric space is insufficiently general and likely to mislead. In a crystal lattice, there are right particles (right degrees of freedom, see Lecture 5) that are not the atoms of the crystal but the vibrations of the lattice of atoms as a whole. Considered as particles, the vibrations are localized by frequency, momentum, and velocity. These crystal vibrations can bounce off (interact with) other vibrations, as billiard balls bounce off each other (Krieger, 1992).

13.4 Machine as Simulacrum

To explain a phenomenon within the machine metaphor is to give an account that is machine-like. This is what it means to provide a *mechanism* for the phenomenon. Although the account might be phrased mathematically by way of symbols the role of those symbols is to represent the nature of every object or event in the machine that is modeling the phenomenon. The intent is that *the symbols pass as replicas of the details and properties* of the simple machines whose summed effects constitute the phenomenon. A prominent Victorian physicist, William Thompson (Lord Kelvin), wrote (Cassirer, 1950):

> I am never content until I have constructed a mechanical model of the object that I am studying. If I succeed in making one, I understand; otherwise, I do not.
>
> (p. 115)

Thompson's words express the desire, common to the physicists of his time, to make things plain, to express them in a sensible form, a form that is easily visualized (March & Freeman, 1963; Lecture 3). To this end, the symbols in a mechanism's corresponding mathematical formulation must connect to the hypothesized material objects composing the mechanism. Arthur Eddington (1928/1958) summarized the likes of Thompson in these terms:

> It was the boast of the Victorian physicist that he would not claim to understand a thing until he could make a model of it; and by a model he meant something constructed of levers, gears, wheels, squirts, or other appliances familiar to an engineer. Nature in building the universe was supposed to be dependent on just the same kind of resources as any human mechanic; and when the physicist sought an explanation of phenomena his ear was straining to catch the hum of machinery. The man who could make gravitation out of cog-wheels would have been a hero in the Victorian age.
>
> (p. 209)

What Thompson desired for the explanation of a physical phenomenon—and what Eddington derided—was a *simulator*. Thompson and his peers were convinced that a mechanical simulation led to an inherent understanding of any given physical phenomenon. In contrast, Eddington and his peers were of the opinion that while a mechanical simulation is a way to visualize or picture a physical phenomenon, it is no guarantor of understanding the phenomenon.[3]

The two quotations just cited are elliptical references to a characterization of machine in terms of simulation. In response to the question of "What is a machine?" they hint that the answer is *machine as simulacrum*. Such an answer is not forthcoming from the consideration of how machines are built. That is to say, it does not follow from an explication of mechanical units—for example, those that compose a clock (Figure 13.2)—and the principle of superposition. A very different tack is required.

The identification of machine as simulacrum is situated at the point of convergence of two 17th-century ideas. One is Hobbes's (1651/1968) insistence that thinking consists of symbolic operations on special brain tokens (Lecture 5). The other is the dualism of system and environment—that is, the dualism of states and dynamical laws—which shaped Newton's mechanics (Lecture 2). The contemporary manifestation of Hobbes's insistence is the "Turing machine." There will be much to discuss when the Turing machine is encountered in earnest in later lectures. For the present lecture, we need only recognize that this machine is a mathematical Hobbesian machine where the parts are symbols that can come in different sizes (strings of symbols) and shapes (syntactic roles) and exhibit different motions (transformations by rule). In a Turing machine, meaningless symbols are analogous to particles in Newton's framework and symbol strings are analogous to configurations of such particles. Further, in a Turing machine, the manipulation of symbols by fixed rules (of arithmetic) that are external to the symbols is analogous to the changes in the states of particles by laws (of forces) that reside in the environment of the particles (Lecture 2). At root, the mathematical machine and the Newtonian formalism for material systems are identical (Rosen, 1988, 1991, 2000). Recursiveness is the core of both (Lecture 2). For both formalisms, conversion of the present to the immediate future exhausts their entailment structure.

What makes the mathematical machine important here is that it is a way of thinking about the syntactic aspect of mathematics—the rules that compose its internal grammar—separately from its semantic aspect—the external matters that it refers to—that is, what it is about or what it means. We recall from Lecture 3 impredicativities or self-referring definitions and the felt need by Russell and Poincaré to prohibit their occurrences in logical and mathematical systems. Those who held similar views, especially the mathematical polyglot Hilbert, believed that the desired prohibition (the vicious circle principle) could be implemented by restricting such systems to their syntactical aspect and adding further syntactic rules as needed to replace the semantic features. Any mathematical system (e.g., Euclidean geometry) stripped of its external referents and encoded strictly by syntactic rules is designated "formalizable." A mathematical system that can be formalized is equivalent, therefore, to the strictly syntactical (by definition) mathematical machine of above. The primary consequence of this equivalence is that a machine can "do" the mathematical formalism. On extending this nexus of ideas we can be led to the following conclusion (Rosen, 1991):

> Simulation is what machines do, and a system (formal or material) *is* a machine if it simulates or can simulate, something else.
>
> (p. 185)

The equations of "machine" with "simulator," "mechanism" with "simulation," and "simulation" with "strictly syntactical" imply that a material system whose phenomena cannot be simulated is a material system that is not a machine. We will have plenty of reasons in future lectures to consider this implication in detail. Here we need only note that Eddington's chiding of Thompson and his fellow Victorian scientists may be interpreted as a reaction against the belief that the natural world can be rendered fully in a strictly syntactic form. Rosen (1988) has stated this possible interpretation more firmly: "Purely syntactical models of material nature are too impoverished in entailment to mirror the causal sequences which can occur in nature" (p. 27).

13.5 Helmholtz's Influential Mechanical View

The mechanical view as a program for 19th-century physics was articulated in clear, uncompromising terms at approximately the mid-point of the century (Cassirer, 1950). Its author was Helmholtz. At its core were the concepts of *force* and *matter*. Newton's controversial action-at-a-distance (Lecture 4) had been accepted for gravitation and was endorsed by Helmholtz as the proper conception for understanding nature more generally. All operations in nature had to be traced to attractive and repulsive forces that acted along the line connecting mutually interacting points and did so with an intensity dependent only on distance (Cassirer, 1950; Einstein & Infeld, 1938/1966; see Figure 13.3). Helmholtz's view was that *simple forces between unalterable objects should explain all material phenomena*. A generic explanation of the preceding kind ought to be the case if all material phenomena were as Descartes had suggested—the manifest behaviors of machines (albeit ones that did not obey the principle of local cause).

Key to the broad application of the mechanical view was the interpretation of "unalterable objects." In respect to the clock of Figures 13.1 and 13.2, the "unalterable objects" are the clock's components. As mechanical units (recall the definition above), they are unchanged by the causal processes in which they participate and persist when those processes stop and when the system to which they belong, the clock, has been taken apart. In the broad application of the mechanistic view that sought to embrace light, heat, electricity and magnetism, the "unalterable object" qua mechanical unit was a *substance*. The notion of substance, introduced by Aristotle, is roughly something that makes a thing what it is, that gives a thing its essential nature. The definitions of Kant, the 19th-century physicist, in the first (1781/1998) and second (1787/1998) editions of the *Critique of Pure Reason* were especially influential: "All appearances contain that which persists (substance) as the object itself, and that which can change as its mere determination, i.e., a way in which the object exists" (p. 299). "In all change of appearances substance persists, and its quantum is neither increased nor diminished in nature" (p. 299).

The defining quality of a substance was conservation. Its total amount (quantum) had to remain unchanged. The mechanical view, therefore, often

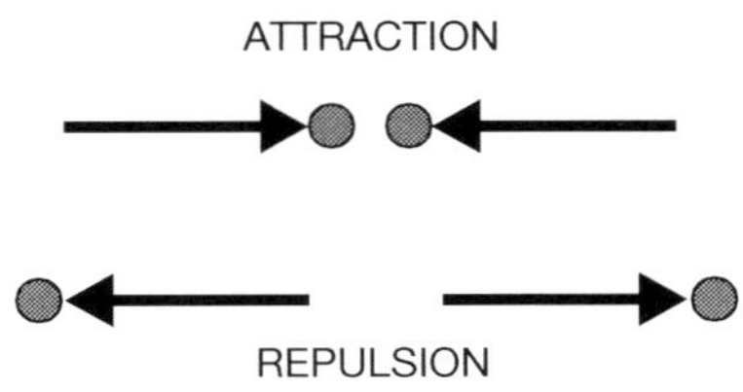

Figure 13.3 Simple forces of attraction and repulsion: force vectors lie on a line connecting the material points.

took the following more revealing form: Explanation of everything must be by means of unalterable things, viz., *substances*, and the simple forces acting between them (Einstein & Infeld, 1938/1966). *Substance ontology* was (and is) the grounding of the mechanical view.

The caloric theory of heat was a prime example. The caloric, like other hypothesized elementary substances, was presumed to consist of unalterable, indestructible atoms. These caloric atoms differed from ordinary atoms in two ways: They lacked mass[4] and (by hypothesis) interacted with each other through repulsive rather than attractive forces. They were presumed, however, to be attracted to ordinary atoms. On the caloric theory, the warming of a cold solid was interpreted as the adding of caloric atoms to the ordinary atoms of the solid. The added caloric atoms, it was argued, attach themselves to the ordinary atoms reducing thereby the forces that attract ordinary atoms to each other. The result is expansion of the solid on heating and the eventual melting of the solid to liquid. With sufficient adding of caloric, the repulsive forces between caloric atoms come to dominate fully the attractive forces between ordinary atoms. Thus, liquids boil to become gases and the strength of the dispersion of the ordinary atoms is realized as pressure on the walls of a container housing the ordinary atoms. Patently, an explanation in terms of two substances and simple forces acting between them is potentially capable of accommodating many heat phenomena.

A similar case could be made for electricity and the phenomena of electrostatics. Like heat and light under the mechanical view, electricity was regarded as a *subtle fluid*—a substance that could move unimpeded through the interstices of solid objects. In fact, electricity was regarded as two kinds of subtle fluids, one called "positive" and one called "negative." Oppositely signed electric fluids were assumed to attract and same-signed electric fluids were assumed to repulse. Rubbing an ebonite rod with fur or flannel seemed to have the twofold effect of separating the fluids and adding to the rod's negative fluid. Figure 13.4 (b and c) shows that the negatively charged ebonite rod located near one end of the bar attracts the bar's positive fluid and repulses the bar's negative fluid. On removing the rod, the fluids of the metal bar mix because of the attraction of unlike fluids. On touching the bar, the repulsed negative fluid escapes. A different outcome is expected if the rod is permitted to contact the metal bar (see Figure 13.4a). Now some of the excess negative fluid is transferred to the metal bar that retains this added fluid (given the good conditions of insulation) following removal of the rod. The metal bar, it should be noted, does not get heavier. The added electric fluid brings no additional weight. Unlike ordinary atoms, but similar to caloric atoms, electric atoms have no mass.

Belaboring these examples of the mechanical analysis of material phenomena that typified the 19th century has been for a purpose. It allows us to appreciate that the mechanical view could be consistently carried out, but only by inventing novel massless substances—new kinds of material agents

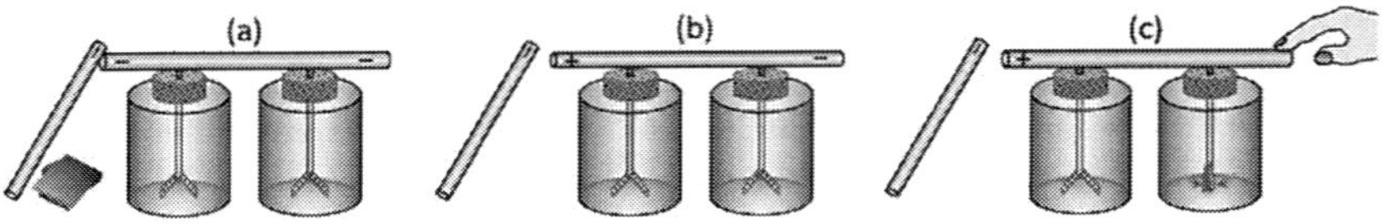

Figure 13.4 The 19th-century theory of two electric fluids (substances). (a) An ebonite rod rubbed with a cloth gains an excess of negative electrical substance and transfers at contact some of the excess to a metal bar and, thereby, to the gold leaves of two electroscopes connected to the bar. The leaves separate because they are of like fluid. If the rod is removed, the leaves stay apart; the excess fluid is retained. (b) A rubbed ebonite rod proximate to the bar attracts the positive fluid in the bar and repels the negative fluid. On removal of the rod, the fluids mix and the leaves of both electroscopes return to their normal downward orientation. (c) If in the latter situation the bar is touched, the negative fluid escapes leaving only the positive fluid at the end proximate to the rod.

with their own special material properties. Einstein and Infeld (1938/1966) summarized the state of affairs thusly:

> In the attempt to understand the phenomena of nature from the mechanical point of view, throughout the whole development of science up to the twentieth century, it was necessary to introduce artificial substances like electric and magnetic fluids, light corpuscles, or ether. (p. 120)

To belabor the lesson further, what is brought out by the analysis of light is the sheer multiplicity of substances if light is viewed mechanically in terms of corpuscles and the sheer complexity of the single substance *ether* if light is viewed mechanically in terms of waves. In the corpuscular theory, each color behaves as an unchangeable substance. To explain light's properties requires as many substances as colors. If, to the contrary, light is a wave, and colors are the component frequencies of that wave, then light is a transfer of energy, not a transfer of substances. However, for this energy transfer to occur, for the light wave to travel, a transparent air-like or water-like substance that lacks mass must pervade the vacuum between luminous and illuminated bodies. Waves cannot exist separate from material media in which they can vibrate. A primary challenge of the hypothesized ubiquitous substance, the ether, was to understand how it could be constructed mechanically in terms of simple forces acting between its constituent particles. The ether's properties seemed extraordinary and contradictory. For example, the ether had to be sufficiently rigid to transmit the extremely rapid vibrations of light and, at the same time, sufficiently rarefied as not to impede the motions of planets. Further, the simpler interpretation of the ether as air-like transmitting longitudinal waves could not be sustained in the face of evidence that light is a transverse wave. To transmit transverse waves, the ether would have to be more jellylike than airlike and, therefore, considerably more complicated in construction.[5] All the issues pertaining to the mechanical perspective articulated by Helmholtz came to a point in the ether. The eventual failure to provide a sensible, mechanically consistent model of the ether and the failure to detect the ether in experiments were of major consequence. Einstein and Infeld (1938/1966) drew the following conclusion:

> Science did not succeed in carrying out the mechanical program convincingly, and today no physicist believes in the possibility of its fulfilment.
>
> (p. 121)

In later lectures, we will need to appreciate the demands placed upon a replacement for the mechanical view.

13.6 Mechanistic Order

In summary, the notion that the order in living things and the universe at large is mechanistic is the notion that order arises from material parts that are: (i) independent and unalterable, (ii) specified uniquely by their properties, and (iii) superposable in indefinitely many ways. Said differently, mechanistic order is the summed quantitative changes in a small number of basic entities that themselves never change qualitatively (Bohm, 1958).

Notes

1 The neuron doctrine represents nerve cells as polarized structures that contact each other at specialized (synaptic) junctions and form the developmental, functional, structural and trophic units of nervous systems. See Guillery (2005) for a contemporary view.

2 The most useful general definition of *topography* for present purposes is that it refers to the physical and natural features of a region or object and their structural relations.

3 Discussion of enhanced understanding at the price of picture-ability is to be found in Hanson (1969) and March and Freeman (1963).

4 Lavoisier and Laplace showed this toward the end of the 18th century by burning chemicals such as carbon and phosphorous in sealed containers. The reactions produced large quantities of heat that escaped the containers and chemical products that remained in the containers. If caloric atoms had mass, then their escape from the containers should have lowered the masses of the containers. To the contrary, the masses of the sealed containers were unchanged. This absence of mass characterized other hypothesized substances, referred to collectively as "imponderables" (Cassirer, 1950, p. 94).

5 Stokes in the 1840s observed that glue and water together form a stiff jelly with the contrasting properties of acting like a solid for rapid repetitive motions but

providing limited resistance to a slowly translating object (Schaffner, 1972). An analogous jellylike ether might transmit light at 186,000 miles per second and simultaneously allow the planets easy travel on their orbital paths at 3 miles per second (Zajonc, 1993).

References

Bohm, D. (1958). *Causality and chance in modern physics*. New York: Harper.

Boring, E. G. (1950). *A history of experimental psychology*. New York: Appleton-Century-Crofts.

Cassirer, E. (1950). *The problem of knowledge*. New Haven, CT: Yale University Press.

Cottingham, J., Stoothoff, R., & Murdoch, D. (1985). *The philosophical writings of Descartes*. Cambridge, UK: Cambridge University Press.

Eddington, A. (1958). *The nature of the physical world*. Ann Arbor: University of Michigan Press (original work published 1928).

Einstein, A., & Infeld, L. (1966). *The evolution of physics*. New York: Simon & Schuster (original work published 1938).

Guillery, R. W. (2005). Observations of synaptic structures: Origins of the neuron doctrine and its current status. *Philosophical Transactions of the Royal Society B*, *360*, 1281–1307.

Hanson, N. R. (1969). *Patterns of discovery*. Cambridge, UK: Cambridge University Press.

Hobbes, T. (1968). *Leviathan*. London: Penguin Books (original work published 1651).

Kant, I. (1998). *Critique of pure reason*. (P. Guyer & A. Wood, Trans. and Eds.), Cambridge, UK: Cambridge University Press (original work published 11781/1787).

Köhler, W., & Wallach, H. (1944). Figural after-effects: An investigation of visual processes. *Proceedings of the Philosophical Society of America*, *88*, 269–357.

Krieger, M. H. (1992). *Doing physics: How physicists take hold of the world*. Bloomington: Indiana University Press.

March, A., & Freeman, I. M. (1963). *The new world of physics*. New York: Vintage Books.

Pastore, N. (1971). *Selective history of theories of visual perception, 1650–1950*. Oxford, UK: Oxford University Press.

Rosen, R. (1991). *Life itself*. New York: Columbia University Press.

Rosen, R. (1988). The epistemology of complexity. In J. A. S. Kelso, A. J. Mandell, & M. F. Shlesinger (Eds.), *Dynamic patterns in complex systems* (pp. 7–29). Singapore: World Scientific.

Rosen, R. (2000). *Essays on life itself*. New York: Columbia University Press.

Russell, B. (1903). *Principles of mathematics*. Cambridge, UK: Cambridge University Press.

Schaffner, K. (1972). *Nineteenth century aether theories*. Oxford, UK: Pergamon Press.

Stokes, G. (1972). On the aberration of light. In K. F. Schaffner (Ed.), *Nineteenth-century Aether theories* (pp. 136–143). New York: Pergamon Press (original work published 1848).

Zajonc, A. (1993). *Catching the light*. New York: Bantam Books.

Lecture 14

Gestalt Theory II: Fields, Self-organization, and the Invariance Postulate of Evolution

In Lecture 13 our focus was on the reasons that the scientific investigation of perception would be drawn to the claim that the whole (any given system, inanimate or animate) is no more than the sum of its parts, the sum of its substances. We confronted Descartes' machine metaphor and its offshoots—mechanism and mechanistic order. In the present lecture, our focus is on the reasons that the scientific investigation of perception might be drawn to a different claim: The whole is *different* from the sum of its parts. The latter phrase would be the clarion call of Gestalt[1] theory and is very much the source of the adopted use of the word *gestalt* in English. Gestalt is German for form or shape and, more broadly, manner or even essence (Boring, 1950, p. 588). In English usage, "gestalt" means "organized whole." The clarion call just noted is for scientific emphasis upon the wholes rather than the parts. This emphasis in Gestalt Theory was made manifest as a concern for (a) fields and field theory, (b) emergent properties, and, most broadly (c) the commonality of principles governing order in living and behavioral things. Quite specifically, these are the concerns of the present lecture.

14.1 Faraday's Lines of Force, Maxwell's Fields

Let us revisit the notion of action at a distance (Lecture 3), this time with the specific examples provided by electricity and magnetism. Looking at Figure 14.1, the question is that of how a force can act between two electric charges or two magnets separated by apparently empty space. The answer given by Faraday (1791–1867) and Maxwell (1831–1879) was that an electric charge or magnetic pole produces in its vicinity an electric field or magnetic field, respectively. This invisible field, diffusing outward in the space surrounding the charge, is inferred from the action that it has on other electric charges or magnetic poles that come into contact with it. The action, therefore, is that of local contact, between one charge and the field of another charge or one pole and the field of another pole.

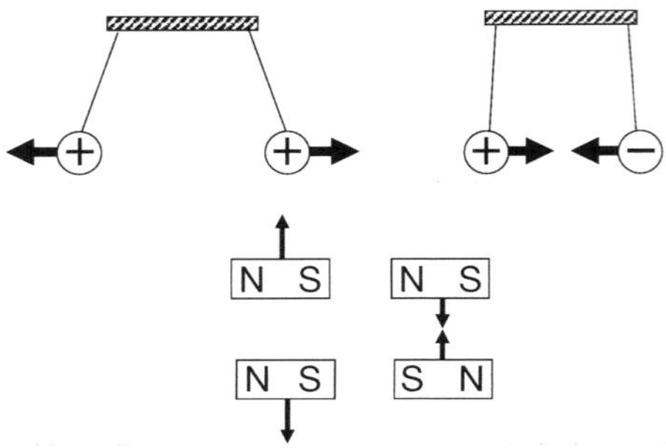

Figure 14.1 Action-at-a-distance in electricity (*top*) and magnetism (*bottom*; where N is north and S is south). Like charges (e.g., both positive) on suspended spheres push them apart, unlike charges pull them together. Like magnetic poles of metal bars repel, unlike magnetic poles attract. Action-at-a-distance in both cases diminishes as the inverse square of the distance between the objects.

One of our intents in this lecture, as noted, is to lay hold of the important concept of *field*. It plays a key role in Gestaltism. Köhler (1947, 1969) argued for neural brain fields in accounts of perception. Koffka (1935/1999) claimed that human acts were to be understood in terms of a behavioral field. And in the domain of social psychology Lewin (1936) introduced the conception of a life-space as a field within which the individual lives and strives. Additionally, as we will come to see in later lectures, the concept of field plays a prominent role in contemporary thinking about how to define the optical support for knowing about one's surrounding through vision. In terms of our immediate concern with the development of ideas that shaped Gestalt Theory, the emergence in the 19th century of classical field theory through the work of Michael Faraday and James Clerk Maxwell was a major departure from the mechanical point of view. The cornerstones of the mechanical view—unalterable objects (substances, mechanical units) and simple forces (acting along a line and dependent only on distance)—were not the cornerstones on which Faraday and Maxwell built the field perspective.

The philosophical antecedents are worthy of our consideration, if only briefly. Of most direct significance are the conceptualizations of Kant and Schelling (Berkson, 1974; Cassirer, 1950; Williams, 1966). In *Critique of Pure Reason*, Kant (1781/1787/1998) amplified the causal entailment of Newton's mechanics (Lectures 2 and 3). His thesis was that the relation among the members of a sequence must be known in addition to the sequence—a desideratum that inheres in Figure 3.4. Kant advocated looking to the form and structure of processes and not solely to the transitions of state. In *Metaphysical Foundations of Natural Science*, Kant (1786/2004) reduced reality to two opposing forces—namely, attraction and repulsion—that fill all of space. In place of corpuscles carrying force, he envisaged a continuum of force through which light and gravitation are propagated. Kant's ideas were the departure point for Schelling (1799/2004). He saw a binary opposition (Lecture 2), a polarity, of attractive and repulsive forces as the foundation of all physical phenomena and dismissed explanations that required the invention of new imponderable substances (Lecture 13). For Schelling, the indefinitely many physical phenomena constituting the world are simply manifestations of the basic forces in different contexts. This important thesis was a major tenet of the influential movement referred to as *nature philosophy*. If the right experimental conditions could be identified, then it should be possible to convert any one manifestation of force (light, heat, electricity, magnetism, gravitation) into any other (Williams, 1866/1989). The mechanical view, with its emphasis on separate fluids of distinct entities, did not give reason for thinking in such terms. There were no theoretical grounds for expecting that corpuscles of light, caloric, positive and negative electricity, north and south magnetism should be convertible, one into the other.

In the spirit of nature philosophy, Faraday entertained the hypothesis that all physical properties were the result of forces (how they configured under this or that set of constraints) and that the corpuscles were best understood as the geometrical foci or centers of those forces. He favored a force-ontology over a substance-ontology. Figure 14.2 introduces us to his intuition that the image of how iron filings are configured on a sheet of paper by an underlying magnet was an archetypal image. Perhaps the universe was densely filled with such *lines of force*. If so, then any given object does not react to a distant force but, rather, it reacts to the strength of the lines of force at its location. There is only nearby action (Lecture 4). The answer to the question above of how a force can act attractively or repulsively in empty space (between charged

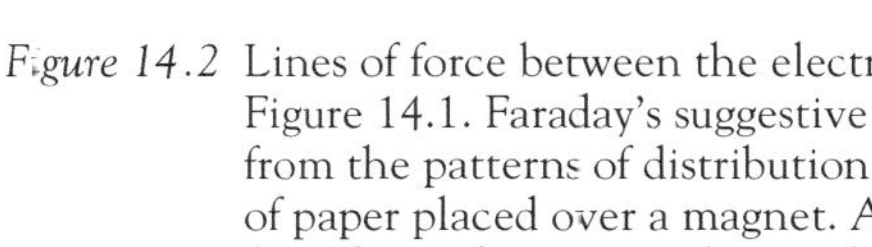

Figure 14.2 Lines of force between the electric charges depicted in the upper panel of Figure 14.1. Faraday's suggestive picture of lines of force was developed from the patterns of distribution assumed freely by iron filings on a sheet of paper placed over a magnet. At each point along its length a line of force has a direction—that is, there is a vector at each point (suggested by the arrows) so the lines of force are an example of what is mathematically a vector field. Faraday envisaged the lines as having a tension along their lengths and a mutual sidewise repulsion.

pith balls and magnets, Figure 14.1) can be framed in terms of the lines of force of Figure 14.2 and their dependence on circumstance (e.g., like charges versus unlike charges).

The patterns made by the lines of force in Figure 14.2 are clearly complicated even for the relatively simple physical case that they are meant to represent (the two electrically charged and suspended pith balls of Figure 14.1). There is much that is evident from inspection of these patterns. First, the lines of force evolve, changing direction from one point to the next in the space around the charges. Second, the lines of force splay, diverging from or converging to a charged location. Third, the lines of force curve, curling gradually toward, or away from, a charged location. Fourth, the lines of force spread, decreasing gradually in proximity to each other with increasing distance from a charged location. Quantification of the patterns of Faraday's lines of force requires mathematical tools that can systematize these qualitative features of direction, directional change, divergence, curl and gradient. This quantification spawned Maxwell's equations, a universal means to specify how electric and magnetic fields are generated and modulated by each other and by charges and currents.

14.2 Order Arises from Dynamics, not Anatomy

Figure 14.3 is a classic set of diagrams that evince invariable experiences among observers. In each case, they are intended to elucidate primacy of the whole[2] pictorial arrangement as opposed to its parts.[3] When considered in light of the constancy hypothesis (portrayed in Figure 11.4), they suggest that perceptual order is not *anatomical order* derivative of isolated conduction and the machine metaphor but *dynamical order* pursuant to general principles. In the terminology introduced in Lecture 13, the perceptions fostered by the line and dot patterns of Figure 14.3 are suggestive of interaction-dominant dynamics as opposed to component-dominant dynamics. And they are suggestive of the field-like phenomena of Faraday and Maxwell. As Köhler (1925) remarked (cited by Stadler & Kruse, 1990):

> The somatic processes underlying static visual fields are stationary equilibrium distributions developed from the inner dynamics of the optical system itself.
>
> (p. 32)

Within the field-theoretic perspective, one might say that the interaction-dominant dynamics of the optical system realizes a homogeneous conductor of bioelectric forces (Nunez, & Srinivasan, 2006; Stadler & Kruse, 1990).

Explanation by reference to anatomy (i.e., components) and explanation by reference to dynamics can invite two very different forms of reductionist argument. Reasonable labels are *morphological* and *strategic*.

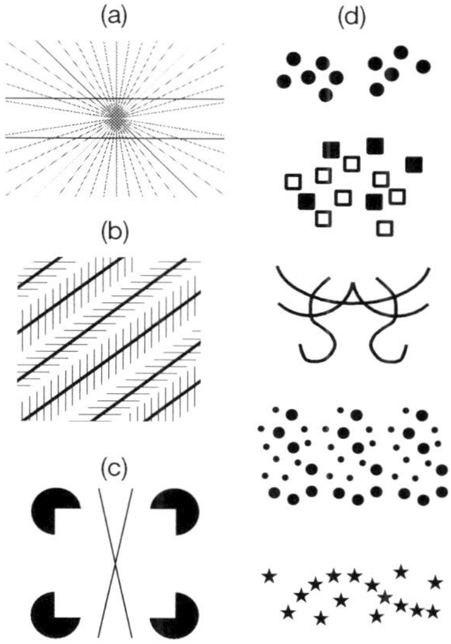

Figure 14.3 Field, not atomisms: (a) Wundt–Herring illusion; (b) Zolner illusion; (c) whole different from sum of its parts. (d) *Pragnanz*: evolution to greatest simplicity in terms of, from top to bottom, proximity, similarity, symmetry, periodicity, good continuation

Morphological (classical) reductionism (Figure 14.4a) entails levels of components that differ in their basicness, with the lowest level the most basic level. Each level is a particular morphology, a class of property types and interaction kinds specific to the property types. The reduction, therefore, is from the property types and interaction kinds at one scale to the property types and interaction kinds at a putatively more basic scale.

Strategic (or methodological) reductionism (Figure 14.4b) entails a common, single set of physical principles or strategies that apply with equanimity to each level (each of Nature's length and time scales). These common strategies produce event regularities and morphological objects that are oftentimes unique to the scale (Iberall, 1977; Soodak & Iberall, 1987; Yates, Marsh & Iberall, 1972). Where these strategies have been identified by physics they constitute, in principle, a repertoire of methods by means of which nature, at any scale, can be investigated. For example, Haken's *Synergetics* (Haken, 1983, 1990) and Iberall's *Homeokinetics* (Soodak & Iberall, 1987; Yates, 2008).

The two kinds of explanations and the two kinds of reductionism associated with them were foreshadowed in Kant's argument in *The Critique of Judgment* (1790/2000, Sections 64–66) that an organism is not a machine. His grounds essentially were those of self-construction. Machines neither produce nor reproduce themselves. Kant's machine-organism distinction is

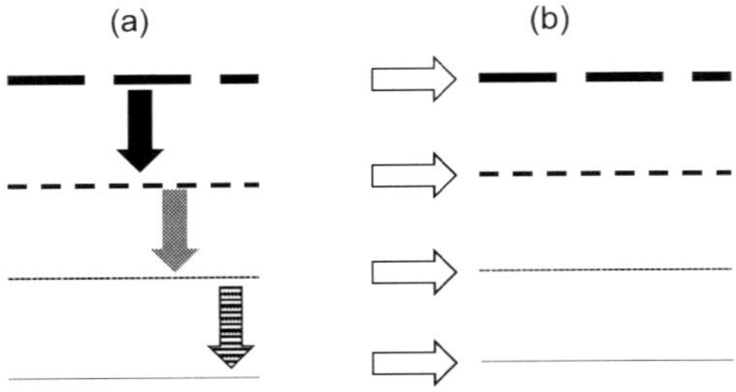

Figure 14.4 (a) *Morphological reductionism*: reduction to forms of a more fundamental, privileged level. (b) *Strategic reductionism*: a common set of physical strategies; no privileged level; level-specific phenomena (regularities).

elaborated in the following paraphrase of his argument. The elegant simplicity of the argument has to be admired.

For any given thing recognized as a machine, for example, a clock or an airplane, the following characteristics seem to hold:

1 The parts of the thing exist for, but not by means of, each other.
2 The parts act together to meet the thing's purpose; their actions, however, have nothing to do with the thing's construction.
3 The thing and its parts rely upon efficient causes arising from outside themselves for their origin and function.

For any given thing that we recognize as an organism, for example, a fly or a tree, the following characteristics seem to hold:

1 The parts of the thing are both causes and effects of the thing; they are not only the means but also the ends.
2 The parts construct and maintain themselves as a unity, each existing by virtue of, and for the sake of, the others and the whole.
3 The thing and its parts are themselves the source of the efficient causes for their origin and function.

It is this self-causing nature of living things that led Kant to describe them as having "natural ends" or Aristotelian final causes and "inner purposefulness," and as such requiring teleological explanation.[4]

14.3 Invariance Postulate of Evolution

Empiricists emphasize constraints from personal history. Nativists emphasize constraints from species history. *Gestaltists emphasize laws invariant to histories.*

The Gestalt perspective on the scientific challenges posed by perception was guided by what Köhler (1930, 1950) would aptly come to call the *Invariance Postulate of Evolution*—the primacy and continuity of the laws of dynamics. When spelled out, the postulate is that all biological facts and events are understandable in terms of the laws and principles responsible for the facts and events in the inanimate world (Köhler, 1969). The postulate is grounding for Section 14.2, the claim that the order in perception arises from the brain's dynamics, not its anatomy. The following two quotations bring the invariance postulate into sharper relief:

> This must suffice as an extremely abbreviated and rough description of what physics and the principle of evolution permit or do not permit the evolutionist to postulate. *No new laws, forces, or elementary processes* are to be used in his thinking.
>
> (Köhler, 1969, p. 86, italics added)

> Under no circumstances should we forget that any processes in our brains, including those which go with psychological facts, must, *qua* processes, be realizations of universal dynamic laws, and to this extent be quite unrelated to evolution and inheritance. I repeat, this follows from the principle of evolution itself.
>
> (Köhler, 1969, p. 90)

Given the invariance postulate, the question then arises as to what changes could evolution have wrought? The answer, Köhler (1947, 1969) suggested, can only be this: Evolution must have introduced particular anatomical or topographical constraints. The question and answer reintroduce an issue identified in Lecture 7 (Section 7.6.2): that explanation and understanding of many phenomena of the kind expressive of perception may necessarily require two formally incompatible descriptive modes. For Köhler's question and answer, one mode is the full set of universal dynamic laws. *The other (seemingly) is not.*

A constraint is any condition that limits the motions, reduces the degrees of freedom, of a dynamical system. A constraint can be referred to as hard or soft, integrable or non-integrable, holonomic[5] or non-holonomic. Mathematically, a constraint may be given in terms of one or more algebraic equations that connect coordinates, or in terms of one or more differential equations that restrict coordinates and components of velocities (Goldstein, 1950/1980). The former constraint is typically referred to as geometric, the latter as kinematic. Kinematic constraints, that cannot be integrated, that cannot be reduced to a holonomic constraint, are called (unsurprisingly) nonholonomic—*not wholly by law*.[6]

We should assume that whereas both integrable and non-integrable constraints fall within Köhler's anatomical class, it is the non-integrable that deserve most theoretical attention. This attention must be directed to the physics of the systems to which Gestalt Theory refers—namely, biological systems qua thermodynamic systems. We address each charge in turn, with a synopsis of thermodynamic systems and their implications prefatory to an elaboration of non-integrable constraints.

14.3.1 From Isolated to Open Thermodynamical Systems

Behind the classical interpretation within Gestalt Theory of the patterns experienced in viewing Figure 14.3 is the so-called *principle of final equilibrium* (Köhler, 1947), a stationary dynamics resultant to the physics of systems isolated from energy and matter. Figure 14.5 contrasts *isolated* systems with *closed* and *open* systems. In the parlance of thermodynamics, a non-isolated system is said to be closed if it exchanges energy with its environment, but not matter, and open if it exchanges both energy and matter. Closed and open systems in respect to process are non-linear and irreversible, isolated systems are linear and reversible.[7] Closed and open systems are self-organizing (see Figure 7.2 for *closed*), isolated systems are not. Closed and open systems are both consonant with the *CES* model (Lecture 1) and befitting the thesis and goals of Gestalt Theory, isolated systems are not (as Köhler, 1955, makes clear). Of particular significance is the highly ostensible fact, depicted in Figure 14.5, that living things (e.g., a plant) are open systems.

A key aspect of the dynamics of closed and open systems is the production of entropy—roughly, a reduction in energy "quality," its availability for doing work (e.g., Atkins, 1994). A plant constructs itself from (a) water in the soil embedding its roots and diffused or suspended in the air, (b) carbon dioxide in the air, and (c) solar radiation (see Figure 14.5). The photosynthesis attendant to (c) drives the synthesis of multiple large biomolecules (e.g.,

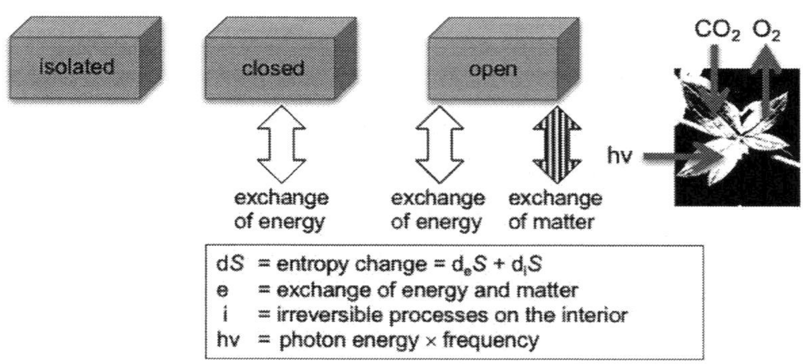

Figure 14.5 Isolated, closed and open thermodynamical systems with the entropy change equation for the open system and a plant as an exemplary example.

glucose, $C_6H_{12}O_6$) from CO_2, H_2O and other small molecules, releasing O_2 in the process. In brief, the plant constructs itself. The means by which it does so comprises a rich network of biochemical reactions driven by affinities,[8] where a nonzero affinity implies thermodynamic disequilibrium requiring continuation of chemical reactions until thermodynamic equilibrium is attained (Kondepudi, 2008). The loss of Gibbs free energy with each reaction is an entropy-generating irreversible process. Hopefully, one can discern from the preceding that an irreversible process ought not to be identified as a progenitor of disorder. Its role, simply put, is constructive: It increases system complexity (Kondepudi & Prigogine, 2007).

14.3.2 On Anatomical Constraints as Non-integrable Constraints

We are now better positioned to evaluate Köhler's anatomical constraints. Their special significance has been cast as follows:

> Evolution requires the genotype–phenotype distinction, a primeval epistemic cut that separates energy-degenerate, rate-independent genetic symbols from the rate-dependent dynamics of construction that they control.
>
> (Pattee, 2001, p. 5)

In these latter terms, anatomical constraints are "rate-independent genetic symbols" and the entropy-producing plant thermodynamics just described are "rate-dependent dynamics of construction." Cast in this manner, the issue at hand is inclusive of (a) the generalized M (mediating) principle encountered in Lecture 3, and (b) the Central Dogma introduced in Lecture 12 and characterized in Figure 12.2.

The *control* referred to in the quotation has a converse: *measurement*, interpreted as the coding of a rate-dependent dynamical state into static symbols (Pattee, 2001). For the issue at hand, the examination of this measurement-dynamics relation by von Neumann (1955, p. 352) is a pedagogically valuable exercise. It illuminates the general problem.

Designate the measured system and the measuring system as σ and μ, respectively. Let μ's task be provision of the initial conditions for σ's dynamic laws, answering the question "What is σ's current state?" μ is a non-integrable constraint. It is also, by definition, a physical system abiding the same laws as σ. In principle, therefore, σ and μ can be combined into the larger system $\sigma + \mu$. To apply the laws of dynamics to this larger system requires a measure of its initial conditions. Another μ system is mandated. An infinite regress is implied.

The option of describing μ in detail through the universal laws is not open. To take the option would mean the loss of μ's function as a measuring device. This is so, as Pattee (2001, 2005) highlights, because laws *cannot express the pragmatic function of measurement* despite their evident capability to describe μ's dynamics in full. The same argument can be made for control, such as the presumed genetic control of protein construction. Let C be non-integrable control constraints. To include them within the larger system C + σ would mean the loss of C's function as a controller because laws *cannot express the pragmatic function of control.*

On elaboration (Pattee, 2001), von Neumann's (1955) argument suggests that the genotype–phenotype distinction is a necessity of the evolutionary process. It is a primeval solution to the problem of constraining and monitoring the self-ordering thermodynamic processes (e.g., those of the Belousov–Zhabotinsky reaction, those of plant growth) in innumerably specific ways, sufficient to encompass the wide variety of phyletic forms, and more. It is an "epistemic cut" that separates inert genetic symbols from the rate-dependent entropy-producing dynamics of construction.[9]

In sum, one interpretation of Köhler's anatomical constraints is that they are non-integrable constraints that satisfy a necessary condition for bridging the epistemic cut when measurement, control, and coding are called for. Pattee (2001) muses:

> Is it not plausible that life was first distinguished from non-living matter . . . by local and unique heteropolymer constraints[10] that exhibit detailed behavior unlike the behavior of any other known forms of matter in the universe?
>
> (p. 19)

14.3.3 Coda

We should not depart this lecture without the observation that the epistemic implications of the Central Dogma are at odds with the primary lessons of Lecture 12 (e.g., probabilistic epigenesis). They are also at odds, but in a much less self-evident way, with the primary conception introduced in Lecture 3, that of informationL. By the latter, the "bridge" between organism as "observer" ("measurer," "controller") and environment as "observed" ("measured," "controlled") is fundamentally a matter of lawfulness at nature's ecological scale. To detect informationL is to perceive the behavioral-relevant dimensions ("measures") of environment and body and the strategies ("controls") for relating environment and body in the satisfaction of intents. At some juncture, we might expect to entertain the possibility that a generalization of informationL applies to genes and proteins.[11]

Notes

1 This term was introduced into psychology and science in general with the essay "On gestalt qualities" by Christian von Ehrenfels in 1890 (reproduced in English in Smith, 1988).

2 Einstein recognized the challenges posed by the concept of "whole." In a Foreword to a book of Wertheimer's essays, he wrote, "Behind these essays lies above all an epistemological requirement which derives from the gestalt–psychological point of view: beware trying to understand the whole by arbitrary isolation of the separate components or by hazy or forced abstractions (see Miller, 1975, p. 75)."
3 Maxwell (1873) observed that Faraday's method was contrary. It began with a whole and proceeded to discern the parts by analysis. The standard method was to begin with the parts and to fashion a whole by synthesis.
4 Kant's intuitions are given a fuller expression in the arguments of Rosen (1991, 2000).
5 From the Greek ὅλος meaning whole and νόμ-ος meaning law.
6 For one who has not encountered the challenges constraints pose to applying the laws of mechanics, pages 11–16 in Goldstein (1950/1980) are an eye-opener.
7 Reversibility is possible only in the limit of infinite slowness. The closer to perfect reversibility, the closer to zero is the speed of the process. Planck (1917/1969, pp. 85–86) remarked: "Whether reversible processes exist in nature or not, is not a priori evident or demonstrable."
8 Affinity is the driving thermodynamic force, the difference in the Gibbs energy of the reactants and the products. For elaboration on the concept of affinity, see Kondepudi & Prigogine, 2007, Chapter 4.
9 For Pattee, this epistemic necessity does not imply ontological dualism. One should expect it to be manifest in any circumstance in which a distinction must be made between a subject and an object, a symbol and its referent.
10 A heteropolymer is a compound formed from subunits that are not all the same, such as a protein composed of various amino acid subunits.
11 We will do so in Lecture 19 when considering the immune system.

References

Atkins, P. W. (1994). *The 2nd law: Energy, chaos, and form*. New York: Scientific American Books (original work published 1984).

Berkson, W. (1974). *Fields of force: The development of a worldview from Faraday to Einstein*. New York: Halsted Press.

Boring, E. G. (1950). *A history of experimental psychology*. New York: Appleton-Century-Crofts.

Cassirer, E. (1950). *The problem of knowledge: Philosophy science, and history since Hegel*. New Haven, CT: Yale university Press.

Einstein, A., & Infeld, L. (1966). *The evolution of physics* New York: Simon & Schuster (original work published 1938).

Faraday, M. (1991). *Experimental researches in chemistry and physics*. London: Taylor & Francis (original work published 1859).

Goldstein, H. (1980). *Classical mechanics*. Reading, MA: Addison Wesley (original work published 1950).

Haken, H. (1977). *Synergetics: An introduction*. Berlin, Germany: Springer-Verlag.

Haken, H. (1983). *Advanced synergetics*. Berlin, Germany: Springer-Verlag.

Haken, H. (1990). Synergetics as a tool for the conceptualization and mathematization of cognition and behaviour—How far can we go? In H. Haken & M. Stadler (Eds.), *Synergetics of cognition* (pp. 2–31). Berlin, Germany: Springer-Verlag.

Iberall, A. S. (1977). A field and circuit thermodynamics for integrative physiology: I. Introduction to the general notions. *American Journal of Physiology/Regulatory, Integrative, Comparative Physiology*, 2, R171–R180.

Kant, I. (1998). *Critique of pure reason*. (P. Guyer & A. Wood, Trans. and Eds.), Cambridge, UK: Cambridge University Press (original work published 1781/1787).

Kant, I. (2000). *The critique of judgment*. Amherst, NY: Prometheus Books (original work published 1790).

Kant, I. (2004). *Metaphysical foundations of natural science*. Cambridge, UK: Cambridge University Press (original work published 1786).

Koffka, K. (1999). *Principles of Gestalt psychology*. London: Routledge (original work published 1935).

Köhler, W. (1930). The new psychology and physics. *Yale Review, 19*, 560–576.

Köhler, W. (1947). *Gestalt psychology*. New York: Mentor Books.

Köhler, W. (1950). Psychology and evolution. *Acta Psychologica, 7*, 288–297.

Köhler, W. (1955). Direction of processes in living systems. *The Scientific Monthly, 80*, 29–32.

Köhler, W. (1969). *The task of gestalt psychology*. Princeton, NJ: Princeton University Press.

Kondepudi, D. (2008). *Introduction to modern thermodynamics*. Chichester, UK: Wiley.

Kondepudi, D., & Prigogine, I. (2007). Modern thermodynamics: From heat engines to dissipative structures. Chichester, UK: Wiley.

Lewin, K. (1936). *A dynamic theory of personality*. New York: McGraw-Hill.

Maxwell, J. C. (1873). *A treatise on electricity and magnetism, Vol. 1* (pp. x–xi). Oxford, UK: Clarendon Press.

Miller, A. L. (1975). Albert Einstein and Max Wertheimer: A gestalt psychologist's view of the genesis of special relativity theory. *History of Science, 13*, 75–103.

Nunez, P. L., & Srinivasan, R. (2006). *Electric fields of the brain: The neurophysics of EEG*. Oxford, UK: Oxford University Press.

Pattee, H. H. (2001). The physics of symbols: Bridging the epistemic cut. *BioSystems, 60*, 5–21.

Pattee, H. H. (2005). The physics and metaphysics of biosemiotics. *Journal of Biosemiotics, 1*, 223–238.

Planck, M. (1969). *Treatise on thermodynamics*. New York: Dover Publications (original work published 1917).

Rosen, R. (1991). *Life itself*. New York: Columbia University Press.

Rosen, R. (2000). *Essays on life itself*. New York: Columbia University Press.

Schelling, F. W. J. (2004). *First outlines of a system of the philosophy of nature*. (K. R. Peterson, Trans.). Albany, NY: SUNY Press (original work published 1799).

Soodak, H., & Iberall, A. (1987). Thermodynamics and complex systems. In F. E. Yates (Ed.), *Self-organizing systems: The emergence of order* (pp. 460–469). New York: Plenum Press.

Stadler, M., & Kruse, P. (1990). The self-organization perspective in cognition research: Historical remarks and new experimental approaches. In H. Haken & M. Stadler (Eds.), *Synergetics of cognition* (pp. 32–52). Berlin, Germany: Springer-Verlag.

Turvey, M. T. (2004). Space (and its perception): The first and final frontier. *Ecological Psychology, 16*, 25–29.

von Ehrenfels, C. (1988). On gestalt qualities. In Smith, B. (Ed.) *Foundations of gestalt theory*. Munich, Germany: Philosophia Verlag GmbH (original work published 1890).

von Neumann, J., (1955). *The mathematical foundations of quantum mechanics*. Princeton, NJ: Princeton University Press.

Williams, L. P. (1989). *The origins of field theory*. New York: Random House. (original work published 1866).

Yates, F. E. (2008). Homeokinetics/homeodynamics: A physical heuristic for life and complexity. *Ecological Psychology*, *20*, 148–179.

Yates, F. E., Marsh, D. J., & Iberall, A. S. (1972). Integration of the whole organism: A foundation for a theoretical biology. In J. A. Behnke (Ed.), *Challenging biological problems: Directions toward their solutions* (pp. 110–132). New York: Oxford University Press.

Lecture 15

Gestalt Theory III: Experience Error, CNS Error, Psycho-neural Isomorphism, Behavioral Environment

Lectures 13 and 14 on the nature of Gestalt theory were necessarily lengthy and detailed. We needed to appreciate the origin of the theory in the burgeoning physics and philosophical rethinking at the cusp of the 18th and 19th centuries. And we needed to gain appreciation for the degree to which Gestalt theory, in its developing and mature (*c.* 1950s) forms, differed from the Establishment perspective on perception and on its relation to physical and biological sciences. This lecture is considerably shorter than Lectures 13 and 14. Its concerns are the themes of Gestaltism that have come to portray the theory in the field of psychology.

Figure 15.1 is Gestaltism's radical revision of the conventional man in the inner room (of a mobile home). It allows us to see fairly immediately where Gestaltism stands in relation to the theoretical perspectives covered in prior lectures. The absence of "man" and the absence of "TV screen" make evident the non-inferential nature of Gestaltism. They bring to the forefront the challenge of formulating the sense in which a psychological state (e.g., perceived cylinder) can be isomorphic with a physical state (cylinder). In Figure 15.1, the second grade of sense is depicted as a heterogeneous array of point activities and the third grade of sense is depicted as a molar brain state—self-organized from the point activities—that does not exhibit any obvious resemblance to the distal cylinder. Lecture 15 is a conceptual unpacking of Figure 15.1.

15.1 Why Do Things Look as they Do?

Gestalt psychology warned against the *experience error* (e.g., Köhler, 1947, p. 95; see Pastore, 1971): attributing the organization of perceptual experience to the proximal stimulus when it should be attributed to the organizing tendencies of the nervous system. Simply, it is an error that arises when the result of organization is mistaken for the cause of organization (Koffka, 1935/1999).[1]

The error's context is the question of "Why do things look as they do?" (Koffka, 1935). Three possible answers can be given:

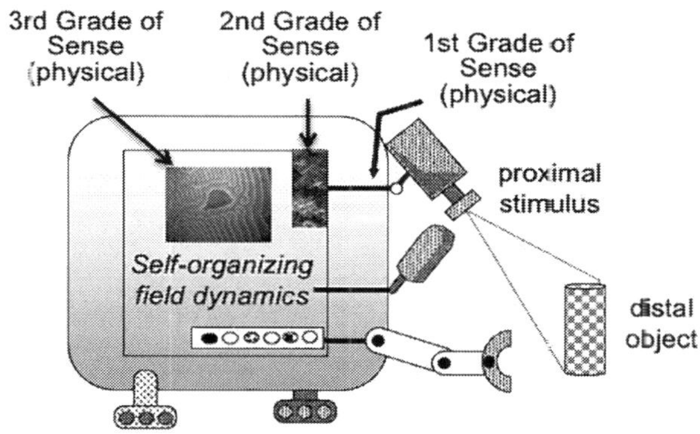

Figure 15.1 "The man in the inner room according to Gestalt theory." Field dynamics of inner room impose a molar spatio-temporal organization on unorganized punctate stimulation. There is no TV screen. There is no "man."

(From Figure 1 in Turvey, 2004, adapted with permission, *Ecological Psychology*.)

1 Because the distal objects are what they are.
2 Because the proximal stimuli are what they are.
3 Because the brain processes are what they are.

To avoid the experience error is to reject possible answers (1) and (2), which amounts to a rejection of realism through the creation of an unbridgeable gap between perceiver and environment. In the present lecture, we will pursue the counter to the experience error suggested by (3): the *CNS error*—attributing the orderliness of perceptual experience to the organizing tendencies of the central nervous system when it should be attributed to informationL's specificity to the environment, to the organism, and to the environment–organism relation (see Lecture 3). Substituting CNS error for experience error brings explanatory challenges that are, technically speaking, not minor, as the celebrated phi-phenomenon makes apparent.

15.2 The Whole is Prior to its Parts: Movement is Movement

Max Wertheimer's pre-eminent discovery can be prefaced in the following manner (after King & Wertheimer,[2] 2005, p. 101). Ehrenfels viewed the whole as *more* than the sum of its parts. It equals the sum of its parts *plus* another element, the Gestalt quality. Wertheimer, in contrast, viewed the whole as entirely *different* from the sum of its parts. It is *prior to* the parts. A whole is an integrated system with an inherent structure of its own that determines the nature of its parts.

Wertheimer investigated apparent movement between two stationary, separately presented geometric figures (two lines or two curves) situated some distance apart in the observer's frontal plane. His pre-eminent discovery (Wertheimer, 1912) was that, for particular conditions of presentation, the observer experienced "pure movement" that connected the two figures but was not in itself a figure. Movement was seen without seeing anything that moved. It was seemingly evidence that motion as such is a fundamental dimension of experience independent of sensations of successive locations. In this latter sense, it is prior to its parts.

Wertheimer labeled this discovery the "phi phenomenon." It is manifest when conditions closely approximate fast alternation with both figures visible simultaneously (Steinman, Pizlo, & Pizlo, 2000). Boring (1942) summarized the discovery and highlighted its historical significance in these words:

> Wertheimer pointed out—essentially—that this finding shows that movement is movement . . . He insisted on the validity of movement as an immediate experience without reference to basic constituents, on the "giveness" of ϕ and its irreducibility to terms of space and time. Out of such an intransigent phenomenology arose Gestalt psychology.
>
> (pp. 595–596)

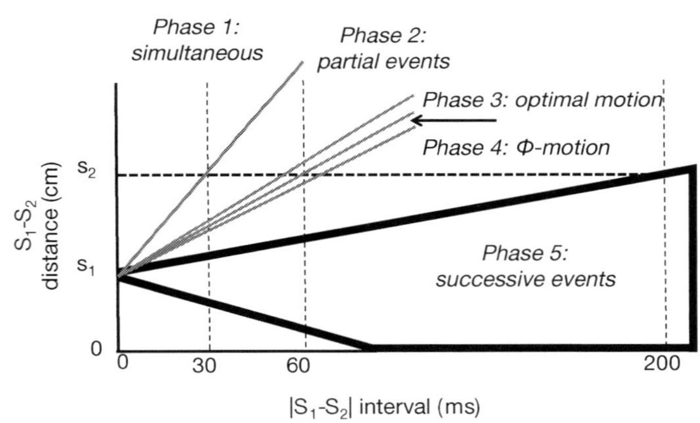

Figure 15.2 A *Minkowskian-like geometry for* ϕ. The five perceptions of two stationary and separately presented geometric stimuli (S_1 and S_2) as a function of the time between their individual presentations (the $|S_1$-$S_2|$ interval). Each upward diagonal line expresses a velocity (the presentation rate of S_1 and S_2). The region within bold lines is a region in which the two events cannot interact.

(From Figure 10.24 in Shaw, Flascher, & Mace, 1996, adapted with permission, Elsevier.)

How should the ϕ-phenomenon be understood? It is a phenomenon emergent from the values assigned to (1) the *duration* of figure exposures, (2) the *spatial* separation of the figures, and (3) the *interval* between exposures. It is a phenomenon that likely falls into the class of non-linear dynamics and the systems that exhibit them—a phenomenon that is potentially addressable in terms of an order parameter (alias, collective variable) and one or more control parameters (Haken, 1983; Kelso, 1995). It is, additionally, a phenomenon that invites critical examination of the geometry within which motion and its perception should be formally articulated. Figure 15.2 is motivated by Minkowski space–time event-geometry (Shaw, Flascher & Mace, 1996). It identifies the categorical changes in motion perception with the category boundaries indexed by velocity (the latter obtained by fixing the distance separating two lights and dividing by the time elapsing between their onsets). It suggests how future work on the ϕ-phenomenon might proceed, treating velocity or rate as the control parameter and motion classification as the order parameter.

15.3 Doctrine of Intractable Nonspecificity Motivates the Experience Error

Despite Gestaltism's goal to address perception in the modern lawful physical terms of its era, it did not pursue this goal beyond the brain. The Faraday-Maxwell field perspective was not brought to bear on the challenges posed by the stationary and time-varying light distributions that immerse organisms. Rather, light to the eye was described in the classical Alhazen tradition of Euclidian points (Lecture 4) within the context of organism-environment dualism (Lecture 2). In consequence, Gestalt psychology cleaved to a doctrine of incommensurability of natural kinds qua descriptors—a misfit between the descriptors of the reflecting surfaces of the environment and one's body (commonly termed distal stimuli) and the descriptors of reflected light (commonly termed proximal stimuli) (Fowler & Turvey, 1982; Shaw & Turvey, 1981; Turvey & Shaw, 1979). To quote Koffka (1935/1999):

> for each distant stimulus there exists a practically infinite number of proximal stimuli; thus the "same stimulus" in the distal sense may not be the same stimulus in the proximal sense; as a matter of fact it seldom is. (p. 80)

And to quote Köhler (1925/1947):

> Thus in the reflected light no trace is left of the units which actually exist in the physical world . . . Thus in countless instances sensory organization means a reconstruction of such aspects of physical situations as are lost in the wave messages which impinge upon the retina. (p. 95)

The claim is that the function that maps the layout of environmental surfaces into the light distributions available to the eye is one-to-many and destructive. The function equivocates on the surrounding environment and fails to preserve the relations and properties of its nested surface layout. This time-honored understanding (Lecture 6, Section 6.2) of the distal–proximal relation, termed the *doctrine of intractable nonspecificity* (e.g., Turvey & Shaw, 1979), gives rise to a paradox, as Koffka (1935/1999) recognized:

> And that raises at once the problem: how the enormous richness and variety of our visual behavioral environment can be aroused by such a mere mosaic of light and shade and color. I think, when formulated in these terms, the problem must appear thrilling by the very paradox which it seems to involve. How can such rich effects arise out of such poor causes, for clearly, the "dimensions" of our environmental field are far more numerous than those of the mosaic of stimulation?
>
> (p. 75)

With a few exceptions, the paradox has rarely been met with disapproval, and the severity of the paradox has rarely, if ever, been met with skepticism. Its backdrop is an implicit organism-environment dualism (Lecture 2). In terms of the *CES* model (Lecture 1), the question posed on the origin of "such rich effects" seems to expect an answer strictly in terms of $C(s)$, ignoring $E(s)$ and $S(s)$—that is, in terms of the causal powers of an (evolving) animal's mind or brain. If such is the case, then it is difficult to make a case for the evolution of an adaptive relation between biological visual systems and their environments. On reasonable grounds, it can be assumed that the sine qua non for that adaptive relation is a necessarily specific relation between reflected light distributions and the layout of reflecting surfaces. A *doctrine of necessary specificity* (Lecture 3) is implied diametrically opposed to the commonly accepted (establishment) doctrine of intractable nonspecificity (e.g., Shaw & Turvey, 1981; Turvey & Shaw, 1979).

15.4 Behavioral Environment, Geographical Environment, and the Isomorphism Principle

For Koffka (1935/1999) the framework for behavior is the behavioral (or phenomenal[3]) environment not the geographical (or noumenal) environment—that is, behavior is with respect to how the environment appears to an organism, not how it is described by physics. Behavior, of course, must occur in the geographical, physical environment (physical laws cannot be compromised). Koffka proposed that its means of doing so is through the mediation of the behavioral environment.

The depicted lake's snow-covered surface in Figure 15.3 is (i) *geographically* $H_2O \leq 0°C$, and (ii) *behaviorally* a surface that can support quadruped

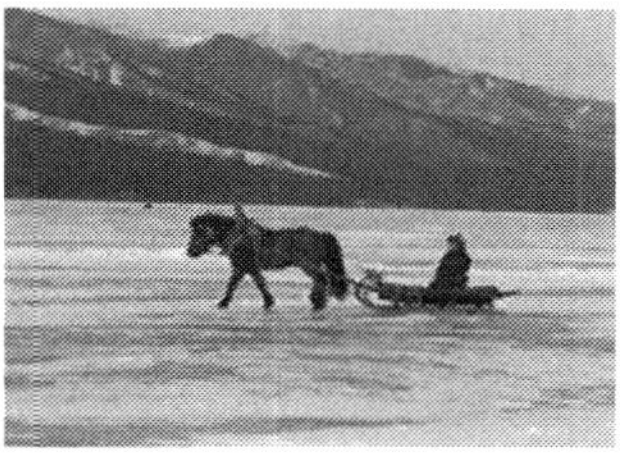

Figure 15.3 Behavioral versus geographic environments. Geographically, the lake is water at or below freezing ($H_2O \leq 0°C$). Behaviorally, the lake is a surface of support.

(Reprinted with permission, François Robin; available at: www.e-mongol.com/mongolia-travel-itineraries)

locomotion with a load. For the locomotion to be manifest, two conversions are implied for the rider and for the horse. The first is a mapping from the geographical environment to the behavioral environment; the second is a mapping from the behavioral environment to behavior. The differences between the geographical and behavioral "languages" should be noted. Whereas the predicates of the geographical are animal-neutral, physical, and meaningless, the predicates of the behavioral are animal-referential, mental, and meaningful. The two languages are separate and irreducible, the one to the other. We have a dualism (Shaw & Turvey, 1981).

A primary driving force for Gestalt theory was abhorrence of dualism. Of similar rank was the desire to work out the facts of psychology so that these facts would be continuous with those of physics and biology (recall Lectures 13 and 14). The formulation of the behavioral environment could not be sustained. The dualism had to be resolved. The resolution entailed eliminating the semantic animal-referential predicates ("surface of support") while preserving their molar qualities. The resolution substituted the physical reality of the perceiver's physiology for the concept of the behavioral environment and it promoted an interpretation of the physiology as molar processes rather than molecular processes. This step was articulated as an isomorphism between perceptual states and neural states—a *psychoneural isomorphism*.[4] Mathematically, given two things, either one of them can provide insight about the other if an isomorphism holds between them. If things A and B are isomorphic, then any property that is preserved by the isomorphism that is true of A is also true of B, and vice versa. Figure 15.4 shows a familiar isomorphism, that between logarithms and anti-logarithms. Figure 15.5 provides appreciation that what seem to be very different structures (e.g., G as perceptual states, H as brain states) can prove to be isomorphic.

The upshot of this reformulation of the behavioral environment was an isomorphism with respect to physical descriptors. Gestaltism pursued

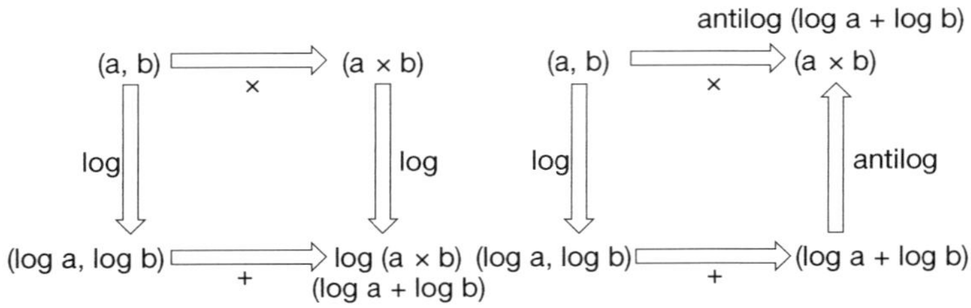

Figure 15.4 *Morphism and isomorphism.* (*Left*) Morphism between multiplied numbers and summed logarithms. (*Right*) Isomorphism identified by the reversibility (antilog) of summed logarithms to multiplication.

a thorough-going physicalism, but it can be argued that its goal (most certainly Köhler's) was not so much epistemological problems (organism–environment relations) as it was a concern for uniformity across the modes of discourse, across the disciplines of physics, biology, and psychology conceived as three different phases of matter. In its bold efforts to dispel unbridgeable gaps in the causal process defined over matter's different phases Gestalt psychology accepted gaps in the epistemic relation between organism and environment. That acceptance licenses unwelcome modern day conclusions of a kind that might have made Köhler (certainly) and Wertheimer and Koffka (possibly) grimace:

> The central message of Gestalt theory is that the primary function of perceptual processing is the generation of a miniature, virtual-reality replica of the external world inside our head, and that the world we see around us is not the real external world but is exactly that miniature internal replica.
>
> (Lehar, 2003, p. 404)

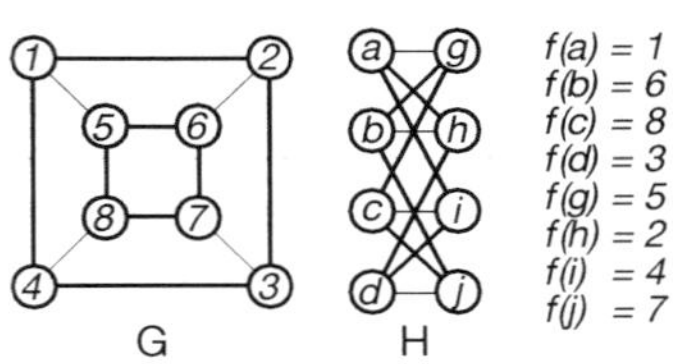

Figure 15.5 *An isomorphism of structures.* The structures G and H are isomorphic in that any two vertices in G are adjacent in G if and only if $f(u)$ and $f(v)$ are adjacent in H. The function f is a bijective (one-to-one) function that preserves edges: Every element in set G is paired with exactly one element in set H, and every element in set H is paired with exactly one element in set G.

> The world we see around us can only be an elaborate, though very compelling, illusion, which must in reality correspond to perceptual data structures and processes occurring actually within our own heads.
>
> (Lehar, 2003, p. 404)

15.5 Token Physicalism versus Type Physicalism

By way of concluding our foray into Gestalt theory we will find it helpful to note the distinction between so-called *token* physicalism and so-called *type* physicalism (see Fodor, 1975). The former is the simple claim that all the events discussed by the various sciences are physical events. The latter is the doctrine that every *property* mentioned in the laws of any science is a physical property. The latter is much stronger than the former. The move made by Gestalt theory—that of replacing behavioral environment by the perceiver's physiology/neurology—was a matter of token physicalism. For every predicate kind of the behavioral environment, the assumption is that there is a coextensive predicate kind of the perceiver's neurology. Simply, each mental token has a corresponding physical token. It is not hard to recognize the immediately preceding statement as a commonplace construal of the reductionist program in perception. It is a version of the morphological form of reductionism identified in Figure 14.4a. More appealing is the strategic form of reductionism identified in Figure 14.4b. Its appeal is that the orderliness observed at all of nature's scales is presumed to follow from a common set of scale-independent principles. In respect to Gestalt theory, strategic reductionism would suggest that the hypothesized events of the behavioral and neural levels would be forged in like manner.

Notes

1 Its predecessor was the *stimulus error*, Titchener's (1902) warning against the danger of confusing knowledge about the physical conditions of a perceptual experience with this experience as such (see Boring, 1921, p. 451). Said slightly differently, the *stimulus error* is attributing the perceptual experience to the physical stimulus when it should be attributed to the mental state the physical stimulus gives rise to.

2 Michael Wertheimer, Max Wertheimer's son.

3 From Kant: Phenomenal is thing-as-perceived; noumenal is thing-in-itself.

4 For a contemporary appreciation, see *Philosophical Psychology*, 1994, Vol. 7, No. 2.

References

Boring, E. G. (1921). The stimulus-error. *The American Journal of Psychology, 32*, 449–471.

Boring, E. G. (1942). *Sensation and perception in the history of experimental psychology*. New York: Appleton-Century-Crofts.

Fodor, J. A. (1975). *The language of thought*. Cambridge, MA: Harvard University Press.

Fowler, C. A., & Turvey, M. T. (1982). Observational perspective and descriptive level in perceiving and acting. *Cognition and the Symbolic Processes, 2*, 1–19.

Haken, H. (1983). *Advanced synergetics*. Berlin, Germany: Springer-Verlag.

Kelso, J. A. S. (1995). *Dynamic patterns*. Cambridge, MA: MIT Press.

King, D. B., & Wertheimer, M. (2005). *Max Wertheimer & Gestalt theory*. New Brunswick, NJ: Transaction.

Koffka, K. (1999). *Principles of Gestalt psychology*. London: Routledge (original work published 1935).

Köhler, W. (1947). *Gestalt psychology*. New York: Mentor Books.

Lehar, S. (2003). Gestalt isomorphism and the primacy of subjective conscious experience: A Gestalt Bubble model. *Brain and Behavioral Sciences*, 36, 357–408.

Maxwell, J. C. (1873). *A treatise on electricity and magnetism, Vol. 1*. Oxford, UK: Clarendon Press (pp. x–xi).

Pastore, N. (1971). *Selective history of theories of visual perception 1650–1950*. Oxford, UK: Oxford University Press.

Shaw, R. E., Flascher, O. M., & Mace, W. M. (1996). Dimensions of event perception. In W. Prinz & B. Bridgeman (Eds.), *Handbook of perception and action, Vol. 1* (pp. 345–395). London: Academic Press.

Shaw, R. E., & Turvey, M. T. (1981). Coalitions as models for ecosystems: A realist perspective on perceptual organization. In M. Kubovy & J. Pomerantz (Eds.), *Perceptual organization* (pp. 343–415). Hillsdale, NJ: Erlbaum.

Steinman, R., Pizlo, Z., & Pizlo, F. (2000). Phi is not beta, and why Wertheimer's discovery launched the Gestalt revolution. *Vision Research*, 40, 2257–2264.

Titchener, E. B. (1902). *Experimental psychology: A manual of laboratory practice*. New York: Macmillan.

Turvey, M. T., & Shaw, R. E. (1979). The primacy of perceiving: An ecological reformulation of perception for understanding memory. In L.-G. Nilssen (Ed.), *Perspectives on memory research: In honor of Uppsala University's 500th anniversary* (pp. 167–222). Hillsdale, NJ: Erlbaum.

Wertheimer, M. (1912). Experimentelle studien uber das sehen von bewegung. *Zeitschrift fur Psychologie, 61*, 161–265.

Part 2

Computational–Representational Perspective

Lecture 16

The Computational–Representational Perspective: Preliminaries

At this juncture, it will be to our advantage to revisit Hobbes and Malebranche in respect to the third grade of sense, and to reappraise the Cartesian Program. On first blush, it will seem somewhat anomalous to let Hobbes and Malebranche serve as a springboard for what follows given what has brought us to this point. That they serve this function well will become evident.

Hobbes saw the third grade of sense as performing symbol manipulations. It was computer-like. Malebranche saw the third grade of sense as making an infinite number of inferences at an instant. It was God-like. Jointly, one might say, they envisioned the third grade of sense as minimally language-like. Given a suitable but finite number of symbols, and given a suitable but finite number of rules, Descartes' third grade of sense could, in principle, produce an infinite number of sequences representing an infinite number of situations.[1]

We can recall from the concluding remarks of Lecture 6 that the third injunction for the Cartesian Program was "discover and explicate the symbol-manipulating procedures employed by the third grade of sense in using the secondary qualities (the second grade of sense) and the endowed knowledge to make successful inferences about the world." The computational–representational perspective to be addressed in Lecture 16 is the contemporary response to that injunction.

16.1 The Representational Medium

The following scenario motivates language's special relevance (Fodor, 1975). Consider an agent *A* in situation *S*. *A* believes that a number of behavioral options B_k are available in *S*. *A* computes: "If B_i is in *S*, then consequence C_i is attainable with probability $p(C_i)$." (The choice of hypothetical B_k depends on what *A* knows about *S* and *B*. The C_i are ordered preferentially. *A*'s behavioral choice is a function of preferences and $p(C_i)$.) What does the preceding assume? Most notably the following: that *A* has a rich means of representing its behaviors to itself and that *A*'s decision making is a matter of computation. The implication is twofold. Without representation there can be no computation. Without computation there can be no means of determining which B_i to enact in S.

For mental functions in general, and perception in particular, the suggestion is that the representing medium must be language-like. For any given organism viewing at a glance any given natural scene the number of shape, size, distance, color, lightness and motion states exhibited at multiple scales of length and time implicate an infinitude of inferences, an infinitude of representations.[2] The infinitude implies that there must be a *productive* or *generative* process much like the rules or grammar of language. The role of the process in respect to the aforementioned states to be perceived is to render intensional[3] the logical formulae (akin to the sentences of language) that convey the reference, truth-value, and connotation of each state.

In the scenario of agent A in situation S, the aforementioned productivity confers on A the ability to generate representations of B_i appropriate to S in those many cases when S has never yet been encountered. Characteristic of sentence production in everyday life is that the sentences produced are largely novel, formulated specifically for the situation at hand. Generalizing to agent A in situation S, productivity bestows novelty of representations and, perforce, novelty of perceptions and actions.

16.2 What Concept Learning Entails

A language-like basis to perception allies with Plato (Lecture 4) and not with Locke and Hume (Lecture 7). The alliance is most evident in respect to concept learning in which Plato's paradoxes of learning and knowing are seemingly at play. The paradoxes are, respectively, that one cannot learn anything *new* unless one already knows it (by some other means), and one cannot know *anything* unless one has already learned (come to know) it (Weimer, 1973). We will recall from Lecture 4 that Plato saw the general resolution of the learning paradox in terms of a process by which episodic experiences unfold universal pre-exiting forms. The lecture anticipated that his general resolution would have broad appeal over the ages. A contemporary variant follows.

Intuitively, to have a concept is to have something that exceeds the particular experiences that gave rise to the concept. The experiences do not *make* the concept as much as they *confirm* it. Contrary to the predilections of Locke and Hume (and latter day proponents of mind as associations), concept formation seems to be essentially a matter of hypothesis formation and confirmation (Fodor, 1975). As such, it demands (i) available relevant hypotheses or a means of generating relevant hypotheses, (ii) a means of representing hypotheses, (iii) a means of representing experiential data, and (iv) a means of assessing the data in relation to the hypotheses. Absent (i)–(iv) Helmholz's doctrine of unconscious inference (Lecture 11) is hamstrung.[4]

16.2.1 Problem of Projectible Predicates

The major formal challenge to a "process of hypothesis formation and confirmation" is that of inductive extrapolation, alias the problem of projectible predicates.[5] Consider yet again the man in the inner room of a mobile home with the added understanding that the home requires energy for its varied functions. At some point when moving from place to place, the mobile home passes close to a post and receives an energy boost. It does not occur with every pass, but it occurs sufficiently often for the man in the inner room to ask what it is about that situation that matters in respect to the delivery of energy. The scenario with some candidate descriptors of the situation, that which can be predicated of the situation, is depicted in Figure 16.1. The challenge for the man in the inner room is resolving which predicate should be projected into a statement of fact. Coming up with possible predicates is typically a relatively trivial exercise, as in the case of Figure 16.1. Coming up with the proper natural kind—that specific predicate whose projection expresses the regularity the man in the inner room seeks to identify—is typically not.

Goodman (1965) provided the classic argument. For any given number of observations of green emeralds made up to some point in time t_i, the hypothesis that all emeralds are green and the hypothesis that all emeralds are *grue* are equally appropriate. The *grue*-predicate can be defined as follows: An emerald is *grue* if and only if it is ((in the set of observations thus far and green) or (not in the set of observations thus far and blue)). There is nothing special about *grue*; predicates of the *grue*-type can be constructed in indefinitely many ways (Goodman, 1965). They illuminate the problem that, given more than one hypotheses compatible with the available data, the data themselves will not suffice to differentiate the hypotheses. Something more is needed. Fodor (1975) suggests that a simplicity metric must be at play, selecting "all *x*s are green" over "all *x*s are *grue*." The basic idea is that for every predicate there is a unique syntactic form such that any one predicate might differ from

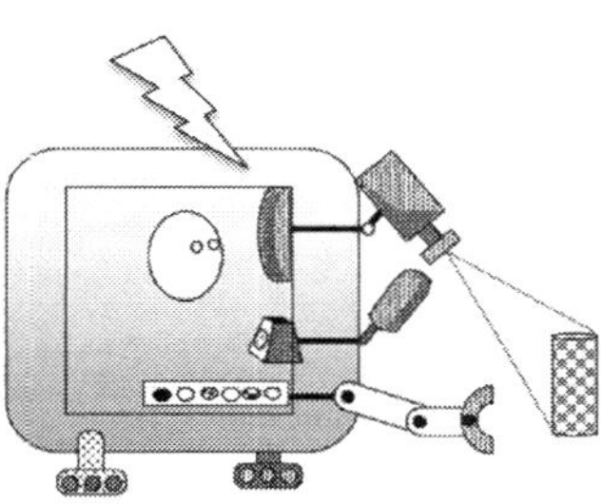

Figure 16.1 Which descriptor is causally related to the occurrence of the energy injection (lightning icon)?

(From Figure 1 in Turvey, 2004, adapted with permission, *Ecological Psychology*.)

another (related) predicate in degree of syntactic simplicity. For an intuitive example, we might note from above that fewer parentheses are needed to give syntactic shape to the predicate green than to the predicate *grue*.

As we will come to appreciate, this basic idea can be elevated to the hypothesis that mental operations (of the kind, for example, that Alhazen and Helmholtz assumed for perception) are formal operations on the shapes of internal representations (e.g., Fodor, 1981; Williams, 1999). The hypothesis to become apparent is that the epistemic relations (e.g., between perceiver and environment) comprising the "knowing about" introduced in Lecture 1 are purely formal, purely syntactic.

16.2.2 Innateness Argument for Language

It has been argued (Fodor, 1975) that "One cannot learn a 1st language unless one already has a system capable of representing the predicates in that language and their extensions" (p. 64). This is Saint Augustine's linguistic-take on Plato. One cannot learn a language whose expressive power is greater than the language one already knows. Given that learning to perceive within the tradition of empiricism is of like kind with learning a language, consideration of language learning provides insight into what that tradition entails.

There are two cases of learning a language. The one expressed in the above quotation implicates a known language that was *not* learned (alias, inherited). The other implicates a known language that was learned. The previous inventory (i)–(iv) can be deemed necessary to both cases. In paraphrase, both cases require a format for representing the data (one's experiences, linguistic and otherwise), a source of hypotheses for predicting future data, and a means for determining the data-to-hypothesis fit (e.g., a simplicity metric). That said, the formatting, the hypothesizing, and the fitting are not the same in the two cases.

It will be to our benefit to begin with the second case, focusing on a simple detail such as learning the meaning of a word in the second language. Of particular concern are the processes of forming and confirming hypotheses. Consider a native speaker of Portuguese attempting to learn the English word "influential," fully competent in regard to conceptualizing the problem and in recognizing its epistemic demands (cf. Bruner, 1997). In learning this English word she must pursue a strategy of determining the defining properties of "influential" in the terms of her native language. Her first charge is to fully grasp the kind of predicate that "influential" is. For example, she must discern that—when used in reference to a man or a woman—the predicate is *social relational* and not *personal attributive* (Williams, 1999): "[A]ge, economic status, and religion matter rather than height, weight, or body temperature" (p. 92). The point of this example is that our would-be-learner is mindful of the workings of modern society. But there is much more. Beyond a system of concepts granted by learning Portuguese, our would-be-learner of English is also mindful of what counts in general as reasonable criteria to be satisfied in predicate selection and what counts as good evidence for adjudicating among candidate criteria.

Let us now consider the case of learning a 1st language on the presumption identified previously that it must necessarily involve a known but unlearned language. There are two closely related questions: What must be true of the known but unlearned language? What are the implications of 2nd language learning (e.g., English after Portuguese) for 1st language learning?

Fodor's (1975) apt label for the unlearned language is *language of thought* (LOT). This language comprises operations on forms (syntactically structured objects). Strategies and knowledge of the kinds (just discussed) that guide the learner of a 2nd language are, by definition, absent from LOT. What LOT has is the formal capability to express any and all the predicates of the 1st language and their extensions. Its role in respect to word learning, for example, is the provision of representations for the words of the 1st language. A new word's meaning is in terms of a truth rule[6] that links a predicate in the 1st language to a predicate in LOT with the fit evaluated in terms of a simplicity metric. The background for theorizing about LOT in this manner is the nature of computation understood as transformations of syntactically ordered symbol strings that leave the strings' truth rules invariant. The very physics of a canonical computing device ensures that the device's state sequences and operations are respectful of the truth rules that the strings of symbols abide (Fodor, 1975, 1994).

The distinction between LOT and 1st language has much in common with Pattee's *epistemic cut* discussed in Lecture 14 (see Section 3.2). In learning the 1st language, LOT's rate-independent symbols are separate from the rate-dependent learning dynamics that they direct. They stand in relation to each other as genotype and phenotype, respectively.

For later lecture topics, we may find it helpful to note here the opposition between the logic of the LOT-first language distinction and Gottlieb's *probabilistic epigenesis* discussed in Lecture 12. For the latter, the contributing factors in 1st language learning are unlikely to be those identified deductively from the formal analysis of language within the disciplines of linguistics, philosophy, and psychology, and are unlikely to include LOT or equivalents. To paraphrase the last sentence of Lecture 12 (Section 2.3), we should expect 1st language learning to include, in significant degree, both pre- and post-natal experiences that have no patent relation to language.[7] First language from the perspective of probabilistic epigenesis is emergent from non-obvious interaction-dominant dynamics.[8]

16.3 Computational and Representational Assumptions

Our development of the computational–representational approach follows Von Eckardt's (1993) explication of so-called substantive assumptions that constrain answers to the basic questions defining Cognitive Science.

Von Eckardt claims that these questions are not why-questions but what-questions and how-questions, with two questions of each kind.

The substantive assumptions are termed "linking" and "system." A linking assumption claims that the domain of inquiry is substantially like a system of type X; a system assumption claims that, substantially, a system of type X has such-and-such properties. These assumptions in respect to computation and representation are characterized in Figure 16.2. As depicted in the top panel, the brain/mind—an assumed data processor, data filer, and data manipulator—is linked to a computational device, a system that possesses a number of data-processing, filing, and manipulating capacities. As suggested in the bottom panel, the brain/mind as an assumed medium for representing data is linked to a representational device, a system with varied capacities for representation. Figure 16.2's lower panel shows four aspects that, pursuant to Peirce (see Von Eckardt, 1993), are deemed essential to the capacity to represent. The *bearer* is a formal structure or process (depicted in the figure as symbols). The *content* is the semantic properties of the bearer. The *ground* is a relation that determines the content. And the *interpretant* is the significance of the content for the agent qua interpreter.[9]

Perhaps the most important feature of Figure 16.2's lower panel is the explicit distinction between data in the semantic sense (what is represented) and symbols and representations in the bearer sense (what is doing the representing). As Von Eckardt (1993) argues, for the computational–representational perspective to be a viable enterprise, it must address the following question:

> *In virtue of what* do mental representations have the informational content they have?
>
> (p. 114)

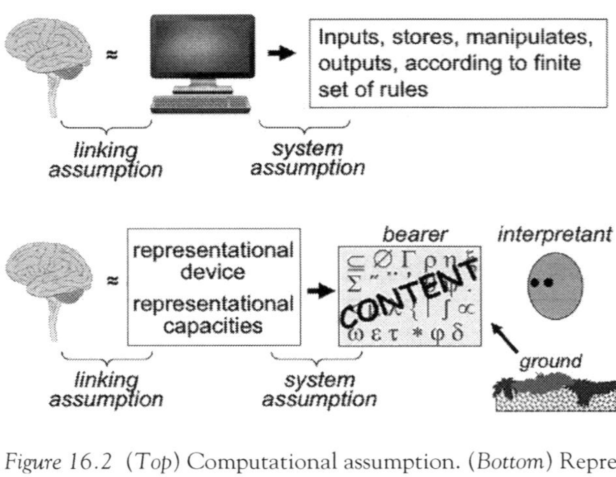

Figure 16.2 (*Top*) Computational assumption. (*Bottom*) Representational assumption.

Absent a distinction between the data (in the semantic sense, so-called informational content) and the data bearer, this fundamental question, in Von Eckardt's view, cannot even be raised. The proposed answer, as noted, is *the ground*. Following Peirce, the ground in Figure 16.2 can be iconic, indexical, or symbolic (conventional), singly or in combination. The arguments we entertained in Lecture 3 that led us to informationL point to the indexical as the ground that most warrants our attention.

The relation between an index and its object or event is of two kinds, causal and spatiotemporal. For causal examples, Peirce suggests that a rap on the door is an index of someone being at the door and a weathervane's orientation is an index of the wind's current direction (Von Eckardt, 1993). For both, the index's signifying property is a causal effect of a property of the event. An exemplary human case of a spatial index is a pointing finger. An exemplary human case of a temporal index is the utterance "now."

What the causal cases in particular make clear is that the indexical ground is existential, meaning, the representing properties of the sign-bearer are what they are because the object or event is what it is The former does not exist without the latter. Further, the indexical ground exists independent of whether there is an interpreter or interpretant. In overview, Peirce's ruminations were directed toward a strictly naturalistic way of grounding representations—that is, one that excludes semantic or intentional properties or relations (Von Eckardt, 1993). Let R be representation, O object, I interpretant, and A agent. Then the schema for the R–O relation can be formulated as:

> R is a representation of O with respect to I (in A) only if R is related to O by an appropriate ground.

Representation for Peirce is triadic. There is, in addition, an R-I relation:

> R is a representation of O for A only if R has the power to produce an I in A.

That is to say, R is a representation of O only if there currently exists an interpreter in the right relation to R. For continuity of conceptual development, we can situate the R–O relation and the R–I relation within the familiar territory of the man in the inner room (Figure 16.3). This move is pedagogically helpful. It makes explicit an otherwise implicit dimension in the long tradition of conceptualizing the man in the inner room (Lectures 7–12). To understand the image of O on the screen, the man in the inner room must know (a) that there is a causal relation and a similarity relation between the image and O, and (b) in what exact respects the image is causally due to O and similar to O. That is, establishing the right relation of the man in the inner room to R requires at the outset that the image of O be considered in conjunction with its ground (causal or spatiotemporal in the case of indices, but resemblance in the case of icons, and conventions in the case of symbols).[10]

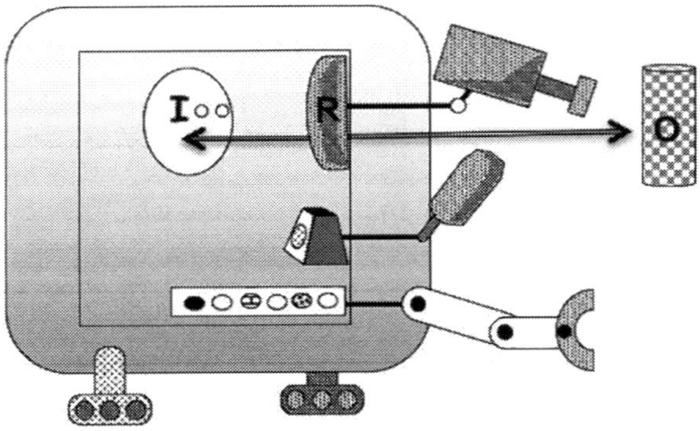

Figure 16.3 Peirce's triadic relation of object (O), representation (R), and interpretant (I) in the man-in-the-inner-room perspective.

(From Figure 1 in Turvey, 2004, adapted with permission, *Ecological Psychology*.)

Armed with the foregoing Peircean distinctions, let us now attend briefly to the computational and representational capacities implicit in Figure 16.2—capacities such as perceiving, recalling, classifying, etc. They possess all or most of the following properties. They tend to be about something (they are *intentional*), they are exercised with varying degrees of success (they can be evaluated in a *pragmatic* sense as more or less befitting the circumstances), when fully exercised, their end states and beginning states relate in a well-defined specific manner (they are *coherent*), they tend to be exercised successfully (they are *reliable*), and they can be exercised in very many different ways (they are *productive*). Collectively, the foregoing defines the *property assumption* (Von Eckardt, 1993).

A charge for a theory of computational and representational capacities would be that of accommodating the aforementioned defining properties. In the process of so doing, the theory would be expected to address the question of whether the capacities and their properties form a whole, a system. Specifically, do they constitute a natural kind, a projectible predicate? A positive answer would imply that capacities abide laws and that a unified theory of the capacities is possible. The foregoing defines the *grouping assumption* (Von Eckardt, 1993).

16.4 Shannon Information

Arguably, the single most important progenitor of the computational–representational perspective is information theory (e.g., Shannon & Weaver, 1949). Computation and computers are what they are because Shannon information is what it is.

At the outset, one must appreciate that Shannon's theory is not with respect to "information" as that word is commonly understood.[11] Rather, it is with respect to *data* "the raw material from which information is obtained" (Devlin, 2001, p. 20). Shannon's theory deals with data quantification in terms of signals expressed as bits (binary digits). What matters is the signal's size (the number of 0s and 1s), not what it denotes.

The centrality of Shannon's information theory to the conception of computation is highlighted in Landauer's (1991) answer to the question of "What is a computer?" "It is basically an array of bits—0s and 1s—with machinery that maps one configuration of bits into another configuration" (p. 23).

One might conjecture on the basis of the preceding that a reasonable test of whether a substantial linking assumption can be made between human and computer is whether or not human behavior is expressible in terms of bits. Although the original forays into this topic were favorable, subsequent inquiries indicated that the range of cognitive behaviors reflecting a dependence on bits is narrow.

The original phrasing of the question by Hick (1952) and Hyman (1953) was in terms of Shannon's depiction of communication (see Seow, 2005). The *transmitter* of information was a visual display; the *message* was an individual stimulus item in the display; the *channel* was the visual perceptual system; the *receiver* was the participant; and the *destination* was the appropriate response. In Hyman's experiment, participants learned to associate a single syllable name with each of eight lights—the four lights which made up the corners of an outer square of lights and the four corners of the next inner square of lights in a matrix of 36 lights (6 rows by 6 columns). On each trial, following a ready signal, one of the lights flashed (one of 7, 6, 5, 4, 3, 2, or 1 on-lights corresponding to 2.81, 2.58. 2.32, 2.00, 1.58, 1, and 0 bits, respectively). The participant named the flashing light as quickly as possible. The naming latency increased linearly as the number of bits increased, and did so at a rate suggestive (to some) of an information capacity (rate of gain of information) of 7 bits/s (Pierce, 1961).[12]

Questions of the generality of the increasing relation between latency and bits were raised by experiments in which participants received ample practice in Hick and Hyman's task (Mowbray & Rhoades, 1959). The practice eliminated the latency dependency on bits. Questions of a cognate nature were also raised by investigations of memory span[13] that showed closely similar spans for strings of digits, strings of letters, and strings of monosyllabic words despite the very large differences in number of alternative possibilities (digits, one of 10; letters, one of 26; words, one of many thousands). Results of the preceding kind, summarized in the terms of a "magical number seven plus or minus two" (Miller, 1959), introduced a contrast between the objective *bit* and a subjective cognitive unit of measure—the *chunk*. The common span of memory was said to be 7 ± 2 chunks.

The understanding that *bit*, the Shannon information measure, is not befitting matters psychological has wide implications that are yet to be fleshed out. One is a rethinking of the substantive linking assumption. In his transformative volume *Cognitive Psychology*, Neisser (1967, pp. 7–8) suggested that the link should be to "program" not "computer." The link of brain/mind is made, not to the machine or device, but to the program as a series of instructions for dealing with symbols. Another is a rethinking of the information measure itself (e.g., Devlin, 1991; Garner, 1962; Luce, 2001; Vigo, 2011, 2013). In information theory, the elements of choice are absolutely neutral and lack any internal structure. Luce (2003) pinpoints the problem in these words: "[T]he probabilities are on a pure, unstructured set whose elements are functionally interchangeable" (p. 185).

Consider the set of lights in the Hyman experiment. There were no relationships among the lights in the sense that any one light could be exchanged with any other. The unstructured Hyman case is not the general case, however. In the more typical psychological experiment, the visual displays, the auditory sequences, etc., are structured, with their elements non-interchangeable in a fundamental way. As Luce (2001) notes, in a typical evaluation of short- or long-term verbal memory, it is a challenge to avoid associations among the words. Stimulus similarity in general, although ill defined and poorly understood, is a widely influential structural aspect of experimental psychology.

In sum, on consideration of the information measure *bit*, a case can be made that the linking assumption in cognitive science is between brain/mind and program (rather than computer) and that the information said to be selected, stored, recovered, manipulated, etc., is not Shannon information[14] but something quite different. The "quite different information" in question is yet to be defined within the context of assumptions comprising the computational-representational perspective.

16.5 Cognition as Disembodied and Propositional

A prominent manifest form of the computational–representational perspective is artificial intelligence (AI). Its guiding assumptions articulated more than two decades ago (Kirsch, 1992) exerted a strong influence on how cognition can be conceived and studied. Here are four that are particularly worthy of note. Contemporary developments must be considered in light of them.

1. Disembodiment (cognition and knowledge can be studied abstractly outside of perception and action and absent the grounding problem, as schematized in Figure 16.4).
2. Pre-eminence of knowledge and conceptualization (emphasis on declarative knowledge and reasoning-like computation).

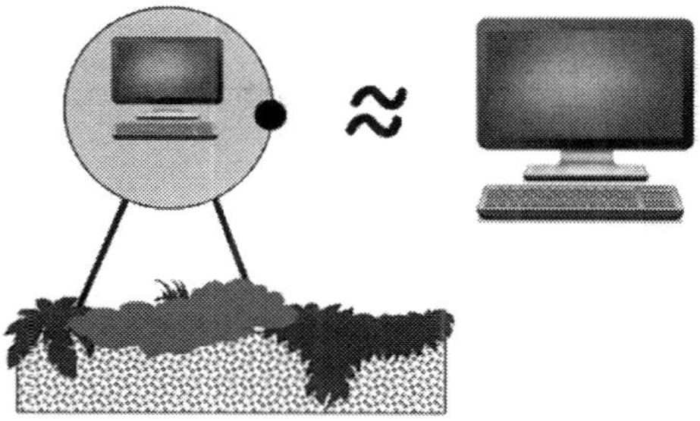

Figure 16.4 The disembodied assumption. Organism conceived as just a computational–representational device. There is neither body nor ground; compare with Figure 16.2.

(From Figure 6.1, Turvey, 2013, adapted with permission, MIT Press.)

3 Cognitive processes as language-like.
4 One and the same architecture for all varieties of cognition.

A fifth assumption sits behind Assumptions 1–4—namely, that learning, concept formation, and the like are complete. The implicit proposal is that the study of how the computational and representational capabilities are acquired can be delayed till later, once the lessons learned from pursuing Assumptions 1–4 are in place. We can help set the stage for Lectures 17–19 by addressing, in the manner of Kirsch (1992), the disembodied processes that disembodied concepts are proposed to explain.

16.5.1 *Inferring and Inferential Breadth*

The success of an inference engine (of the kind intimated by the third injunction of the Cartesian Program, Lecture 6) will be dictated by (a) the number of concepts at the engine's disposal, and (b) the degree to which they are interconnected. The two requirements are seemingly best approached formally. Such would be the disposition of the logical approach to AI, the so-called logicist program. Its goal, prefaced in Figure 16.4, is to identify appropriate conceptualizations of computational-representational desiderata independently of issues of grounding and implementation (Kirsch, 1992; Minker, 2000). The significance of inferential breadth can be communicated bluntly (Kirsch, 1992):

> [T]o prevent ridiculous displays of irrationality it is necessary to postulate an elaborate tissue of underlying conceptualizations and factual knowledge. The broader this knowledge base the more robust the understanding, and more reasonable the action.
>
> (p. 12)

16.5.2 Perception's Propositional Nature

The abductive form of inference favored by the Alhazen and Helmholtz variety of perceptual theory, and similarly favored by AI, is a matter of perceptual conjecture conjoined with perceptual evidence (Josephson & Josephson, 1996). Evidence and the related notions of confirmation and falsification derive from relations between propositions, the latter understood as abstract objects to which an organism is related by psychological attitudes (such as belief, hope, expectation; Audi, 1999).[15] To conjoin perceptual evidence with perceptual conjecture requires that the evidence be propositional like the conjecture, that is, in the form of a composition of concepts.[16]

16.5.3 Learning as a Conceptual Advance

AI likens knowledge of any given domain to a theory, to a system of axioms linking basic concepts. Learning is then understandable as a conceptual advance in the sense of movement along a trajectory of theories. Defined as formal principles of "conceptual advance," principles of learning can be studied in the context of Figure 16.4. A presumption of invariance of learning principles over different conditions of grounding (different CES systems in the terminology of Lecture 1) has been the norm (see Hilgard & Bower, 1966). Its proof may require the abstract approach of disembodiment.

16.5.4 Decay of Knowledge

Degradation of rational performance of the kinds symptomatic of a number of diseases and disorders of the central nervous system are addressable. As an example, a formalization of the network of concepts undergirding inferential breadth promises the ability to follow and explicate the course of Alzheimer's disease, from the early unsystematic, erratic memory mishaps to its prototypical pattern. The promise stands independent of identifying the disease's grounding.

16.5.5 Portability of Knowledge

An everyday cognitive achievement is the carry-over of one domain of knowledge unto another. The notion that knowledge is propositional, that it consists of compositions of concepts, allows the possibility that knowledge drawn from any one microtheory can be combined, in principle, with that drawn from any other. Ordinary decision-making ostensibly rests on the ability to draw on, and compose from, knowledge available in multiple domains. "Compositionality would explain portability (Kirsch, 1992, p. 14)."

Notes

1 These infinities of language, however, are not at an instant. They are not fully what Malebranche had in mind.
2 It is an observation made repeatedly in Malebranche's *Last Elucidation* (the *Elucidation on Optics*; Malebranche, 1997, pp. 720–753).
3 Roughly interpreted as "to give meaning to."
4 A reasonable quip with respect to any proponent of empiricism in regard to perception is the following: "Scratch an empiricist and you will find a nativist." Helmholtz's empiricism presumes that (i)–(iv) are given.
5 Predicate is a term designating a property or a relation.
6 A truth rule in LOT is somewhat special. It is of the form: "*x* is *F*" is true iff *x* is G (where an arbitrary singular term can take the place of *x* and, significantly, G is a predicate in LOT coextensive with *F*). Typically, a truth rule is of the form "*x* is *F*" is true iff *x* is *F*. The latter would apply, for example, in the case where one's perceptual state "*x*" is (of) *F*, and *F* is a property of the environment.
7 That such could be the case is suggested by research reviewed in "The child's path to spoken language" (Locke, 1995).
8 Efforts to characterize adult language dynamically are limited. Petitot (1995, 2011) provides one strategy.
9 The lower panel of Figure 16.2 expresses interpretant in the image of Peirce's theory of representation, as a mental effect of the content in the mind of the content's interpreter.
10 For elaboration, see Section 4.4 in Von Eckardt, 1993.
11 The common-sense intuition is that for something to be informative it must, at a minimum, increase one's knowledge about itself and, where possible, about other things. The greater the knowledge increase, the more informative is the thing that induces the increase. This *naïve informationalism* (Vigo, 2013, p. 2) holds information to be partly subjective.
12 Consonant with the conclusion that follows, Garner (1962, p. 93) observed "there are psychological factors involved in carrying out any timed task which are quite independent of information variables." And further, "measurements of information rate can be meaningful for determining transmission rates for very specific situations—so specific that little psychological generality is possible."
13 Given a single presentation of a string of things, whatever their nature, the memory span is defined by how many are recallable immediately upon termination of the presentation.
14 Luce (2003) identifies one notable exception to the incompatibility of psychological structure and information theory. This is when the number of stimuli in information theory and the number of hypotheses being considered in a Bayesian analysis is two. In this particular case, the influence of stimulus structure is much diminished, and the possibility arises of treating the two stimuli as without structure beyond probabilities of choice.
15 To ensure circumspection, a summary statement from the contribution on *proposition* in Audi (1999, pp. 753–754) is that the characterization of psychological attitudes as propositional is at best one component of "a more refined, largely unknown account" and that "a satisfactory doctrine of propositions remains elusive."
16 For an overview of research on the topic of conceptual combinations, see Hampton (1997).

References

Audi, R. (1999). *The Cambridge dictionary of philosophy*. Cambridge, UK: Cambridge University Press.

Bruner, J. S. (1997). *The culture of education*. Cambridge, MA: Harvard University Press.

Devlin, K. (1991). *Logic and information*. New York: Cambridge University Press.

Devlin, K. (2001). Claude Shannon, 1916–2001. *Focus: The Newsletter of the Mathematical Association of America, 21*, 20–21.

Fodor, J. A. (1975). *The language of thought*. Cambridge, MA: Harvard University Press.

Fodor, J. A. (1981). *Representation*. Cambridge, MA: MIT Press.

Fodor, J. A. (1994). *The elm and the expert*. Cambridge, MA: MIT Press.

Garner, W. R. (1962). *Uncertainty and structure as psychological concepts*. New York: Wiley.

Goodman, N. (1965). *Fact, fiction and forecast*. Indianapolis, IN: Bobbs-Merrill.

Hampton, J. (1997). Conceptual combination. In K. Lamberts & D. Shanks (Eds.), *Knowledge, concepts, and categories* (pp. 133–159). Cambridge, MA: MIT Press.

Hick, W. E. (1952). On the rate of gain of information. *Quarterly Journal of Experimental Psychology, 4*, 11–26.

Hilgard, E. R., & Bower, G. H. (1966). *Theories of learning*. New York: Appleton-Century-Crofts.

Hyman, R. (1953). Stimulus information as a determinant of reaction time. *Journal of Experimental Psychology, 45*, 188–196.

Josephson, J. R., & Josephson, S. G. (1996). *Abductive inference: Computation, philosophy, technology*. Cambridge, UK: Cambridge University Press.

Kirsch, D. (1992). Foundations of AI: The big issues. *Artificial Intelligence, 47*, 3–30.

Landauer, R. (1991). Information is physical. *Physics Today, 44*, 23–29.

Locke, J. (1995). *The child's path to spoken language*. Cambridge, MA: Harvard University Press.

Luce, R. D. (2003). Whatever happened to information theory in psychology? *Review of General Psychology, 7*, 183–188.

Malebranche, N. (1997). Elucidation on optics. In T. M. Lennon & P. J. Olscamp (Eds.), *Search after truth: With elucidations of the search after truth* (pp. 687–719). Cambridge, UK: Cambridge University Press (original work published 1678).

Miller, G. A. (1956). The magical number seven, plus or minus two: Some limits on our capacity for processing information. *Psychological Review, 63*, 81–97.

Minker, J. (2000). Introduction to logic-based artificial intelligence. In J. Minker (Ed.), *Logic-based artificial intelligence* (pp. 3–33). Dordrecht, Netherlands: Kluwer Academic Publishers.

Mowbray, G. H., & Rhoades, M. V. (1959). On the reduction of choice reaction times with practice. *Quarterly Journal of Experimental Psychology, 11*, 16–25.

Neisser, U. (1967). *Cognitive psychology*. New York: Appleton-Century-Crofts.

Petitot, J. (1995). Morphodynamics and attractor syntax: Constituency in visual perception and cognitive grammar. In R. Port & T. van Gelder (Eds.), *Mind as motion* (pp. 227–282). Cambridge, MA: MIT Press.

Petitot, J. (2011). *Cognitive morphodynamics: Morphological models in perception and syntax*. Bern, Switzerland: Peter Lang.

Pierce, J. R. (1961). *Symbols, signals, and noise: The nature and process of communication.* New York: Harper & Row.

Seow, S. E. (2005). Information theoretic models of HCI: A comparison of the Hick-Hyman law and Fitts' law. *Human–computer Interaction, 20*, 315–352.

Shannon, C. E., & Weaver, W. (1949). *The mathematical theory of communication.* Urbana: University of Illinois Press.

Turvey, M. T. (2004). Space (and its perception): The first and final frontier. *Ecological Psychology, 16*, 25–29.

Turvey, M. T. (2013). Ecological perspective on perception-action: What kind of science does it entail? In W. Prinz, M. Beisert, & A. Herwig (Eds.), *Action science: Foundations of an emerging discipline* (pp. 139–170). Cambridge, MA: MIT Press.

Vigo, R. (2011). Representational information: A new general notion and measure of information. *Information Sciences, 181*, 4847–4859.

Vigo, R. (2013). Complexity over uncertainty in generalized representational information theory (GRIT): A structure-sensitive general theory of information. *Information, 4*, 1–30.

Von Eckardt, B. (1993). *What is cognitive science?* Cambridge, MA: MIT Press.

Weimer, W. B. (1973). Psycholinguistics and Plato's paradoxes of the Meno. *American Psychologist, 28*, 15–33.

William, M. (1999). *Wittgenstein, mind, and meaning.* London: Routledge.

Lecture 17

Pattern Recognition and Representation Bearers

The later parts of Lecture 16 highlighted the values of disembodied cognition. Those values were in respect to the progress that could be made in regard to classes of problems that seem to call out for universal formal solutions. One such problem, of exceptionally wide scope, is pattern recognition. We can introduce ourselves to the problem by means of Figure 17.1.[1]

We can say of Figure 17.1a that the person on seeing the dog expects that it will bark, given that the person knows barking is what dogs do. It is seemingly a simple matter of associating "dog" and "barks." With a little more scrutiny, however, we realize that the person must first recognize that the optical pattern projected by the object being looked at is that of a dog and not one of indefinitely many other kinds of actual or possible things. The person must then refer this fact ("it is a dog") to his or her record of past encounters with dogs. One of many things that the person will discern in the record is that the

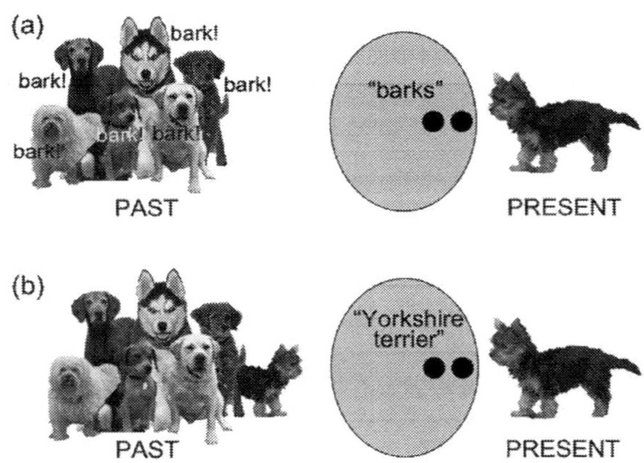

Figure 17.1 (a) Recognizing that the present thing barks is a matter of determining which class of past things the present thing best fits. (b) Recognizing that the present dog is a Yorkshire terrier is a matter of determining which template of past dogs the present dog best fits.

majority of dogs in the person's past tended to bark. That a person (or an organism in general) cannot take advantage of a thing's past associations without first recognizing (classifying, identifying, categorizing, etc.) the thing in question was brought to prominence by Höffding (1891). It has come to be referred to as the Höffding step (or function) (see Köhler, 1940; Neisser, 1967).

17.1 The Höffding Step: Definition and Problems

Patently, Figure 17.1a implies two distinct phases. Phase 1 is describing the thing in the world in terms of descriptors or predicates[2] that define the kind *dog*. Phase 2 is using this kind description to access the class of dog memories.[3] Figure 17.1b similarly implies two distinct phases but in this case the descriptors in Phase 1 are those that define an individual (*Yorkshire terrier*) in the kind *dog*. Phase 2 is using this individual description to find a match in the class of dog memories so that the individual can be identified (e.g., named). Of the two phases, the emphasis—theoretical, experimental and technical—is most typically given to Phase 2. Pattern recognition is usually equated with Phase 2. What makes the two phases so different intellectually that inquiry is likely to neglect Phase 1?

One's perceptual systems must deliver the base descriptions of the environment. Could these descriptions be provided in a singular vocabulary? Is there a universal set of descriptors (predicates) that could accommodate all circumstances? As we learned in Lecture 11 (see Figure 11.4) the responses of the specific nerve fibers to the proximal retinal stimuli are historically taken to be the necessary occasions for visual perception. From the Müller–Helmholtz perspective, the base visual sensations, singly and in association, comprise a vocabulary sufficient, in theory, to support the descriptions of all visible things. They could not do so, however, qua sensations. Mean light intensity as such, for example, would enter into a description of every pattern but would not serve as a designator of any pattern.

Let us suppose that pattern recognition is not achievable by any single, universal set of descriptors or predicates. And let us suppose, more boldly, that the number of sets of predicates needed for pattern recognition is indefinitely many, corresponding to the indefinitely many things that an organism commonly relates to in its lifestyle behaviors. These suppositions bring to light the highly problematic nature of Phase 1. The problem can be articulated in terms of Figure 17.1: How does the person know what predicate set to use to characterize the object in view? To take the Höffding step means to realize a description of a pattern (in Figure 17.1, the pattern in question is the optical distribution lawfully generated by a particular surface layout, viz. the dog) that can then be referred to memory for its recognition. In Figure 17.1a the desideratum is the set of predicates that suffice for the category *dog*. In Figure 17.1b the desideratum is the set of predicates needed to distinguish a distinct member of the category *dog*, namely, *Yorkshire terrier*. These will not be identical sets.

Here is the reason that the Höffding step is *highly* problematic: It can be conducted if and only if the recognizer knows beforehand which particular set of predicates is needed. The enactment of Phase 1 always assumes that one knows a priori what one is looking at (e.g., a dog) and with respect to what purpose (e.g., affirming it barks in the scenario of Figure 17.1a, ascertaining its breed in the scenario of Figure 17.1b). *The Höffding step requires an intelligence loan*[4] (as encountered in Lecture 6). For most (and perhaps all) implementations of pattern recognition by machine, and explications of pattern recognition by brain, this intelligence loan is taken. The loan taking is twofold. For dog recognition, the pattern recognizer must borrow from the intelligence bank (1) a set of predicates dedicated to dogs, and (2) prescience about when that set of predicates is to be used.

The specialness of the dog predicates must be noted. They will not apply to the visual skills of reading handwriting, distinguishing among a plumber's tools, determining objects that are reachable and graspable from a seated position, recognizing fungal genera, etc. A different predicate set is required, one that is likely to be unique for each of the aforementioned variants of pattern recognition and, we should suppose, for endless others.

As intimated earlier, the Höffding step is a response to a particular variant of a fundamental question—how do present experiences connect with past experiences? The connection cannot be as Höffding (1891) suggested.

Figure 17.1 depicts dog memories as tokens (of the species type and of the breed or class type). A type is never encountered. Only individuals or tokens are encountered. To encounter a member of a concept is not to encounter the concept. Patently, the tokens differ on a variety of dimensions while preserving invariant qualities that specify their commonality as "dog" and, for example, as "Yorkshire terrier." Amplifying the earlier allusion, resolving the predicates needed to define type membership and token status presumes, at a minimum, that one can perceive individual dogs and the differences and likenesses among them. In brief, informationL and direct perception are presumed (Lecture 3). It would seem that they must provide the ground for any explication of how an organism's present and past connect.

17.2 Template and Prototype as Representation Bearers

The Höffding step aside, there is Peirce's concern (Lecture 16) for the representation bearer. Figure 17.1 depicts dog memories as pictures of dogs. It is in keeping with a commonplace assumption of memories (representation bearers) as images or copies (see Sections 4 and 5 of Bennett & Hacker, 2003). Remembering a previously seen dog is like matching the current view of the dog to a copy of it in memory. Early in the history of pattern recognition research the latter came to be dubbed "template matching" (e.g., Uhr, 1963).

The dictionary definition of a template is a shape or pattern that is cut out of some material (e.g., metal, plastic) for the purpose of making replicas with the same or other material. In the present context, a template is that to which something can be fitted or not. Figure 17.1b has seven templates. Recognizing the presently viewed dog (a Yorkshire terrier) is a matter of determining which of the seven templates provides the best fit to the viewed dog's image. One means of doing so is to compute a point-wise cross-correlation between $(x, y)_{image}$ and $(x, y)_{template}$ for each of the seven templates. Other things being equal, the higher the cross-correlation value, the better the fit (cf. Brunelli, 2009).

Further consideration of how the fitting of image to template might work is informative. A classical formulation of the retinal image to template matching problem is in terms of the law of isolated conduction (the constancy hypothesis) encountered in Lecture 11, Figure 11.3. Suppose that the template for the letter K is a particular connection among neurons based upon original learning of just one instance of K under highly standardized conditions of presentations of K, retinal stimulations by K, and visual experiences of K. For example, *this* K, with size, distance and orientation held constant. Then any deviation from the preceding would result in a failure to fit the presented K (its retinal image) to the K template meaning that *this singular stimulus would not be recognized.* To realize a fit, to achieve that which defines recognition, requires that the man-in-the-inner-room (Figure 17.2) perform operations that adjust any current image of K in the direction of normalcy—e.g., resizing and reorienting the image to fit the template's size and orientation. That this may have to be done on an individual template basis is apparent from the simple fact that the templates of the individual dogs in Figure 17.1b cannot be of equal size without eliminating a primary distinction among them.

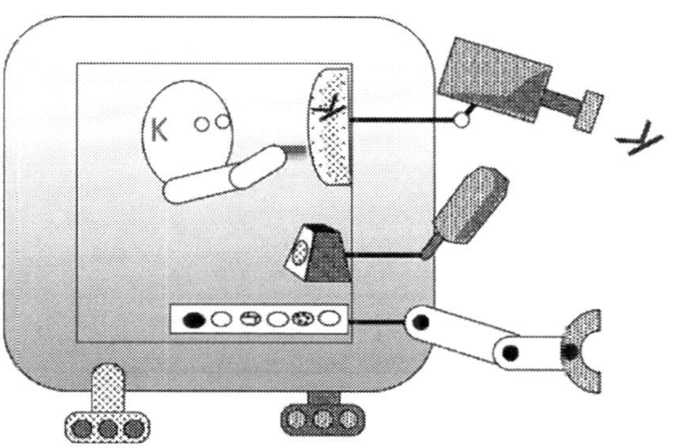

Figure 17.2 Man-in-the-inner-room resizing and reorienting the image K on the screen to fit the size and orientation of the template K in his memory.

(From Figure 1, Turvey, 2004, adapted with permission, *Ecological Psychology*.)

A further general demand on size renormalization is that it must be respectful of an image's group symmetry. In the case of K, it is the set[5] of transformations (such as displacements, rotations, reflections) that when performed on K, leave K as it was before (invariant, in its canonical form). There is no universal group symmetry for the problems of template matching. The symmetry group for K is not, for example, the symmetry group for M.

The normalization issue is, unfortunately, larger than the preceding problem suggests. There is no necessary relation between the template of the Yorkshire terrier in memory and its present image. How one sees the terrier now is not necessarily how one saw it previously. Focusing on two minimal differences, in comparison to the past Yorkshire terrier (Figure 17.1b) the present Yorkshire terrier may be in an upright posture and the viewer's perspective may be more anterior. To cut to the chase: The normalizing procedure for the image must be locked into the symmetry of the template that is being sought in memory.[6] However, a template matching pattern recognition system can normalize successfully, and make a fair measure of similarity (e.g., cross-correlation), only with foreknowledge of the image's template.

Templates are appealed to in another guise, namely, exemplar models of categorization (Hintzman, 1986; Medin & Schaffer, 1978). Historically, and commonly, *category* (e.g., dog) is equated with *concept*. The equation intimates that the representation bearer of a category is a definitional structure. For "dog" this would be an ordered collection or list of distinguishing properties or features that are both necessary (every dog has property or feature *x*) and sufficient (each dog expresses every *x* in the definition). To capture the variation over dogs in compliance with the definitional structure, proponents of exemplar models assume a template for each dog experienced to date with recognition of a current dog determined by the degree of similarity between it and the templates. The minimal number of templates needed to conduct a successful comparison and the means of computing similarity from the ensemble of templates are, however, open questions.

The exemplar theory is typically advanced in response to the interpretation of category representations as prototypes (e.g., Nosofsky & Zaki, 2002). A prototype is defined by some *sufficient number* of the properties that members of the category tend to have rather than *singly necessary* and *jointly sufficient* properties that have been the classical desiderata of concepts (Margolis, 1994).[7] In the theory of prototypes, a category is expressed by a summary representation in the form of a central tendency of all the experienced category members (e.g., Posner & Keele, 1968; Rosch, 1999). Recognizing a pattern is then a matter of determining an item's similarity to the alternative prototypes, selecting that which is most similar.

The significance of prototype is that it is an attempt to capture something ordinary about pattern recognition: One can recognize both type (it's a dog) and token (it's a Yorkshire terrier). How the two kinds of matching are achieved within the prototype formulation is, however, not so straightforward.

The difficulty might follow from what exemplar theory regards as the failings of prototype theory—that it is mute on category size, the specific differences among tokens, and the correlations among properties of the tokens (e.g., lengths of tails, sizes of ears; Medin & Thau, 1992). Implementation aside, the problem raised is how to coordinate an intensional definition (one that identifies the type) with an extensional definition (one that lists all encountered tokens).

17.3 Matrix of Distinctive Features as Representation Bearer

Pattern recognition need not be in terms of wholes. Indeed, our introduction in this lecture to the problem of pattern recognition was in terms of "a universal set of descriptors or predicates." That such could be the case for at least one domain of human perceiving, that of speech, was suggested by the Prague School of phoneticians in the 1930s and 1940s (Malmkjaer, 1991). The original idea was that spoken words of a language are differentiated by oppositions between phonemes[8] with the phonemes kept separate by their distinct features. The latter were phonetic properties such as "voice," "nasality," and so on. In the hands of Jakobson and colleagues (Jakobson, Fant & Halle, 1951), the features replaced the phonemes as the basic units of phonology. One and the same feature set could apply equally to consonants and vowels. In the ideal, and stated generally, distinctive features as a set are the minimal number of features that distinguish maximally among the members of a class.

Table 17.1 is a phonetic feature matrix for *dog* with "+" and "–" representing the presence or absence of the feature in question. Roughly, to detect the positively valued phonetic features is to perceive the spoken word *dog*. Table 17.1 expresses a mapping from one pattern (input) to another pattern (output). It is obvious (but in need of saying) that the input pattern for the word *dogs* is very similar to that for *dog*. This plain fact would seem to identify a principle:

Table 17.1 Fully specified feature matrix for the spoken English word *dog*

Feature	*/d/*	*/ɒ/*	*/g/*
vocalic	–	+	+
consonantal	+	–	+
compact	–	+	+
grave	–	+	–
flat	–	+	–
nasal	–	–	–
tense	–	–	–
continuant	–	+	–
strident	–	–	–
voice	+	+	+

Similar input patterns generate similar output patterns. As will become apparent, this principle is often (perhaps typically) violated.

17.3.1 Lessons from Speech

Table 17.1 is intended as a representation of the spoken word *dog* derived from the acoustical structure by a bank of phonetic feature detectors. The challenge posed by the acoustical structure for phonetic feature detectors should be noted. We do so by means of Figures 17.3 and 17.4. Each displays the characteristic component of the quality of speech sounds, namely, resonance bands that are commonly considered to determine the phonetic quality of consonant–vowel complexes.

Figure 17.3 is a speech spectrogram. It identifies fundamental aspects of real speech, most notably the frequency regions in which there are relatively high concentrations of acoustic energy (the resonance bands). They are commonly referred to as *formants*. They index vowels and the so-called resonant consonants (as represented by the letters *l*, *m*, *n*, *r*, etc.). Three formants are visible in Figure 17.3, in their steady states and in their transitions to those states. Also visible is a burst and a fricative (a type of consonant made by the friction of breath in a narrow opening, producing a turbulent air flow).

Figure 17.4 shows schematic variants developed for the purposes of experimental investigations by means of a device known as the pattern-playback, a means for synthesizing speech from hand-painted facsimiles of actual spectrograms (for its developmental history, see Liberman, 1996). For our current focus on pattern recognition based in features, we may wish to note the lessons of Figure 17.4. The upper panel summarizes an experiment by Liberman, Delattre, Cooper and Gerstman (1954) involving schematic first

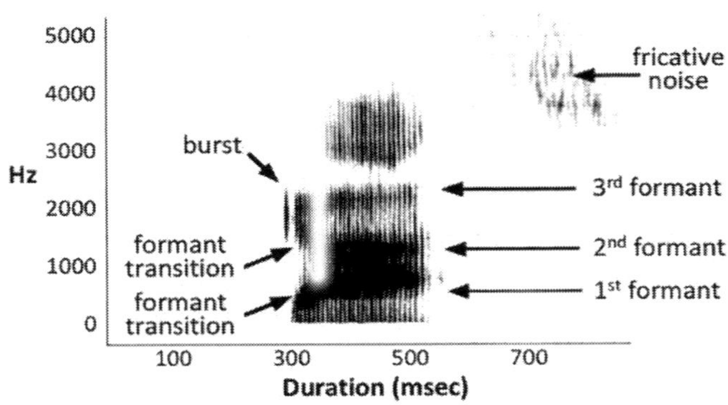

Figure 17.3 Spectrogram of the utterance /ga/, showing the phonetically important parts of the sound pattern.

(From Figure 1, Liberman, Delattre, Cooper, & Gerstman, *Psychological Monographs*, 1–13, 1954, APA, adapted with permission.)

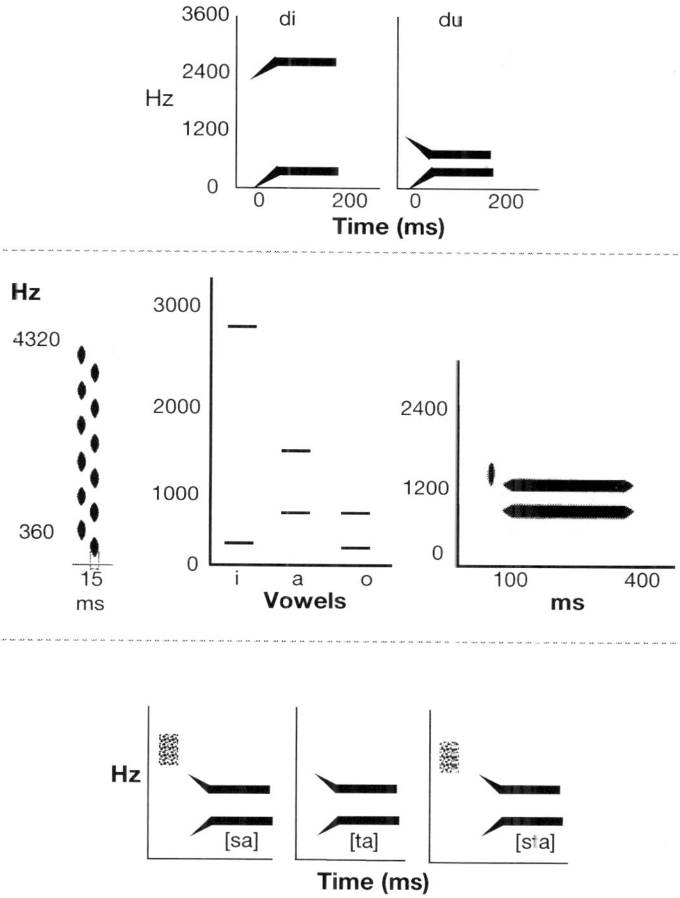

Figure 17.4 (*Upper*) Different things mean the same thing. (*Middle*) The same thing means different things. (*Lower*) Nothing means something. See text for details.

Upper: (From Figure 1, Liberman, Cooper, Shankweiler, & Studdert-Kennedy, *Psychological Review*, *74*, 431–461, 1967, APA, adapted with permission.)
Middle: (From Liberman, Delattre, & Cooper, *American Psychologist*, 1952, APA, adapted with permission.)
Lower: (From Figure 1, Liberman, Isenberg, & Rakerd, *Perception & Psychophysics*, *30*, 133–143, 1981, adapted with permission, Springer.)

(lower) and second (higher) formants. As indicated, the spectrograms of the upper panel are heard as the syllables /di/ and /du/. This difference originates in the transitions to the second formant conveying the difference in the time-varying consonants, rising upward from a high region in the case of /di/ and falling downward from a low region in the case of /du/. The lesson of the upper panel is: *Different things (transitions to the steady-state vowels) are heard as the same thing (the phoneme /d/)*.

The middle panel of Figure 17.4 summarizes an experiment by Liberman, Delattre and Cooper (1952). It teaches a second lesson: *The same thing (a given schematic stop) is heard as different things*. The leftmost part of the middle panel shows schematic stops of 15 minutes' duration at 12 different frequencies. The central part of the middle panel shows three of the seven vowels used in the experiment, with each vowel defined by its first and second formants. Each schematic vowel was preceded by each schematic stop, in the manner depicted in the rightmost panel. The individual participant's task was to listen to each syllable and report whether the initial stop consonant was *p*, *t* or *k*. Identification did not depend solely on the schematic stop's frequency. For *p* and *k* it varied with the following schematic vowel.

The third lesson follows from the bottom panel of Figure 17.4 summarizing an experiment by Liberman and Pisoni (1977). The lesson is: *Nothing (an interval without sound) is heard as something* (more precisely, *gives rise to something*).[9] For schematic first and second formants heard in isolation as /ta/, a preceding burst of noise followed by a brief interval of silence gives rise to the perception /sa/. The same preceding burst of noise followed by a slightly longer interval of silence (50 minutes) gives rise to the perception /sta/.

In sum, what we have learned from this brief excursion into speech perception phenomena is the context-conditioned variability of phonetic features and the potential pervasiveness of variables of relevance to perception that are non-obvious (see Lecture 12) prior to their exposure through experimental manipulations. Figure 17.5 reinforces this lesson. It suggests that

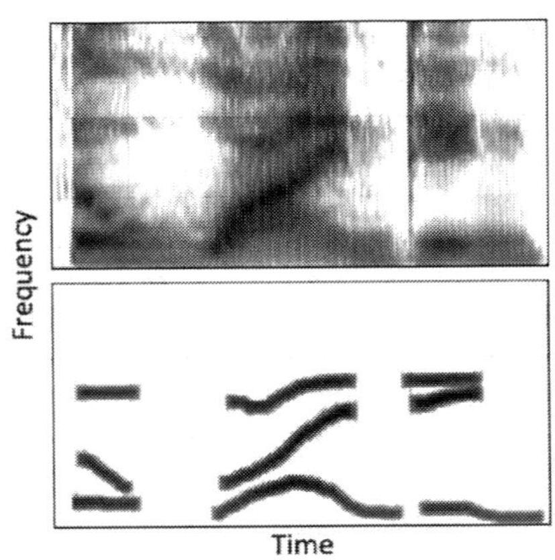

Figure 17.5 (*Top*) Spectrogram of a natural utterance and (*bottom*) a three-tone sinusoidal analog. Both depict "the winding" taken from the sentence "Take the winding path to reach the lake."

(From Figure 2, Remez et al., 2013, adapted with permission, Springer.)

phonetic features may not be necessary; speech is perceptible in the absence of canonical acoustic correlates of phonemes in the spectrum (Remez, Rubin, Pisoni, & Carrel, 1981). The upper panel of Figure 17.5 is the spectrogram of the naturally uttered sentence, "Where were you a year ago?" The lower panel is a time-varying sinusoidal analog. It follows the changing formant center frequencies—the natural resonances of the supralaryngeal vocal tract. One hears it as "Where were you a year ago?" simultaneous with the awareness that what one is hearing is not speech. It seems that speech perception is constrained by time-varying acoustic properties that are at a deeper level of abstraction than the spectra and the speech cues typically studied in speech research.[10]

17.3.2 Lessons from the Perceptron

Discussions of feature-based pattern recognition, both past and present, benefit from a consideration of a particular kind of computer, the perceptron, implemented by Rosenblatt (1962) and critically evaluated by Minsky and Pappert (1969; see Dewdney, 1989). As depicted in Figure 17.6a, a perceptron has a "retina" in the form of a grid. The perceptron's task is to classify retinal (grid) patterns. The local pattern detectors of the perceptron are referred to as predicates (three are shown in Figure 17.6a.). Each predicate ϕ examines a finite number of locations in the grid (referred to as the predicate's support). Each ϕ is a logical function of its support, and each transmits a 0 or 1 to the main component. To recognize a pattern at the scale of the retina, the main component compares a weighted sum of the predicate values to a threshold θ. If the threshold is exceeded, then the retina-sized pattern is recognized. Consider a perceptron Π of the kind $\Sigma(-1)\phi_i(x){:}0$. Its task is to determine whether a retinal pattern comprises non-rectangles of the kind depicted in Figure 17.6b. For the *ith* intersection point on the retina there are four tangent

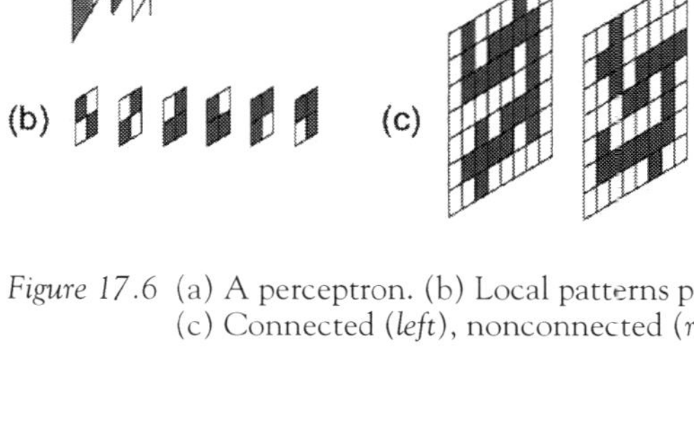

Figure 17.6 (a) A perceptron. (b) Local patterns predicated as *nonrectangles*. (c) Connected (*left*), nonconnected (*right*).

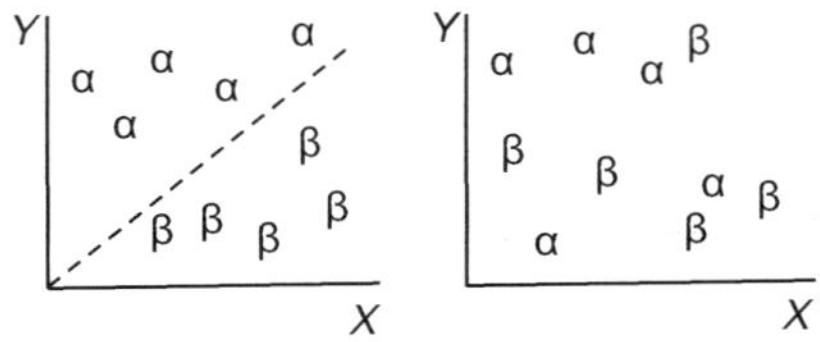

Figure 17.7 Examples of two-dimensional cases of linearly separable categories (*left*) and nonlinearly separable categories (*right*), where α and β are members of categories α and β. No straight line can partition the members of the two categories in the right panel.

cells and a predicate ϕ_i that examines them and no others. For any pattern in Figure 17.6b, $\phi_i = 1$.

Perceptrons were shown by Rosenblatt to be good learners and provided a springboard for future efforts to equate "understanding" with "pattern recognition" (cf. Winograd & Flores, 1986). They were, however, fallible in a particular, highly informative way. Figure 17.6c shows two patterns that differ in connectedness. By the mathematical principles of connectedness the left pattern is connected, the right pattern is not. Each pattern could be realized by a single predicate (like a template) but that seems to defeat the purpose of the perceptron concept. To evaluate fully the perceptron's capabilities Minsky and Pappert (1969) limited the predicates definable on the mesh of Figure 17.6c in either diameter (a square k units on a side) or order (k units). Their investigations revealed that no diameter-limited or order-limited perceptron could respond differentially to the patterns of Figure 17.6c. Behind this failure in respect to connectedness was a fact contrary to the simple fact identified above: There are cases, probably many, in which similar input values do not map to similar output values. These cases are ones in which the patterns are not linearly separable (Figure 17.7). They abide the exclusive OR function (Figure 17.8).

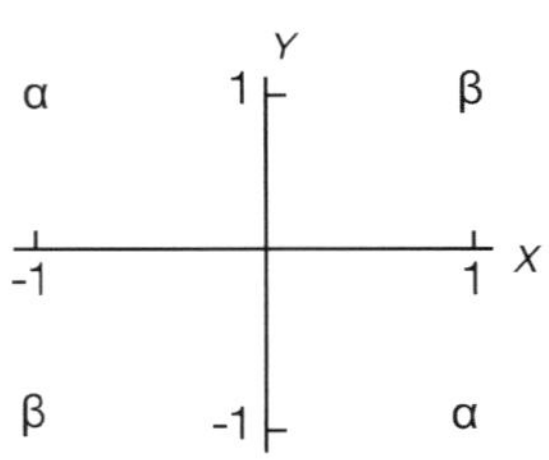

X	Y	XOR
1	1	β
1	-1	α
-1	1	α
-1	-1	β

Figure 17.8 The XOR function. It takes two binary inputs and generates one binary output. The output is β if either input but not both inputs is 1. The output is α if both inputs are 1 or both inputs are –1. Note that the most dissimilar inputs (X, Y values) map to the same output (β) and the exact opposites map to the same output (α).

The exclusive OR (alias XOR) function affords a further comment on the prototype versus exemplar issue. Prototype theory, unlike exemplar theory, assumes linear separability because construction of prototypes requires that all examples be closer to their own category prototype than to the prototype of a contrasting category (Medin & Thau, 1992). XOR also affords appreciation of a potentially fundamental aspect of biological pattern recognition—namely, nonlinearly separable categories are no more difficult to learn than linearly separable categories (Medin & Thau, 1992). To the extent that ill-defined categories are nonlinearly separable categories, then, we may suppose that they may be no more difficult to learn than well-defined categories.

Patently, there are several important lessons to be learned from the perceptron. The largest lesson followed from its failure. Whereas the elegant simplicity of the perceptron's learning algorithm was admirable, its inability to learn a mapping for nonlinearly separable problems rendered the perceptron as a nonviable model of natural pattern recognition. Obviously, two levels are too few. Would more levels solve the problem? And if so, what would be the minimal number? A theorem of Kolmogorov (see Caudill & Butler, 1990) suggested that one other layer—a layer hidden between input and output—would suffice in principle. Thus, the inquiry into neural networks (Lecture 18) was born.

17.3.3 *Lessons from Pandemonium*

Elaborating on the predicate idea of perceptron recognizing a spoken word can be conceived as (a) beginning with its speaker-idiosyncratic acoustic form, (b) proceeding to the predication of possible consonants and vowels (Table 17.1), (c) assembling the possible combinations of these consonants and vowels, and finally (d) achieving a match to that word in memory that best fits that combination of predicates. In the colorful language through which it is commonly conveyed, the foregoing is the basic pandemonium architecture (Selfridge, 1959; Selfridge & Neisser, 1960): from an image, to feature demons, to cognitive demons, to the decision demon—a sequence that maps onto the preceding (a)–(d). "Pandemonium" refers to the feature demons and the cognitive demons screaming simultaneously for attention. The feature demons when stimulated scream at the cognitive demons, the cognitive demons when stimulated scream at the decision demon.

In respect to Figure 17.1, the cognitive demons are memories of dogs that one has seen. They are portrayed as templates. In pandemonium, they would each be represented as a matrix of features. A closed universal set of visual features, however, has yet to be identified, and the quest for them, for any given category (such as dogs and handwritten words), may well be misguided. Consider Figure 17.9. It hints at multiple dimensions of variation, none of which are especially basic. Larsen and Bundesen (1996) suggest that whatever might be the significant dimensions of variation for the handwritten digits 0–9 in Figure 17.9 (a small sample from a set of 4,000), they are not mutually orthogonal and not likely to be universal. Larsen and Bundesen (1996) suggest a *template-matching pandemonium* pattern recognition system. In this system "feature" demons or analyzers store individually a particular template that is a copy of a digit presented previously.[11] When a handwritten digit is presented to the pandemonium system for recognition, it is first normalized in spatial position and size and then smoothed. Each "feature" demon then determines the degree of match between the digit and the digit template that it stores. The degree of match is a measure of the maximum correlation that can be found between the two patterns by permitting some displacement between their centroids. This degree of match provided by one template constitutes a "feature," functionally defined. As in the original pandemonium, these "features" are used as evidence (either positive or negative) in the

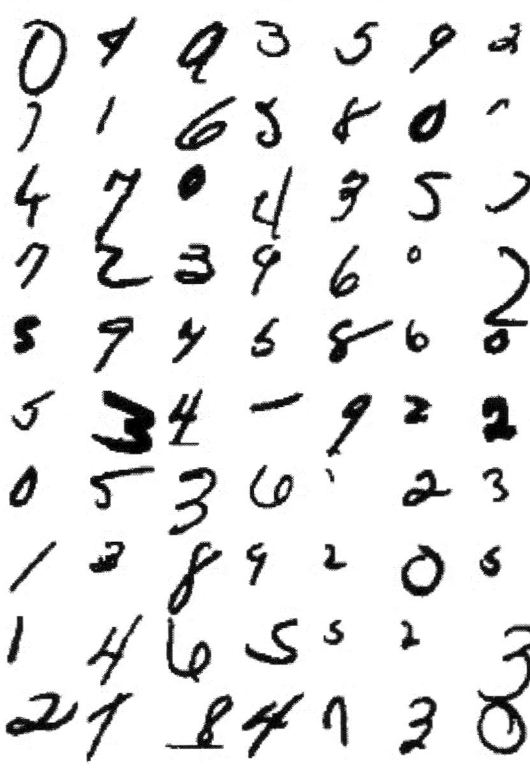

Figure 17.9 Digits from zip codes collected by the U.S. Postal Service from dead letter envelopes. (Figure 1 in Larsen & Bundesen, 1996, reprinted with permission, Springer.)

determination of a presented digit's identity mediated by the cognitive demons, one for each type of character. The net inflow to a cognitive demon is a weighted sum of the degrees of match determined by the "feature" demons. Each cognitive demon's activation increases with its net inflow.[12]

The lesson from this case of template-matching pandemonium resides in the repeated placing of "features" in quotes. There are no a priori features. More bluntly, *there are no features*. For each novel pattern from a given set, "features" are generated that are quantifications of that pattern's degree of fit to each of the previously stored patterns from that set, where fit is in terms of wholes, not parts.

17.4 An Atomistic Theory of Patterns and Concepts?

Our examination of the template-matching pandemonium notion allows us to confront an issue of some significance. The convention of defining a thing X through features or predicates amounts to a definitional account of X. The thesis underpinning Larsen and Bundesen's (1996) template-matching pandemonium contradicts this convention. For the general case of pattern recognition, it implies that there may be no truly definitional account of a thing X in the form of "X is what it is because it has property *i*, property *j*, property *k*, and so on." Recognition of X is not a matter of having a definition of X.

If the latter is the case, then recognition of X is strictly insular in the sense that recognizing X has nothing to do with recognizing anything else. The theory of pattern recognition so implied may be termed an "atomistic theory." It would parallel the atomistic theory of concepts (e.g., Fodor 1998, 2008) that has emerged in refinements and elaborations of the Language of Thought (see Lecture 16). Viewed in this atomistic sense, both patterns and concepts can refer because they stand in a causal relation to their referents.[13] The lingering question is whether this accommodates the Höffding step.

17.5 Representation and Reality: Straight Lines and the In-ness Problem

The notion of features and feature detection has figured prominently in the present lecture. The preceding section and Section 17.3.1, however, should give us pause in respect to the ontological status of features. As will become evident, the "pause" is fully justified.

Dodwell (2000, p. 113) attributes to Koffka (1935/1999) the question "Why does a tree look like a tree?" to McCulloch and Pitts (1943) the question "Why does a square look like a square?" and to Andrews (1964) the question "Why does a straight line look straight?" The foregoing questions refer obliquely to a problem that is a conceptual relative of the out-ness problem (Lecture 9, Section 9.3.3). We will take the liberty of calling it the *in-ness problem*. It is given expression through questions of the kind: "Why should the thing in here (the brain) be taken to look like the thing out there (in the environment)?"[14]

The straight-line question is the most relevant to our current deliberations. The discovery of so-called line detectors by Hubel and Wiesel (1962)—single cells in the visual cortex with simple receptive fields selective (putatively) for environmental straight lines—gave ascendancy to the notion of features as foundational to pattern recognition. More particularly, the discovery gave license to explain the everyday perception of "a straight line" by reference to an internal neural representation of straightness. The license is invalid, however, for a variety of reasons (Dodwell, 2000). A single-cell straight-line detector responds to lines in other orientations. Visible straight lines experienced by humans and other members of the phylum *craniata* are often in the scale of tens of meters (possibly continuing across the entire visual field) in contrast to the millimeter scale confining the stimuli activating single cells. The question is how individually coded line segments combine to represent extended line segments, be they straight or curved—an aspect of the so-called binding problem.

The severity of the straight-line question is worsened by consideration of how such a line maps from the visual field to the retina. In approximate terms, the mapping is from a plane surface (perpendicular to the line of sight) to a hemisphere. A straight line in the visual field becomes a curved line on the retina with larger or smaller size. The relation is one (a straight line of length L) to many (non-straight lines of lengths other than L). Here's the in-ness problem: Why should a curved line detected *in here* (the brain) be taken to be a straight line *out there* (in the environment)? Or, in the trialism terminology, *why should a curved line registered by the second grade of sense be taken to be a straight line by the third grade of sense*? By what means would this abduction (recall Lecture 12) from curved line as effect to straight line as cause have arisen?

The foregoing questions are made transparent by the ability to adapt to wedge prisms that cause straight lines to appear curved. With some reasonable amount of prism experience, attendant to self-movement relative to the surroundings, straight lines in the environment distorted by wedge prisms are perceived close to normal (Dodwell, 2000). This evolution from the initial perception of straight lines as curved to the perception of straight lines as straight is shown in Figure 17.10. In contrast, the cortical representation shown in Figure 17.10, dictated as it is by the retinal–occipital neuroanatomy, is unchanged in virtue of the fact that it is true to the unchanging retinal image. As Dodwell (1992, 2000) underscores, the facts expressed in Figure 17.10 undermine arguments for unique brain representations of lines. There is no ready solution to the problem of determining a unique representation for even a single straight line at the retina and, likewise, no ready solution to how the desired property is preserved in the mapping from retina to cortex.

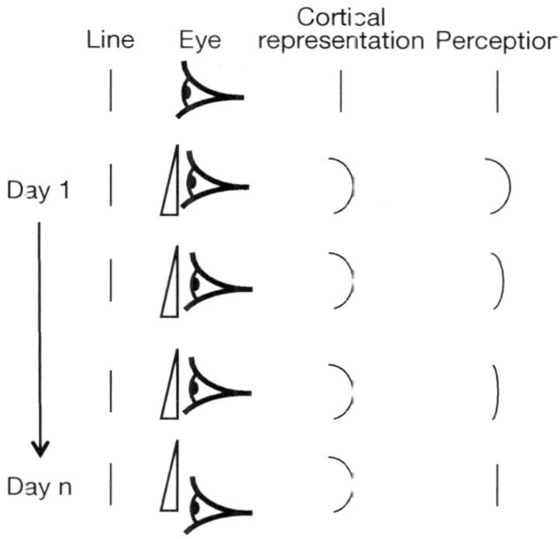

Figure 17.10 The phenomenon of prism adaptation. Wedge prisms distort the retinal image such that for a given straight line the projection on the retina is non-straight. This retinal non-linearity and the retina–cortex linkage are unchangeable by prolonged prism experience. Perception, in contrast, is changeable. Despite the persistent curved image and consequent cortical activity, perception evolves to "straight line" consonant with the environmental straight line.

(From Figure 10 of Turvey, 2015, adapted with permission, Imprint Academic.)

A priori, one cannot demonstrate that there is an internal representation for "straightness" that enters into a simple one-to-many correspondence with the members of the class of entities called "straight lines." On the grounds that the concept "visually straight" cannot be defined in physiological terms, one is led to the claim that the property straightness is "intrinsically foreign to the brain and its physiology" (Dodwell, 2000, p. 117). The implications of the in-ness problem reinforce those of the out-ness problem. Perception does not seem to satisfy locality.[15]

Notes

1 In what follows, the dogs in this figure are first discussed in terms of lists of distinguishing features to make one kind of point and then as whole images to make another, but related, kind of point.
2 For logical propositions a predicate is something that is affirmed or denied of the subject of the proposition. A proposition is a declarative sentence that is either true or false (e.g., all dogs bark).
3 Figure 17.1 identifies the challenge of connecting present states of affairs (e.g., current visual experiences) with past states of affairs (e.g., previous visual experiences). The simulative and projective assumptions discussed in Lecture 4 were motivated by the challenges of vision's physical basis and the principle of

nearby action. The associative theories advanced by Locke, Hume, and Berkeley covered in Lectures 7 and 8 were motivated by the challenges of mental content grounded in experience, specifically, the forms and interrelations of ideas.

4 One might say, more radically, it requires an intervention of God.

5 A set of transformations is called a group if it contains the inverse of each transformation and the product of any two of them—which includes the product of one with itself and with its inverse (Birkhoff & Maclane, 1977).

6 A long-term debate is whether the search of memory is one template at a time (serial) or all at once (parallel) (see Neisser, 1967).

7 In somewhat simpler phrasing, each individual property is necessary, and together as a group they are sufficient.

8 A working definition is the smallest unit of speech that distinguishes one word from another (e.g., the "sounds"/d/ and /f/ distinguish dog from fog).

9 For a more extensive investigation see Liberman, Dorman and Raphael (1979).

10 This sentiment is reinforced by other exotic analogs of speech, such as noise-band vocoded speech (Shannon, Zeng, Kamath, Wygonski, & Ekelid, 1995) and acoustic chimeras of speech (Smith, Delgutte, & Oxenham, 2002).

11 The training set was 4,000 digits presented one at a time in random order. Each digit is stored as a template. After each pass through the training set, performance was measured on a separate test set that consisted of 2,000 digits (200 tokens of each type). No learning occurred during passes through the test set.

12 In overview, the template-matching pandemonium system uses the templates for "feature analysis," strengthens the role of useful templates, and weakens the role of useless ones.

13 This is Kripke's (1980) proposal for the case of proper names.

14 This in-ness problem was encountered implicitly in Lecture 16 in the form of Figure 16.3. For I to take R as representing O requires that I has direct access to O (cf. Judge, 1985).

15 In very rough terms, straight-line perception is not a matter of a straight line *out there* (world) making contact with a straight line *in here* (mind).

References

Andrews, D. P. (1964). Error-correcting perceptual mechanisms. *Quarterly Journal of Experimental Psychology*, *16*, 104–115.

Bennett, M. R., & Hacker, P. M. S. (2003). *Philosophical foundations of neuroscience*. Oxford, UK: Blackwell Publishing.

Birkhoff, G., & Maclane, S. (1977). *A survey of modern algebra* (4th ed.). New York: Macmillan.

Brunelli, R. (2009). *Template matching techniques in computer vision: Theory and practice*. New York: Wiley.

Caudill, M., & Butler, C. (1990). *Naturally intelligent systems*. Cambridge, MA: MIT Press.

Dewdney, A. K. (1989). *The Turing omnibus*. Rockville, MD: Computer Science Press (reissued as *The new Turing omnibus*, 1993, New York: Henry Holt).

Dodwell, P. (1992). Perspectives and transformations. *Canadian Journal of Psychology*, *46*, 511–537.

Dodwell, P. (2000). *Brave new mind: A thoughtful inquiry into the nature of meaning of mental life*. Oxford, UK: Oxford University Press.

Fodor, J. A. (1998). *Concepts: Where cognitive science went wrong*. Oxford, UK: Oxford University Press.

Fodor, J. A. (2008). *LOT 2: The language of thought revisited*. Oxford, UK: Oxford University Press.

Hintzman, D. L. (1988). Judgments of frequency and recognition memory in a multiple-trace memory model. *Psychological Review*, 95, 528–551.

Höffding, H. (1891). *Outlines of psychology*. New York: Macmillan.

Hubel, D. H., & Wiesel, T. N. (1962). Receptive fields and functional architecture in monkey striate cortex. *Journal of Physiology*, *160*, 106–154.

Jakobson, R., Fant, G. C. M., & Halle, M. (1951). *Preliminaries to speech analysis: The distinctive features and their correlates*. Cambridge, MA: MIT Press.

Judge, B. (1985). *Thinking about things: A philosophical study of representation*. Edinburgh, UK: Scottish Academic Press.

Koffka, K. (1999). *Principles of Gestalt psychology*. London: Routledge (original work published 1935).

Köhler, W. (1940). *Dynamics in psychology*. New York: Liveright.

Kripke, S. (1980). *Naming and necessity*. Cambridge, MA: Harvard University Press.

Larsen, A., & Bundesen, C. (1996). A template-matching pandemonium recognizes unconstrained handwritten characters with high accuracy. *Memory & Cognition*, *24*, 136–143.

Liberman, A. M. (1996). *Speech: A special code*. Cambridge, MA: MIT Press.

Liberman, A. M., & Pisoni, D. B. (1977). Evidence for a special speech-perceiving subsystem in the human. In T.H. Bullock (Ed.), *The recognition of complex acoustic signals* (pp. 59–76). Berlin, Germany: Dahlem Konferenzen Life Sciences Research Reports.

Liberman, A. M., Delattre, P. C., & Cooper, F. S. (1952). The role of selected stimulus variables in the perception of unvoiced stop consonants. *American Journal of Psychology*, 65, 497–516.

Liberman, A. M., Dorman, M. F., & Raphael, L. J. (1979). Some experiments on the sound of silence in phonetic perception. *Journal of the Acoustical Society of America*, 65, 1518–1512.

Liberman, A. M., Delattre, P. C., Cooper, F. S., & Gerstman, L. J. (1954). The role of consonant-vowel transitions in the perception of the stop and nasal consonants. *Psychological Monographs*, 68, 1–13.

Malmkjaer, K. (Ed.) (1991). *The linguistics encyclopedia*. London: Routledge.

Margolis, E. (1994). A reassessment of the shift from the classical theory of concepts to prototype theory. *Cognition*, *51*, 73–89.

McCulloch, W. S., & Pitts, W. (1943). A logical calculus of the ideas immanent in nervous activity. *Bulletin of Mathematical Physics*, 5, 115–133.

Medin, D. L., & Schaffer, M.M. (1978). Context theory of classification learning. *Psychological Review*, 85, 207–238.

Medin, D. L., & Thau, D. M. (1992). Theories, constraints, and cognition. In H. L. Pick, P. van den Broek, & D. C. Knill (Eds.). *Cognition: Conceptual and methodological issues* (pp. 165–187). Washington, DC: APA.

Minsky, M., & Pappert, S. (1969). *Perceptrons: An introduction to computational geometry*. Cambridge, MA: MIT Press.

Neisser, U. (1967). *Cognitive psychology*. New York: Appleton-Century-Crofts.

Nosofsky, R. M., & Zaki, S. R. (2002). Exemplar and prototype models revisited: Response strategies, selective attention, and stimulus generalization. *Journal of Experimental Psychology: Learning, Memory, and Cognition*, 28, 924–940.

Posner, M., & Keele, S. (1968). On the genesis of abstract ideas. *Journal of Experimental Psychology*, *77*, 353–363.

Remez, R. E., Rubin, P. E., Pisoni, D. B., & Carrell, T. D. (1981). Speech perception without traditional speech cues. *Science*, *212*, 947–950.

Rosch, E. (1999). Reclaiming concepts. *Journal of Consciousness Studies*, 6, 61–77.

Rosenblatt, F. (1962). *Principles of neurodynamics*. New York: Spartan Books.

Selfridge, O. G. (1959). Pandemonium: A paradigm for learning. In *The mechanization of thought processes*. London: H. M. Stationery Office.

Selfridge, O. G., & Neisser, U. (1960). Pattern recognition by machine. *Scientific American*, *203* (August), 60–68.

Shannon, R. V., Zeng, F.-G., Kamath, V., Wygonski, J., & Ekelid, M. (1995). Speech recognition with primarily temporal cues. *Science*, *270*, 303–304.

Smith, Z. M., Delgutte, B., & Oxenham, A. J. (2002). Chimaeric sounds reveal dichotomies in auditory perception. *Nature*, *416*, 87–90.

Turvey, M. T. (2004). Space (and its perception): The first and final frontier. *Ecological Psychology*, *16*, 25–29.

Turvey, M. T. (2015). Quantum-like issues at nature's ecological scale (the scale of organisms and their environments). *Mind & Matter*, *13*, 7–44.

Uhr, L. (1963). "Pattern recognition" computers as models for form perception. *Psychological Bulletin*, *60*, 40–73.

Winograd, T., & Flores, F. (1986). *Understanding computers and cognition*. Reading, MA: Addison-Wesley.

Lecture 18

Turing Reductionism, Token Physicalism: The Computational System Assumption

In Lecture 6 we encountered proposals that perception is a species of calculation or computation. In Lecture 16 we encountered suggestions that if such were the case, then the study of perception should be formal, in the character of artificial intelligence. The algorithms for conducting perception should be approached as logical truths. In the latter part of Lecture 16, we identified this strategy within the artificial intelligence community as *logicism*. Our primary goal in this lecture is appreciating the formal foundations for the assumption that perception is a species of computation. We inquire whether perception is reducible to the states of a Turing machine.

18.1 Mathematics as a Natural Object

In brief, the primary thesis of the logicistic school of thought is that mathematics in its many forms is derivable from logic. A major proponent of the thesis was the 17th-century scholar Leibnitz. Kline (1980) who summarized Leibnitz's position in these words: "Because mathematical truths are necessary, they must be derivable from logic whose principles are also necessary and hold true in all possible worlds" (p. 217).

In the second decade of the 20th century, the philosopher–mathematicians Russell and Whitehead published *Principia Mathematica* in three volumes. It would become the definitive version of logicism's position. And it would present mathematics as something to be examined and analyzed in the manner of studying a natural object to reveal its properties. Logic could reveal the fundamental laws of mathematics—its "first principles."[1] And just as logic is viewed as a body of truths, the laws of mathematics would also be truths. Paradoxes and inconsistencies within mathematics would be eliminated. As we came to appreciate in Lecture 3, for Russell, the paradoxes arose primarily from the use of impredicative definition: defining a collection of things through use of the total collection itself. As noted in Lecture 3, Russell deemed such definition "meaningless." In *Principia Mathematica*, the law of the excluded middle was taken to task. The law states that all propositions are true or false. The law, however, is itself a proposition. In its assigned role as a basis for affirming a true law of logic, its very status as a proposition means that it itself can be false. For Russell and Whitehead, the law, in the form as stated, was meaningless (Kline, 1980).

18.1.1 Hilbert's Questions

The nature of the system of thought expressed in *Principia* raised a variety of questions. Most notable were those of Hilbert. He wished to know about the limitations of the logicistic scheme defended by Russell and Whitehead. His quest was practical: Is there a way to determine what could and what could not be proven in the theory embodied by *Principia*? To implement the quest required a *formalist* approach, in the sense that all mathematical statements should be expressed in a precise formal language abiding well-defined rules. The game of chess provides an apposite analogy (Hodges, 1983, p. 91). The steps in a proof are like the allowable moves in chess, the axioms are like the allowable starting positions, and doing arithmetic is like playing the game. Statements about chess of the kind "two knights cannot force a checkmate" correspond to statements about the scope of mathematics. The latter was the concern of Hilbert's program for mathematics.

The program consisted of a number of specific questions in dire need of an answer. Each referred to an unsolved problem, the solution of which would significantly advance knowledge of mathematics. Three of these questions in particular would set the stage for formalizing Descartes' grades of sense, particularly the third grade. That is to say, they would define the third grade's modus operandi, viz., computation, and provide hints as to its limitations. The questions were: Is mathematics *complete*; that is, in a technical sense, can every statement be proved or disproved? Is mathematics *consistent*; that is, would statements produced by a sequence of valid steps always be valid? Is mathematics *decidable*; that is, is there a definite method applicable in principle to any statement, one that is guaranteed to adjudicate correctly on whether the statement is true or false? Gödel took on the task of addressing completeness and consistency. Turing took on the task of addressing decidability. Let's see how they went about their respective tasks.

18.1.2 Gödel Numbering and Gödel's Proof

The starting point is the notion of *formal mathematical system* adverted to earlier. Such a system, with designation F, is a collection of abstract symbols together with a grammar, that is, a set of rules that identify how strings of symbols can be combined to generate new strings of symbols. The definition of F also includes (a) symbol strings in the capacity of theorems (adopted without proof), and (b) rules of inference for generating new, grammatically correct, symbol strings (theorems) from prior symbol strings (Casti, 1992a).

Gödel's ingenious strategy was to encode F as integers. If mathematics can be conceptualized as a game played with symbols (to reiterate, a game like chess), then one could play the game just as well with numerical symbols as with any others. Table 18.1 communicates the strategy for the elementary signs employed in logical formulae.[2] Beyond these signs are variables of three types: numerical, sentential, and predicate. Numerical variables range over integers and integer expressions. Sentential variables range over sentences (closed formulae). Predicate variables range over the likes of *prime*, *composite*, *less than*, and *greater than*. The three types of variables are transformed into Gödel numbers according to the following coding rule: Prime numbers greater than 10 code the numerical type, their squares code the sequential type, and their cubes code the predicate type, with all the prime numbers taken in numerical order.

A commonly used example of Gödel numbering is the logical formula for "there exists a number x which is the immediate successor to the number y," namely, $(\exists x)(x = sy)$ (Casti, 1992b; Nagel & Newman, 1958). By the preceding coding rule, the numerical variables x and y are assigned integers 11 and 13 (first two primes larger than 10) and the remaining symbols, for example, (,, =, and s, are coded as identified in Table 18.1. The resultant sequence of numbers for $(\exists x)(x = sy)$ is 8, 4, 11, 9, 8, 11, 5, 7, 13, 9. Although these Gödel numbers uniquely represent the formula, the challenges Gödel hoped to meet required something better, something considerably more efficient. The challenges required a unique number for each and every statement and sequence of statements that could be made about arithmetic. If Gödel could meet the challenge, then he would have a means to express every possible proposition about the natural numbers *as a number*. He would have a means to use number theory, to use arithmetic, "to examine its own truths" (Casti, 1992b, p. 311). In respect to the successor formula, the goal was achieved through the following steps: (i) Take the first 10 prime numbers; (ii) raise each to the Gödel number of the corresponding element in the formula; (iii) multiply them together (Nagel & Newman, 1958). The resultant Gödel number is $(\exists x)(x = sy) \rightarrow 2^8 \times 3^4 \times 5^{11} \times 7^9 \times 11^8 \times 13^{11} \times 17^5 \times 19^7 \times 23^{13} \times 29^9$.

Table 18.1 A minimal example of Gödel numbering

Sign	*Gödel Number*	*Meaning*
~	1	not
v	2	or
⊃	3	If . . . then
∃	4	there exists
=	5	equals
0	6	zero
s	7	immediate successor of
(	8	punctuation
)	9	punctuation
,	10	punctuation

Gödel applied the foregoing strategy to the logical paradoxes, each rooted in self-reference. The classic example is "This sentence is false."[3] Historically, it is identified as Epimenides Paradox. Commonly, it is referred to as the Liar Paradox (Barwise & Etchemendy, 1987), the name under which it was encountered in Lecture 3.[4] To implement the strategy, Gödel rephrased the paradox as "This statement is not provable," a rephrasing that situates the paradox in *F* allowing thereby its translation into arithmetic. The rephrasing is called a "Gödel sentence." Let's designate it as G. If not provable, then G's assertion is true and the implication is that *F* is *incomplete* (no corresponding theorem). If provable, then G is true, implying that what is stated is true and, perforce, not provable, implying that *F* is *inconsistent* (statement and negation both provable). The upshot is Gödel's theorem. Here's a formal-logic version of the theorem: For any consistent formalization of arithmetic, there exist arithmetic truths that are not provable within that formalization. Here's an algorithmic version: There is no algorithm whose end results consist of all true statements of arithmetic and no false ones.[5] For some, Gödel's theorem is sufficient reason to dismiss a formal (computational) perspective on the perception and action capabilities of biological systems (e.g., Penrose, 1989, 1994). For most, the theorem's relevance to the perspective is tangential. There are, however, arguments of a different kind, originating within the formal (computational) perspective, that provide the sufficient reason (e.g., the problem of NP-complete, to be considered shortly).

18.1.3 Turing's Machine

Returning to Hilbert's questions, what did he mean by "decidability"? As Hodges (1983, p. 96) underscores, it was not the determinism of the hard sciences. It was a more abstract notion—*the quality of being fixed in advance*, such that nothing new could arise. The challenge was to abstract the quality in question and apply it to the manipulation of symbols. The standard typewriter of the 1930s was Turing's conceptual point of departure. His joint ruminations on (a) the typewriter's functions and (b) decidability led to the conception exemplified in Figure 18.1: a finite-sized "table of behavior." For all intents and purposes, the table *was* an automatic machine.

The equating of decidable with a mechanical abstraction (in the form of a super typewriter) would come to be termed a Turing Machine (TM). As Figure 18.1 implies, TM in the abstract comprises a device in the form of a tape divided into squares of constant size on which symbols can be written ("inputs") and from which symbols can be read ("outputs"), and a device able to change position rightward or leftward one square at a time that writes and reads the symbols on the tape. To complete the TM picture, an additional device functions as a central processor and a finite memory. It is able to keep track of its current state (out of finitely many states) and the symbol that has just been read. In sum, TM is an input/output device plus a read-write device

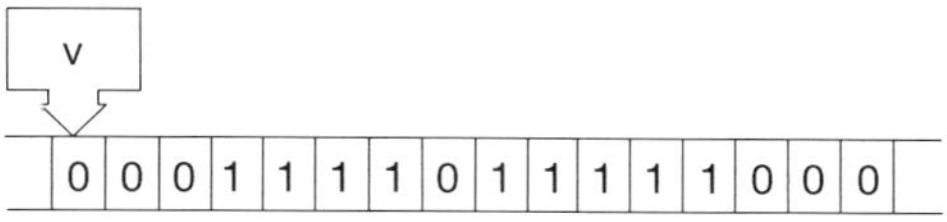

	0	1
C1	Move R; C1	Move R; C2
C2	Write 1; C3	Move R; C2
C3	Move L; C4	Move R; C3
C4	No move; C1	Erase; no move; C4

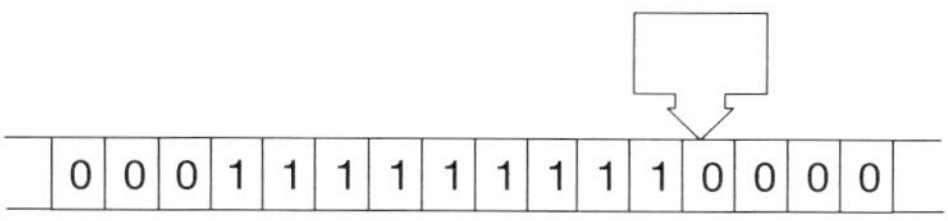

Figure 18.1 Turing's "definite method" rendered as a "table of behavior" (C is configuration, R is right, L is left). The table transforms the upper tape to the lower tape. It has the character of an adding machine. Beginning with the scanner leftward of the two strings of 1s separated by a single blank space, it adds the two strings, and stops. (The essential task is filling in the blank space and erasing the final 1.)

plus a finite-state device with (i) states that come from a finite set Q, (ii) symbols that come from an alphabet S, and (iii) read/write motions or directions that come from a set D = (left, right, stop). To reiterate, TM is a machine that is essentially the same thing as its program—quintuples of the form (q, s, q', s', d) where q' and s' are the next configuration and next symbol, respectively (Dewdney, 1989, p. 187). Of further note, TM provides a computational description without any reference to physical composition. The table of behavior in Figure 18.1 is absent physical constraints. What makes the TM of Figure 18.1 a system for doing addition are strictly the functional relations expressed by (q, s, q', s', d).

TM bears on Descartes trialism, particularly the thesis implicit in Helmholtz's unconscious inference that the third grade of sense (mental states) could be understood as computational states. And given that TM, in principle and in practice, is not bound to any specific material incarnation[6] it could be argued that, in respect to so-called mental states, *it doesn't matter what the matter is*. This so-called multiple realizability of TM allows one to be *both* a materialist and a mentalist—without qualms (Fodor, 1981). The assertions that mental states are distinguished, one from the other, by a functional relation, and that they are realizable in multiple material forms, defines the perspective on the third grade of sense known as functionalism (Putnam, 1975). For a functionalist, the third grade of sense is fully characterized by high-level descriptions, abstracted from (i.e., independent of) its implementation.

18.2 Structural Descriptions and Decision Problems

In Lecture 17 we encountered the notion that individual entities in the environment might be best understood as composed from an alphabet of parts. Specifically, we considered the notion that an entity such as a phoneme or a letter of the alphabet could be equated with a list of distinguishing features. Although reasons were given to be skeptical of such a notion, it is the case that elaborations of the "distinctive features" idea comprise most efforts to understand the perceptual achievements of identification and recognition. Here we introduce ourselves to the general approach of forging structural descriptions of entities in terms of parts and their relations. As will become evident, in so doing we provide an arena within which to engage more fully the implications of Gödel's and Turing's articulations of Hilbert's challenges of completeness/consistency and decidability, respectively. The implications are in the practical domains of *optimization problems* (trying to find the solution with the best possible score according to some scoring scheme) and *decision problems* (deciding whether a statement is true or false).

18.2.1 Constituent Structure

Figure 18.2 returns us to Peirce's conception of representation bearer, the ground for such, and the content of such (Von Eckardt, 1993). Our focus here is on the parts as individual representation bearers. Although representation bearers have multiple instantiations, it is very convenient to liken them to words, as entities that have specific content or meaning which singly or in combinations function as single units (constituents) in a higher order organization. To be succinct: A word or a group of words is a constituent—something that functions as a single unit within a hierarchical structure.[7]

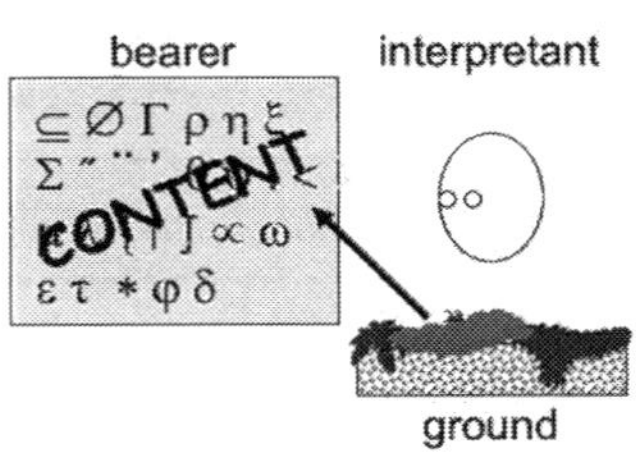

Figure 18.2 Individual representation bearers, the ground that determines their content, and the interpretant for whom they have significance.

Adopting a word (or, more broadly, a linguistic) perspective facilitates appreciation that representation bearers exhibit the properties of compositionality, productivity, and systematicity. *Composition* is the formal relation of parts to each other, with the specifics of how they relate, how they are arranged, determining the specific semantic consequences. *Productivity* is the repeated application of a fixed set of rules to a fixed number of parts to generate an, in principle, uncountable number of compositions (e.g., sentences) of indefinitely varied complexity. *Systematicity* is the intrinsic connections of one composition to multiple other compositions: Given a sentence S, systematic variants of S can be generated by permuting or substituting constituents of the same grammatical category.[8] Within the field of computational vision, the analogy between shape perception and language perception has a long history (e.g., Huffman, 1971; Minsky, 1975).

18.2.2 Geons in the Capacity of Phonemes and Visual Recognition by Components

A particularly attractive aspect of spoken language (and, by implication, written language) is the paucity of phonemes (about 44 in English) and the potentially unlimited number of words they can compose. The transcribed spoken words in the *Oxford English Dictionary* amount to approximately half a million. Perhaps the visual perception of forms follows language perception's lead. An approach to the perception of 2D renditions of 3D objects advanced by Biederman (1987) assumes that such is the case. Figure 18.3 gives examples of vision's hypothesized phoneme analogs, referred to as geons,[9] and the objects they can compose. Essentially, they are a subset of generalized cylinders (e.g., boxes, pillars, cones, spheres). As with phonemes, each geon is expressible by a small number of distinctive features—its edge kind, its symmetry kind, its curvature kind, its axis kind, and its relation kinds in respect to other geons. And further, consonant with phonemes, as few as 36 geons cover the estimated 30,000 recognizable 2D depictions of 3D objects (see Biederman, 1987, pp. 127).[10]

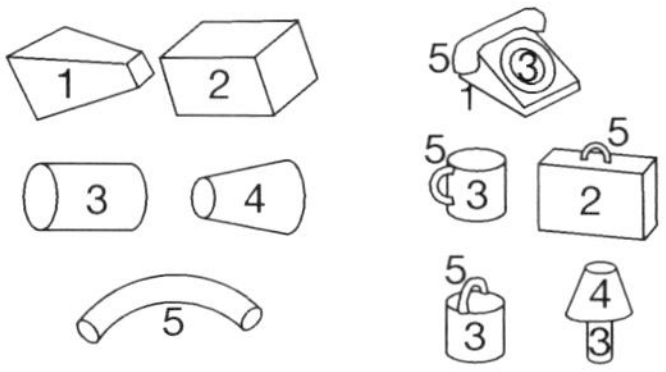

Figure 18.3 Examples of geons (left) and objects they compose (right).

(From Figures 7 and 11, I. Biederman, Recognition by components. *Psychological Review*, 94, 111–139, 1987, APA, adapted with permission.)

18.2.3 Representation as a Formal Symbol System

The conceptualizations in respect to constituent structure need buttressing. A further revisiting of Descartes will be to our benefit (Lecture 6). In his opinion, given imperfections and defects of the retinal image in respect to distal objects (Lectures 5–6), the nature of what was before the eyes could only be derived by the third grade of (visual) sense conceived as a rule-governed, quasi-mathematical process of reasoning (Lecture 6, Section 6.5). For that to be the case, the visual sensations constituting the second grade of sense would have to be represented in the style of a formal symbol system (cf. Marr, 1982, p. 20). Just as a musical score represents the multivarious sound structure of a symphony, the second grade of sense would have to represent the multivarious optical structure of the first grade of sense.

For the issues and theories that hang on structural descriptions, the choice of representation system is far from trivial. Here's Marr (1982):

> [E]ven though one is not restricted to using just one representation system for a given type of information, the choice of which to use is important and cannot be taken lightly. It determines what information is made explicit and hence what is pushed further into the background, and it has a far-reaching effect on the ease and difficulty with which operations may subsequently be carried out on that information.
>
> (p. 21)[11]

18.2.4 P, NP, NP Complete, NP Hard

Hilbert's 10th problem was in respect to algorithms. Given any particular computation problem, was there an algorithm that could solve it? A *yes* as answer would be in need of elaboration. Solvable formally is very different from solvable practically. An algorithm may exist. but time-to-completion for a current computer might be tens of thousands of years. However, given the evolution rate of computers, the latter dismissive doesn't really amount to much. A future computer might execute the algorithm in hours, seconds, or faster. Clarifying the answer "yes" to Hilbert's 10th question must be in terms other than "how long does it take?" The more appropriate focus is efficiency, the question of "how many steps does it take?" with "step" interpreted in the TM sense. The larger the data set, the larger the number of TM steps. A TM program (qua algorithm) runs in *polynomial time* (P) if there are fixed integers A and k such that for input data of length n, the computation is completed in at most An^k steps (for any values of n) (Devlin, 1999, p. 293).[12] The answer to the question posed of an algorithm ("is it efficient?") can now be expressed succinctly. Relative to P-algorithms, algorithms that run in *exponential time* (e.g., 2^n or n^n, etc.) are inefficient (see Figure 18.4).

A problem of some significance, the so-called traveling salesman problem (a minimal variant of which is given in Figure 18.5), does not have an efficient

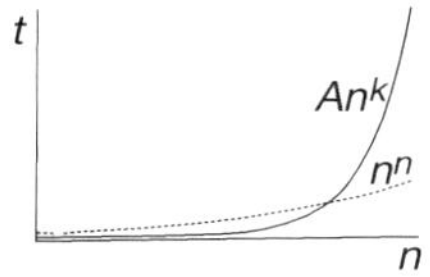

Figure 18.4 Contrast between exponential time algorithm (solid) and polynomial time algorithm (dotted) with *t* as time and *n* as number of steps.

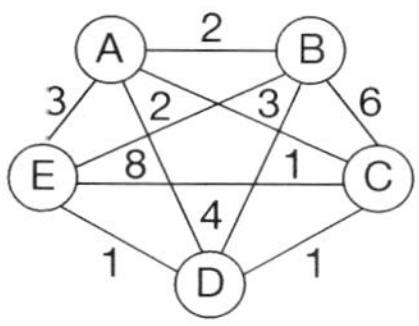

Figure 18.5 Traveling salesman problem. All sites (A–D) with their given intersite distances must be visited. Choose the route requiring the least total amount of travel. For n sites, there are n! possible itineraries. 5! is 120 possible routes; 10! is 3,628,800 possible routes; 25! is $1.551121004 \times 10^{25}$ possible routes. The required algorithm is exponential-time.

general solution. It could be of type P, but there is no proof. The preference is to type it as NP—*nondeterministic polynomial time*. It is instantiated as a TM that makes random guesses in the course of its operation. Each successive location in the N locations of the salesman's travel is guessed right (with probability 1/N! meaning that it is most unlikely). It is most important to appreciate here that we are identifying a super special computer, one with magical powers, a computer that functions as an *oracle*. Its magic is that it can guess the correct solution (at each step of the traveling salesman problem, for example) from among all of a problem's possible solutions. One might want to construe this magical device as a matchless parallel computer: Like no other, it can test all possible solutions simultaneously.

Problems of the NP-type, in a form known as *NP-complete*, act as a benchmark for NP problems. If one NP-complete problem is solvable by a P algorithm, then all NP problems are solvable by P algorithms. It is said that an NP-complete problem is just as hard as every other NP problem. Consequently, proof that *any* problem (e.g., travelling salesman) is NP-complete is proof that it is insoluble by any algorithm of type P. As will become apparent, scene analysis is such a problem.

18.3 TM Scene Analysis and NP-Completeness

The conceptualization of Descartes' trialism entered a new phase with the advent of computer-based perspectives on vision conducted in terms of the

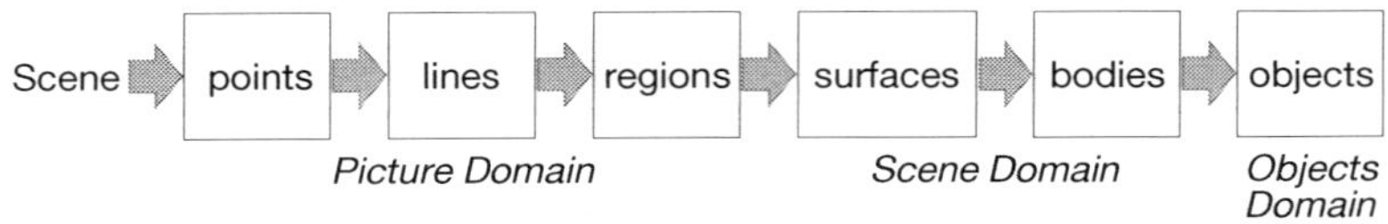

Figure 18.6 Basic structure of scene analysis by machine.

schematic shown in Figure 18.6. As we shall see, we can proceed to equate the second grade of sense with the *picture domain* and the third grade of sense with the *scene* and *object domains*. We can also proceed to consider whether the third grade of sense conceived computationally—that is, as TM—is up to the task.

18.3.1 Domains of Scene Analysis by Machine

The stages depicted in Figure 18.6 mediate between a scene (an environmental layout) and its resulting 3D description. The stages are assumed to abide a principle of graceful degradation: Given failure to achieve a full representational solution at any stage, a partial representational solution is contrived, and suffices for further computation, albeit limited.

We can assume on grounds of historical convention that the scene is projected on the 2D retina as an array of points that is partitioned into sets according to intensity (in the lexicon of physics) or brightness (in the lexicon of psychology). The 3D layout cannot be inferred from this points-representation. The charge of early vision is first to recover the lines that inhere in the initial points representation and second to determine from these lines the regions into which the 2D image can be parsed.[13] Collectively, points, lines, and regions compose the *picture domain*. As of this stage of processing, the constituent representations are indifferent to the 3D structure that the picture represents. Subsequent to the recovery of regions, computation is directed to mapping (a) regions to surfaces, and (b) surfaces to objects, with (a) and (b) defining the *scene domain*. The computation of scene domain from picture domain has been a primary concern since the late 1960s. Efforts to address this concern were directed at constructing systems sufficiently intelligent to infer (as the reader can readily do) the 3D structure from 2D line portrayals of opaque polyhedra. Figure 18.7 gives examples of line drawings of scenes of variously arranged solid geometric objects without shading and with shading, together with examples of vertices and their joinable regions.[14] Investigations of how their implied 3D structure could be recovered were shaped by the hypothesized isomorphism between visual structure and linguistic structure. A brief exposure to the seminal investigations of Guzman (1968) and Waltz (1975) will suffice to convey the gist of scene analysis by machine.[15]

The starting point for Guzman was the regions within the picture domain. Given a line drawing parsed into regions, the program's goal was to discover

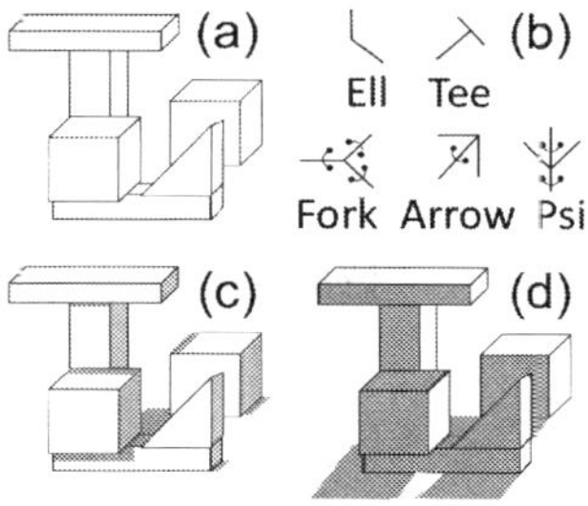

Figure 18.7 (a) A block-world scene consisting of polyhedral objects with (b) examples of their vertices and their implied regional links. (c and d) The block world in shadow under two different lighting conditions.

the number of separate 3D objects depicted in a typical 2D line portrayal. Specifically, the goal was to determine which groups of regions are the faces of a single body, a preliminary step to delivering a 3D account of the 2D portrayal. The grouping of regions can be inferred from the vertices. Consider the arrow-type vertex in 18.7b. In an architected environment, such a vertex would be an aspect of an exterior corner of an object—a site where two plane surfaces form an edge. The implication is that the two regions meeting at the arrow's shaft, and only those two regions, are linked. By connecting regions as a function of where they meet, the Guzman program (albeit with some shoehorning) separates the eight bodies represented in Figure 18.7a.

The introduction of shading in Figures 18.7c and 18.7d is noteworthy for the reduction in possible 3D interpretations of the 2D vertices, a leading feature of what has come to be referred to as "The Waltz Effect" (Winston, 1975, p. 5). By taking the illumination on both sides of the constituent lines into account, Waltz (1975) found that an arrow vertex was reduced from approximately 186,000 possible interpretations (or labels) to 86 possible interpretations, and a psi vertex was reduced from approximately 11×10^6 possible interpretations to 436. Foundational to "The Waltz Effect" were prior demonstrations by Huffman (1971) and Clowes (1971) of how severely environmental layouts constrain the way lines and vertices fit together in line drawings. Given this determinism, deciding on a line's status[16] in the drawings shown in Figures 18.7c and 18.7d is analogous to solving sets of algebraic equations comprising variables (in this case, lines) and constraints (in this case, vertices). The Waltz algorithm typically yields just one interpretation for each line in a drawing, and rapidly converges on the 3D scene that the drawing as a whole represents (Winston, 1975). However, as Waltz (1982, p. 129) made sure to remark, although elegant and efficient for the scenes to which it was tailor-made, it generalized only poorly to scenes composed of entities of a different kind (e.g., curved objects, textures, shiny surfaces).

18.3.2 Scene Analysis is NP-Complete

It is important to underscore that we have been considering a problem that is crafted within the Cartesian trialism—namely, given a specific state of the second grade of sense (a 2D straight-line drawing), the third grade of sense is charged with deciding whether it is the projection of the visible part of a set of opaque 3D polyhedra (e.g., Figure 18.7a). We have been considering this problem, crafted within Descartes' trialism, as a fundamental algorithmic problem (if not the preeminent problem) in computer vision. And we have been introduced to two reasonably successful algorithms for this problem and the problem's multiple extensions. We have not, however, inquired about the problem's status in respect to the computational issues raised earlier in this lecture (Section 18.2.4). Is it P or is it, in fact, NP-complete? The answer is the latter (Cooper, 1998, 2008; Kirousis & Papadimitriou, 1988). *There is probably no polynomial-time algorithm for solving the problem of scene analysis.* This is true even in the relatively simple case of trihedral scenes (no four planes share a point) without shadows and cracks. Determining whether the lines in a drawing of the kinds shown in Figure 18.7 are globally labeled according to the Huffman–Clowes scheme is itself NP-complete (Kirousis and Papadimitriou, 1988). Further, although some drawings that fully satisfy the Huffman–Clowes line-labeling scheme prove to be unrealizable physically (Sugihara, 1986), they nonetheless prove to be NP-complete (Kirousis & Papadimitriou, 1988). Cooper's (2008) summary of this state of affairs is blunt: "Most computational problems corresponding to the interpretation of line drawings (straight lines, parallel lines, planar forms, collinearity) have turned out to be intractable" (p. 229).

One might argue, as Cooper (1998) has, that scenes of the kinds shown in Figure 18.7 are intractable because of the constraints that hold among the interpretations of a scene's many different aspects. There is a great deal of circular dependency among the scene's constituents, and in natural (ecological) scenes this dependency spans multiple scales. Decomposition into "independent non-combinatorial sub-problems (Cooper, 1998, p. 28)" is infeasible. In some sense of the word, the scene and its interpretation must be treated as a whole. One reading of this conclusion is that a set theoretic perspective on scene analysis will not do. A hyperset theoretic perspective may be required. Its immediate appeal is that, like a natural scene's structure, a hyperset graph can have an indefinite number of relations (in the sense of paths, cycles, and loops; Omodeo, 2010).

It will be to our long-term benefit to finish this part of the lecture with Kirousis and Papadimitriou's (1988) musing on their discovery of the NP-completeness of scene analysis:

> In view of our negative complexity result, we must accept at least one of the following hypotheses: either the real problem of vision is much easier, due to "hints" we receive from aspects, such as texture and shadows, not

captured in our formulation; or the probabilistic distribution of the scenes encountered in the natural and artificial world is biased in favor of kinds that yield to ingenious fast heuristics.

(p. 17)

We will have good reason to consider these two hypotheses in later lectures. There is an element of truth in both of them.

18.4 The 2½D Sketch

Keeping the fact of NP-completeness in mind, we turn our attention to a further evolution in TM-based conceptualizations of Descartes' trialism. In the work of Marr (1976, 1978, 1982) and Marr and Hildreth (1980), the trialism passed another threshold, most particularly in regard to the nature of the second grade of sense. Roughly speaking, Marr addressed the question of how far into the visual system should one expect to go before finding a need for epistemic processes, such as memory and inference. He addressed the question of how big is the reach of the second grade of sense. Exactly how much processing tied strictly to retinal data can be conducted before the third grade of sense becomes involved?

Marr's overall TM-based perspective on vision is articulated in Figure 18.8. The 2½D Sketch is the second grade of sense consequent to (a) the input image and (b) the primal sketch (in so-called raw and full forms) that together constitute the first grade of sense. The raw primal sketch[17] is a transformation of the light distribution on the retinae (input images) into an elaborate but primitive description of the patterns of intensity changes. Detection of these changes is by a tunable differential operator capable of taking first or second spatial derivatives at any desired spatial scale, namely, $\nabla^2 G$, where ∇^2 is the Laplacian operator $(\partial^2 / \partial x^2 + \partial^2 / \partial y^2)$ and G is the two-dimensional Gaussian distribution

$$G(x,y) = \exp\left(-\frac{x^2 + y^2}{2\pi\sigma^2}\right) \tag{18.1}$$

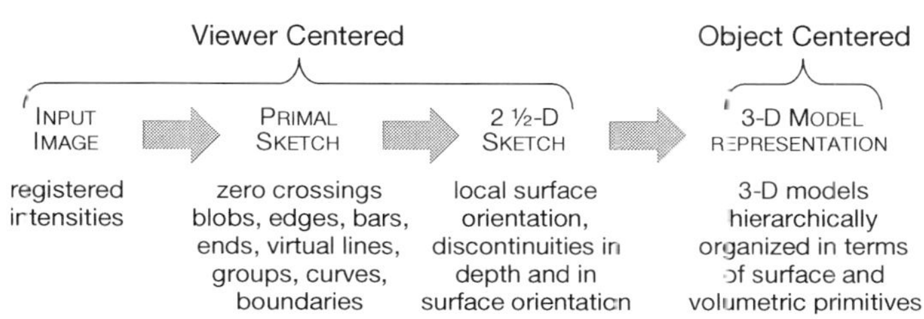

Figure 18.8 Marr's (1982) representational framework.

The parameter σ is the tunable spatial constant. Consider a photo of a plant in front of a chain-link fence (Figure 18.9a). A *raw primal sketch* (Figure 18.9c) is given in terms of the zero-crossings (Figure 18.9b) obtained by application of $\nabla^2 G$ across the image.[18] The resultants for a smaller and a larger value of σ are given by Figures 18.9d and 18.9e, respectively. The *full primal sketch* includes ways of representing intensity changes in the form of blobs (Figure 18.9f), oriented edge segments (Figure 18.9g) and bars (Figure 18.9h) together with ways of marking the geometry local to significant places.

The 2½D Sketch arose, one might say, from the ashes of scene analysis by machine. It arose in particular from the failure, articulated earlier (Section 18.3), to implement segmentation—to divide an image into meaningful regions (Marr, 1982, pp. 270–275). In approximate terms, it proved impossible to recover regions by means of grouping criteria based on local similarity or cues instantiated in visual intensities, that is, by means of analogues of the raw primal sketch. As underscored in our perusal of scene analysis, segmentation rested upon an observer's specialized knowledge of the make-up of the world in terms of meaningful things. As such, it constitutes the wrong problem for

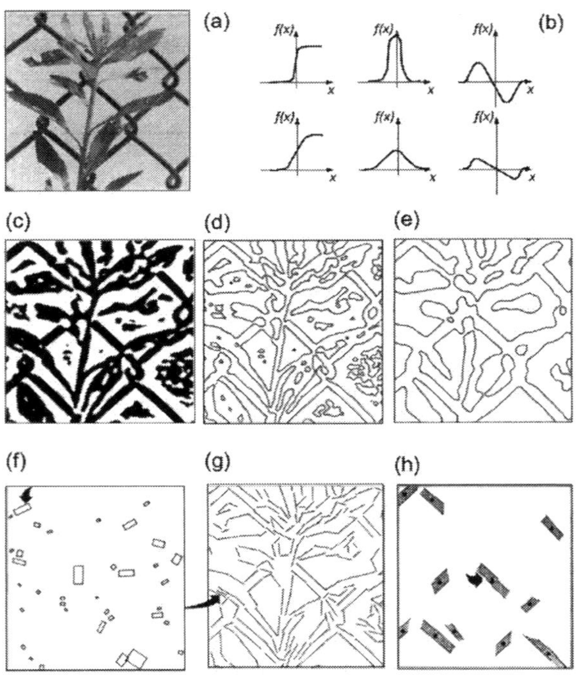

Figure 18.9 *The primal sketch, raw and full.* See text for details. (From Marr & Hildreth, Theory of edge detection, *Proceedings of the Royal Society B*, 1980, *207*, 187–217, adapted with permission, The Royal Society.)

Marr. The right problem for Marr is how visible surfaces are represented without the aforementioned knowledge, either a priori or a posteriori. The right problem's solution must be grounded in the physical conjunction of illumination, surface geometry, surface reflection, and vantage point.[19] The so-called 2½D Sketch is the proposed solution. Its function is to make explicit the orientation and rough depth of the visible surfaces, and the contours of their discontinuities. It does so in a viewer-centered only coordinate frame (hence, it is not fully 3D). Its primitives are local surface orientation, distance from viewer, and discontinuities in depth and surface orientation.

For Marr, the 2½D Sketch is the necessary precursor to perception of shapes and their spatial organization in an object-centered coordinate frame. Marr saw the conjunction of the viewer- and object-centered frames completing (see Figure 18.8) the 3D requirement for a fully functioning visual system. Given the issues just raised (Section 18.3.2), the latent query is whether this hypothesized system is P. The most likely answer is that it is not. The complicatedness of the hypothesized processes, the number and variety of interdependent degrees of freedom, should lead us to suspect (with confidence) that the proposed system is NP-complete.

18.5 Malebranche Redux and Direct Perception

We may recall that Malebranche posed the question of how it was possible to perceive the non-denumerable details of any given everyday scene if the basis for doing so was inference. How should we comprehend the third grade of sense's ability to make an infinite number of inferences, perform an infinite number of calculations, across multiple spatial scales *at an instant?* Malebranche's answer was: By the grace of God. The lesson from this lecture is that Malebranche's bold question can be interpreted as a question of "P or not P?" and his answer can be interpreted as the assertion "N-P complete."

The conclusion that there is no polynomial-time algorithm for solving the problem of scene analysis bears on the variants of Figure 3 and attendant arguments developed in Lecture 3. N-P completeness rules out Figure 3.2 and supports Figure 3.1—that is, the present conclusion is concordant with the direct perception thesis that perception is based on ecological information that is specific to its source. Whatever the organism, informationL is specific to the organism's surroundings (exterospecificity) and the organism's relation to its surroundings (proexterospecificity).[20] Neither the organism's surroundings nor the organism's relation to its surroundings *can be inferred*. More generally, and more prosaically, one can make many inferences about what one sees, but one cannot see by means of inference.

Notes

1 Paralleling the standard reductionist strategy of the physical sciences, mathematics would be reduced to logic.

2 Gödel used only seven elementary signs. Some tables of elementary signs have 15 entries (e.g., Dewdney, 1989). The number depends on how the formal calculus is set up (Nagel & Newman, 1958).

3 The problem becomes apparent when one attempts to decide whether the statement is true or false. Seemingly, it is true if and only if it is, in fact, not true. In preview, paradoxes of this kind matter. They do so because "The significance of a paradox is never the paradox itself, but what it is a symptom of" (Barwise & Etchemendy, 1987, p. 4).

4 See Lecture 3, note 12.

5 Both versions are due to Casti (1992b, p. 313). There are many other (less intuitive) ways of expressing Gödel's theorem, as is made evident by a casual review of the literature.

6 In practice, the currently universal material basis is silicon but expectations are that its future could be the likes of chalcogenide glass (see Loke, Skeltona, Wang et al., 2014) or DNA (see Kahan, Gil, Adar & Shapiro, 2008).

7 In linguistics, the analysis of constituent structure is associated primarily with phrase structure grammars.

8 In the view of some, systematicity is a questionable property of representation bearers: "my view of systematicity is maximally pessimistic: it does not exist; but if it did, languages would not have it; and if it existed and languages had it, systematicity still would not be all that interesting to many of the debates in which it has figured" (Johnson, 2004, p. 112).

9 Geon is a contraction of geometrical ions.

10 Many everyday objects, perhaps most, do not decompose naturally into a union of clearly distinct volumetric parts. And if they do so decompose, it is often only partially. Ullman (1996, p. 30) asks, "What, for example, are the decompositions of a shoe, a loaf of bread, or a sleeping cat?"

11 Marr's use of the term "information" is used here in a colloquial sense not a scientific sense.

12 The standard algorithms for adding by hand two whole numbers and integer multiplication by the standard method are polynomial time algorithms (for details, see Devlin, 1999, p. 293). Changes in the instantiation of TM and details of programming affect only the sizes of A and *k*, meaning that *steps to compute* = An^k is well founded.

13 Computationally, a region can be defined as a set of points with the property that a path drawn between any two points of the set does not cross a line.

14 In this body of work the labeling of vertices and lines has commonly followed the joint formulations of Huffman (1971) and Clowes (1971) (see Winston, 1975).

15 It should come as no surprise that this field of inquiry, in its contemporary highly practical form, is rich in technical issues, methods, and applications.

16 Conceived as a convex edge, an obscuring edge, a crack, a shadow, a concave edge, or as a separable concave edge.

17 The term "sketch" denotes a construction in a viewer-centered coordinate frame (see Marr, 1982, p. 42). It is conceptually similar to an artist highlighting or shading areas of a scene in order to create an impression of depth.

18 Zero-crossings take analogue or continuous representations, with their continuous intensity values, into discrete symbolic representations.

19 On Lecture 3's line of argument, one would say that the solution is grounded in the ecological physics of the layout of surfaces, most particularly in ecological optics. It is grounded in *informationL*, as noted in 18.5.

20 As will be noted eventually, the specificity is inclusive of the organism (propriospecificity) and the surroundings' relation to the organism (expropriospecificity; Shaw, 2001).

References

Barwise, J., & Etchemendy, J. (1987). *The liar: An essay on truth and circularity*. New York: Oxford University Press.

Biederman, I. (1987). Recognition by components: A theory of human image understanding. *Psychological Review*, *94*, 111–139.

Casti, J. L. (1992a). *Reality rules I: Picturing the world in mathematics—the fundamentals*. New York: Wiley.

Casti, J. L. (1992b). *Reality rules II: Picturing the world in mathematics—the frontier*. New York: Wiley.

Clowes, M. B. (1971). On seeing things. *Artificial Intelligence*, *2*, 79–116.

Cooper, M. C. (1998). The tractability of segmentation and scene analysis. *International Journal of Computer Vision*, *30*, 27–42.

Cooper, M. C. (2008). *Line drawing interpretation*. London: Springer-Verlag.

Devlin, L. (1999). *Mathematics: The new golden age*. New York: Columbia University Press.

Dewdney (1989). *The Turing omnibus*. Rockville MD: Computer Science Press (reissued as *The new Turing omnibus*, 1993, New York: Henry Holt).

Fodor, J. A. (1981). The mind–body problem. *Scientific American*, *244*, 114–123.

Guzman, A. (1968). *Computer recognition of three-dimensional objects in a visual scene*. (Tech. Rep. MAC-TR-59). Cambridge, MA: MIT (Tech. Rep. MAC-TR-59).

Hodges, A. (1983). *Alan Turing: The enigma*. New York: Simon & Schuster.

Huffman, D. A. (1971). Impossible objects as nonsense sentences. In B. Meltzer & D. Michie (Eds.), *Machine intelligence 6* (pp. 295–323). Edinburgh, UK: Edinburgh University Press.

Johnson, K. (2004). On the systematicity of language and thought. *Journal of Philosophy*, *101*, 111–139.

Kahan, M., Gil, B., Adar, R., & Shapiro, E. (2008). Towards molecular computers that operate in a biological environment. *Physica D: Nonlinear Phenomena*, *237*, 1165–1172.

Kirousis, L.M., & Papadimitriou, C.H. (1988). The complexity of recognising polyhedral scenes. *Journal of Computer and System Science*, *37*, 14–38.

Kline, M. (1980). *Mathematics: The loss of certainty*. New York: Oxford University Press.

Loke, D., Skeltona, J. M., Wang W-J., Lee, T-H., Zhao, R., Chong, T-C., & Elliott, S. R. (2014). Ultrafast phase-change logic device driven by melting processes. *Proceedings National Academy of Science*, *111*, 13272–13277.

Marr, D. (1976). Early processing of visual information. *Philosophical Transactions of the Royal Society, B*, *275*, 483–524.

Marr, D. (1978). Representing visual information. *Lectures on Mathematics in the Life Sciences*, *10*, 101–180.

Marr, D. (1982). *Vision*. San Francisco, CA: Freeman.

Marr, D., & Hildreth, E. (1980). Theory of edge detection. *Proceedings of the Royal Society, B*, *207*, 187–217.

Minsky, M. (1975) A framework for representing knowledge. In P. H. Winston (Ed.), *The psychology of computer vision* (pp. 211–257). New York: McGraw-Hill.

Nagel, E., & Newman, J. R. (1958). *Gödel's proof*. Oxford, UK: Routledge.

Omodeo, E. G. (2010). Bisimilarity, hypersets, and stable partitioning: a survey. *Rendiconti dell'Istituto di Matematica dell'Università di Trieste*, *42*, 211–234.

Penrose, R. (1989). *The emperor's new mind: Concerning computers, minds, and laws of physics*. Oxford, UK: Oxford University Press.

Penrose, R. (1994). *Shadows of the mind: A search for the missing science of consciousness*. Oxford, UK: Oxford University Press.

Putnam, H. (1975). *Mind, language and reality*. Cambridge, UK: Cambridge University Press.

Shaw, R. E. (2001). Processes, acts, and experiences: Three stances on the problem of intentionality. *Ecological Psychology, 13*, 275–314.

Sugihara, K. (1986). *Machine interpretation of line drawings*. Cambridge, MA: MIT Press.

Ullman, S. (1996). *High-level vision*. Cambridge, MA: MIT Press.

Von Eckardt, B. (1993). *What is cognitive science?* Cambridge, MA: MIT Press.

Waltz, D. L. (1975). Understanding line drawings of scenes with shadows. In P. H. Winston (Ed.), *The psychology of computer vision* (pp. 19–91). New York: McGraw-Hill.

Waltz, D. L. (1982). Artificial intelligence. *Scientific American* (October), 118–133.

Winston, P. H. (1975). Machine vision. In P. H. Winston (Ed.), *The psychology of computer vision* (pp. 1–17). New York: McGraw-Hill.

Lecture 19

Reflections on the Physical Symbol System Hypothesis

Lecture 18 was, essentially, an exposition of the so-called formality condition, that the processes constituting the third grade of sense are formal symbol-manipulating processes. Chess and language are commonplace exemplars of formal systems. The game of chess is *self-contained* in the sense that it is fully independent of the environment that embeds it. The discrete tokens matter—their types, their positions, and their permissible moves—but the embedding environment does not. Additionally, the system of tokens and rules is *perfectly definite*, no ambiguities, no approximations, no indeterminacies. Further, the system of tokens and rules is *finitely checkable*. Determining the validity of each position and each move is a matter of checking a finite list of permissible positions and moves.

The formality condition gives primacy to syntax, to the way in which symbols are arranged to form symbol strings. In everyday language, syntax is the set of rules that arrange words into constituent structures such as phrases and clauses. The thesis that mental processes are syntactical lends itself to a linguistic characterization of a mental representation as a proposition with two degrees of freedom, a propositional attitude and a propositional content. Attitude is denoted by a verb (e.g. "believes") governing an embedded clause beginning with "that": *X* believes that *Y* is *Z*.[1] Multiple verbs of widely different nature can be inserted in the same *X*, *Y* and *Z* frame. For example, expects, hopes, denies, disagrees, hates, remembers, perceives. Content is denoted by the linguistic forms assumed by *Y* and *Z*, also open to indefinite variation.

The formality condition is companion to the physical symbol system hypothesis (PSSH) (Newell & Simon, 1976), namely, *a digital computer has the necessary and sufficient means for intelligent action*. Arguably, PSSH is the dual claim that (i) human thinking and perception–action are kinds of symbol manipulation (because a symbol system is necessary for intelligence) and (ii) machines can be intelligent (because a symbol system is sufficient for intelligence) (Nilson, 2007). On the other hand, as some have suggested, PSSH may imply nothing more than that *intelligence can be digitized* (Touretzky & Pomerleau, 1994)—that is, PSSH is an assertion about the simple abstract 0s and 1s expressing the functionality of a digital computer. In this lecture, we introduce ourselves to some prominent perspectives on, and counterpoints to, PSSH and its intellectual companion.

19.1 The Discrete (Symbolic) and Continuous (Dynamic) Modes

Lectures 16–18 were dedicated to the possibility that the desired understanding of "knowing about" introduced in Lecture 1 could be founded on the exact idea of computation as an integral component of science's formal grasp of information. In those lectures, we examined the idea that "knowing about" is a species of computation over discrete symbol strings as knowledge bearers. The examination found the idea wanting. That is, it found PSSH wanting.

In Lectures 7 and 14 we encountered, respectively, Pattee's defense of the generalized complementarity principle (e.g., Pattee, 1977) and his promotion of the notion of the primal epistemic cut (Pattee, 2001). Their significance here is that they ground Pattee's insistence that a complex system does not have the option of operating in either the symbolic mode or the dynamic mode. It must operate in both modes, and often concurrently (Pattee, 1987). The problem of protein folding is a prime example. It seemingly comprises two qualitatively different phases—one a discrete symbolic process, the other a series of continuous dynamical processes.

In the first phase a genetic code (DNA) synthesizes an amino acid string.[2] Its depiction in Figure 19.1a can be conceived as a linear arrangement of symbols, with each symbol signifying an amino acid. Figure 19.1a is referred to as the primary structure. More complex structures, termed secondary (Figure 19.1b) and tertiary (Figure 19.1c), follow dynamically from the primary structure. They do so by way of weak forces (noncovalent bonds) between individual amino acids within the primary structure. The force types are

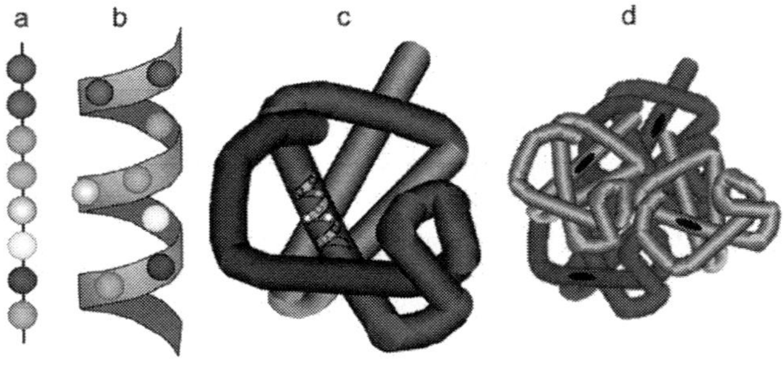

Figure 19.1 (a) *Primary structure*: Symbol string. (b) *Secondary structure:* Alpha helix. (c) *Tertiary structure*: Consequence of combination and interaction of secondary structures (different variants of A). (d) *Quartenary structure*: Structure composed of the joining of multiple protein subunits.

electrostatic forces, hydrogen bonding, van der Wals forces, and hydrophobic interactions (Alberts, Johnson, Lewis, et al., 2002). Even more structural complexity follows when two tertiary structures combine. A resultant quaternary structure is depicted in Figure 19.1d.

For Pattee, the amino acid symbol string is a constraint on the forces responsible for the protein's shape and function. Folding the protein cannot occur without the continuous dynamics. And the dynamics cannot proceed to fold successfully without the discrete symbol string to provide the necessary constraint. If solvents are used to disrupt the noncovalent interactions behind the tertiary structure (Figure 19.1c), then the system reverts to the secondary structure (Figure 19.1b). If the solvents are removed, then the tertiary structure is reinstated (Alberts, Johnson, Lewis, et al., 2002). In paraphrase, remove the dynamics, no shape; restore the dynamics, shape is exactly as it was before, that is, in accord with the symbol string.

The foregoing symbol–dynamics relation can be generalized as follows:

> [S]ymbols act as relatively simple, individual, nondynamical (nonintegrable) constraints on a larger dynamic system.
>
> (Pattee, 1987, p. 334)

> [I]n natural systems, a discrete description can be neither created nor interpreted by the discrete mode.
>
> (Carello, Turvey, Kugler & Shaw, 1984, p. 232)

To gain an appreciation of the generalization we can consider—by means of Figure 19.2—the case of a self-organizing fluid system, *the surface-tension-driven Bénard convection instability*. It is a prime example of a dissipative system, a system that is integrable (i.e., it depends on the rate of flow of energy, or of both energy and matter) and whose emergence from randomness to orderliness follows from fluctuations.

The top panel in Figure 19.2 shows the thermal flow from a heated substrate (an energy source) to the fluid's surface (an energy sink) at air temperature. The middle panel (left) shows fluid motion driven from the liquid-air interface. It shows how spatial variations in the interface's temperature lead to gradients in the surface tension that drive motion in the underlying fluid. Liquid is pulled from the warmer regions to cooler regions by the higher surface tension of the cooler regions. The middle panel (*right*) shows that at a critical source-sink temperature difference, the bulk fluid movement becomes structured as a series of small cells (so-called Bénard cells), with each cell comprising approximately 10^{21} molecules, and with each cell rotating in a direction opposite to its immediate neighbors.

The lower panel of Figure 19.2 is the view from above over successive time scales. In (i), incoherent motion at the microscopic level leads to homogeneity at the macroscopic level. In (ii), two cells are seen emerging within an instant

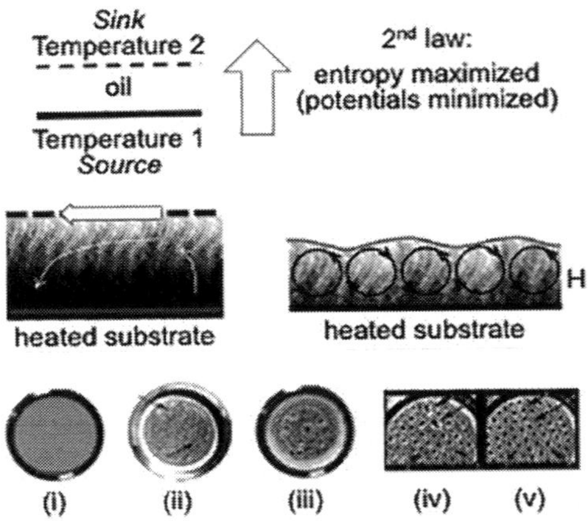

Figure 19.2 An exemplary self-organizing system. See text for details.

(*Top* and *middle*: from Figure 6.3, Turvey, 2013, MIT Press. *Bottom*: from Figures 2, 4 and 5, Swenson, 1989, Wiley. Adapted with permission.)

of the fluid becoming fully cellular.[3] In (iii–v), the developmental process leading to a time-independent organization of regularly arrayed hexagonal cells entails spontaneous fissioning of cells and competitive exclusion.

One gains from Figure 19.2 an intuitive feel for Pattee's (1987) thesis that symbol strings constituted by amino acids act at the same level as that of the fluctuations that generate a dissipative structure but are *radically different in kind from those fluctuations*. The symbol strings are exceptionally stable. They manage to stabilize themselves independently of the statistics or mean values of the macroscopic organizations that embed them.

The lessons pursuant to the preceding are as follows. Symbol systems can be constructed from matter, albeit in ways that await full disclosure. Amino acid strings are proof, as is the computer. The opposite, however, is not the case—that is, matter cannot be constructed from symbols. To do so would be in violation of physical laws. Accordingly, at best, PSSH is a half-truth (Pattee, 1989), a conclusion supplemented by the argument that systems operating strictly in the discrete mode cannot progress to a higher degree of competence—that is, they cannot self-complex.

19.2 Intelligence without Representation or Reason

Since the very early days of what would come to be called computer science there have been multiple ways of instantiating computation. Each instantiation, however, has proven to be equivalent to one of four principal forms differing in their level of generality. Table 19.1 is the (classic) Chomsky

Hierarchy of computational levels (Chomsky, 1958). The systems and issues addressed in Lecture 18 were from the hierarchy's highest level, the place of residence for the physical symbol system hypothesis. Here our focus is on the lowest level, that of Finite State Automata. Why?

Consider Moravec's (1988) sentiments in *Mind children: The future of human and robot intelligence.*

> The deliberate process we call reasoning is, I believe, the thinnest veneer of human thought, effective only because it is supported by this much older and much more powerful, though usually unconscious, sensorimotor knowledge.
>
> (p. 15)

> The fastest progress can made by imitating the evolution of animal minds, by striving to add capabilities to machines a few at a time, so that the resulting sequence of machine behaviors resembles the capabilities of animals with increasingly complex nervous systems.
>
> (p. 17)

> The route is from the bottom up, and the first problems are those of perception and mobility, because it is on this sensorimotor bedrock that human intelligence developed.
>
> (p. 17)

These sentiments are enshrined in the subsumption architecture of Brooks (1991, 1999), a robotics design in which perception is tightly connected to action through multiple incremental layers, with each layer manifesting a very specific competence. Each layer is a network of simple finite state machines with each finite state machine (FSM) characterized by a finite input alphabet, a finite set of states, and a transition function that transforms the present state and current input into a different state (if needed) and a given output. In brief, subsumption is an in-principle strategy for decomposing any intelligent adaptive behavior into multiple layers, each constituted by a collection of relatively simple FSMs, which increase in goal complexity from the lower to the higher layers.[4]

Table 19.1 The Chomsky Hierarchy

Machines	*Grammars*
Turing machines	Phrase structure
Linear-bounded automata	Context-sensitive
Push-down automata	Context-free
Finite state automata	Regular

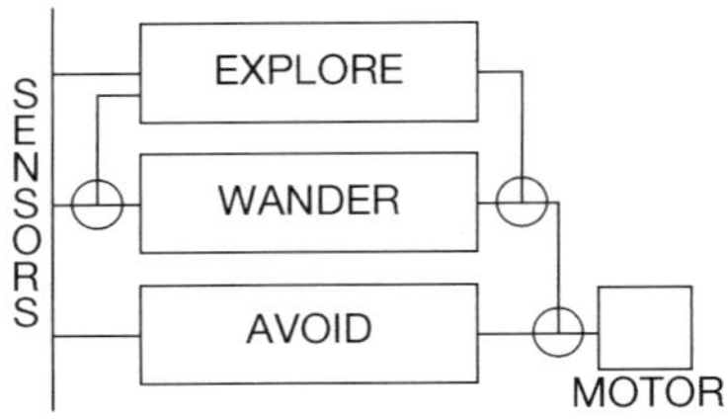

Figure 19.3 A minimal subsumption architecture. See text for details.
(Adapted from Brooks, 1991, Creative Commons.)

Among the earliest examples of the subsumption architecture was a three-layered system (from lowest to highest) of "*avoid* (objects)," "*wander* (widely)," and "*explore* (specific places)" (Figure 19.3; Brooks, 1991). That the functioning of avoid and wander layers never relies on the existence of the explore level, and the functioning of the avoid layer never relies on the existence of the wander layer, is impetus for each layer to have access to all data of all sensors and the ability to suppress (or overrule) inputs and inhibit outputs of the other layers. A major consequence of these design features is an ability of the *avoid* layer—for example, to work reflexively while *explore* pursues the larger goal, with feedback for both layers occurring primarily through the environment.

In sum, and in principle, the subsumption design relates perception to action absent mediation by the formal processes of representation implied by PSSH. The design, in précis form, is (a) no internal simulation of the environment; (b) no central control; (c) no partitioning into categorically distinct perception and action systems, with a central system that links them; (d) deploying layers (comprising FSMs) qua behaviors that operate in parallel; and (e) enriching behavioral competence by the progressive adding of layers. What can such systems do? Brooks (1999) contends that they can make predictions, make plans, and have goals without resorting to PSSH and, perforce, central, manipulable, symbolic representations.

19.3 Epistemically Autonomous Systems

Figure 1.1 of Lecture 1 is our working definition of a system **s**, after Mahner and Bunge (1997). To recall, it comprises C(**s**), the inner degrees of freedom (DF) that compose **s**, *E*(**s**), the outer DF that envelop **s**, and *S*(**s**), the relations, both bonding and non-bonding, among inner DF and between inner and outer DF, that constitute the structure of **s**. As underscored in Lecture 1, because environment is not an entity, it cannot be that *E*(**s**) as a whole acts upon, or interacts with, or is registered by **s**; rather, particulars of *E*(**s**) act upon, or interact with, or are registered by, particulars of C(**s**).

The registration issue is our point of focus in this section of the present lecture. The focus is in terms of the very broad and very deep question of

"How could the perceptual capabilities of organisms have evolved?" They were not engineered in any ordinary sense of that term. As Jacob (1977, 1982) contends and Coen (1999) amplifies, Nature is a tinker, not an engineer.[5]

19.3.1 Evolution's Tinkering

A tinkered pancake-making machine (from the imagination of the early 20th-century artist and illustrator William Heath Robinson) is shown in Figure 19.4. It involves a steam iron, a brick, makeshift stanchions, ropes, wires, a coal-scuttle, carriage wheels, a clothes washtub, and various kitchen items. The human tinker has created the machine through a process of arranging and rearranging the parts, of assigning and reassigning the roles of the parts, of discarding some of the originally selected parts, and favoring the incorporation of other previously untried parts. These manipulations of the parts to contrive contraptions are accompanied by assessments of how well they work. In these latter respects, evolution is like tinkering: It is constrained by what kinds of things are available, and what can be done with them. Like human tinkering, evolution "is an interactive process which does not plan ahead" (Coen, 1999, p. 360). That said, evolution's variant of tinkering departs significantly from that expressed by Figure 19.4. Changes in the parts composing an organism (the analogues of parts in Figure 19.4) are achieved by tinkering at the level of the genes and the success or failure of the tinkering is assessed at the level of the multiple individual organisms comprising the

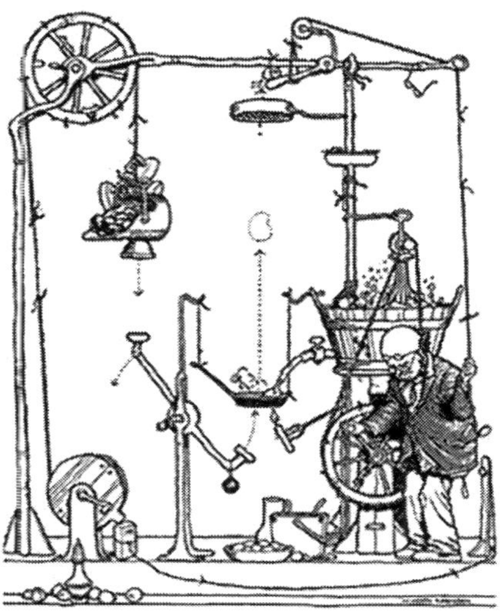

Figure 19.4 A tinkered pancake-making machine.

(Reprinted with permission from the William Heath Robinson Trust.)

species. The tinkering portrayed in Figure 19.4 is direct, at the level of the working parts.[6] Evolution's tinkering is indirect, at the level of DNA[7] (Coen, 1999).

The metaphor of tinkering can only be of value to deliberations on the evolution of perceptual capabilities if DNA is subject to influence from the organism, its environment, and their relation. Established thinking is often expressed through the *selfish gene hypothesis* (Dawkins, 1976/2006) or a simile thereof—that DNA is sealed off from organism and environment and subject only to internal influences that are random and gradual (namely, microscopic stochastic processes). Counter to established thinking, however, are observations and arguments to suggest that physiological function and organism–environment interactions affect both the nature and the rate of DNA change (e.g., Noble, 2006, 2013; Shapiro, 2009, 2011). The so-called central dogma was a focus of Lecture 12. The dogma and rebuttals to it were summarized in Figures 12.1–12.3. In respect to the present concern, one's overall impression from these prior deliberations should be that DNA is tinkerable.

In respect to perceptual function, evolution's tinkering would have to be (a) in regard to the infinitudes of $E(\mathbf{s})$, and (b) founded upon non-Newtonian interactions more so than Newtonian interactions. Let's consider the infinitudes first. It should be apparent that indefinitely, many predicates could be assigned to the pieces, aspects, dimensions, etc. of $E(\mathbf{s})$. Given an a priori partitioning of $E(\mathbf{s})$ into ecological niches (the reciprocals of organisms), one can only know which partitions are in fact niches by the presence of organisms—that is, one can only know a posteriori (Lewontin, 1982).[8] The same holds thematically for those elements of $E(\mathbf{s})$ that are conditions of effective environmental stimulation. They can only be identified and defined in reference to an organism (Bird & Layzell, 2002). The point is that organism and niche co-evolve—that the concepts of organism and niche are co-implicative.

The notion of non-Newtonian interactions is pursuant to drawing a distinction between simple atomisms and complex atomisms (Kugler & Turvey, 1987/2016). The term *simple atomism* can be used for any $\mathbf{s}$ that lacks an internal structure and, perforce, an onboard source of potential energy. The mass of such an $\mathbf{s}$ is the dominant factor in respect to its interactions with $E(\mathbf{s})$. Specifically, the interactions occur through forces and mass-dominated conservations, namely, energy and momentum. The interactions are Newtonian. Conversely, the term *complex atomism* refers to an $\mathbf{s}$ that possesses internal structure and an onboard source of potential energy. Interactions between complex atomisms and $E(\mathbf{s})$ are inclusive of descriptions or observables in which the mass (M) dimension is largely irrelevant, limiting composition of variables to the dimensions of length (L) and/or time (T). As classes, these descriptions or observables are termed *geometric* (L), *spectral* (T), and *kinematic* (L/T) and the interactions that involve them are termed informational (in Gibson's sense, Lecture 3) not forceful[9]—in engineering terms, they are soft couplings rather than hard couplings. Patently, organisms are prime examples of complex atomisms, meaning that their interactions with $E(s)$ are, in significant degree, non-Newtonian (Kugler & Turvey, 1987/2016, 1988).

Does tinkering partake of laws? If it did, it would either have to make use of a revised Newtonian notion of cause or make no appeal to cause at all (cf. Petrusz & Turvey, 2010). The discussion of the structure of reality by Barwise and Perry (1983) eschews the word "cause" entirely in favor of "constraint" (cf. Turvey & Carello, 1985). Of particular significance are *nomic constraints* that provide stabilities to which organisms may become attuned and *conditional constraints* that hold only under certain circumstances. An aspect of the environment sufficiently regular to be a nomic constraint could be an aspect of the environment lawful enough to serve as a basis of tinkering. The evident successes of evolution and adaptation are suggestive of sufficiently persistent nomic constraints. Following Petrusz and Turvey (2010, p. 57), *cause could be a guarantor of the persistence of regularities, but regularity without cause could be sufficient for adaptation through tinkering if it is regular enough.* There is experimental evidence (e.g., Tagkopoulos, Liu & Tavazoie, 2008) to suggest that the progression of naturally coupled environmental changes over billions of years is the primary selection pressure in evolution (Baliga, 2008). Because these natural environmental changes occur in a coordinated manner, they are, from the perspective of organisms, routine and predictable. They are, in short, nomic constraints.

19.3.2 Pask's Ear

It follows from the foregoing that a preliminary step toward answering the question of "How could the perceptual capabilities of organisms have evolved?" entails understanding autonomous selection from the infinitudes of $E(s)$ on the grounds primarily of non-Newtonian interactions. Surprisingly, perhaps, the most celebrated example of the kind of experiment needed to make this preliminary step was conducted more than half a century ago. In the 1950s, Gordon Pask conceived and built a series of electrochemical contraptions designed for the purpose of finding their own "observables" or "relevance criteria" (Cariani, 1993). The most celebrated contraption (Pask, 1958, 1960) has come to be known as "Pask's ear" (see Bird, Layzell, Webster & Husbands, 2003; Cariani, 1992, 1993).

An example is given in Figures 19.5 and 19.6. Figure 19.5 elaborates the "amplifying servomechanism" and the "signal network" segments of Figure 19.6. It depicts a number of small platinum electrodes inserted into a dish of ferrous sulphate and connected to a current-limited electrical source. The electrodes function as either sinks or sources of current depending on the activity of the overall configuration. The passing of current through the array of electrodes leads to the formation of metallic threads between electrodes where current flow is maximal. Specifics of the growth of the dendritic-like

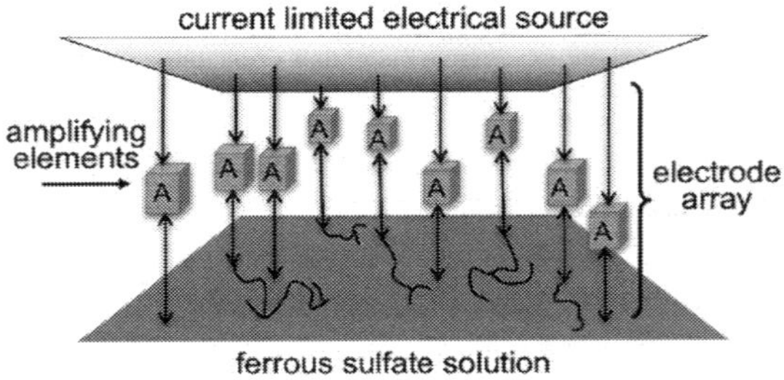

Figure 19.5 *Most prominent example of Pask's electrochemical systems*. Schematic of the relation between the electrode array and the ferrous sulphate solution. **A** is amplitude. See text for details.

(From Figure 4, Pask, 1960, adapted with permission, Elsevier.)

threads depend on which electrodes convey the current. With reduction in current magnitude (the resource for growth), threads that are well formed compete and threads that are unstable amalgamate to form a single cooperative arrangement. There is a trial-and-error dynamic to the growth of any given thread that is subject, additionally, to the influences of threads already developed and threads developing concurrently. Eventually, the network of threads achieves a dynamically stable organization.

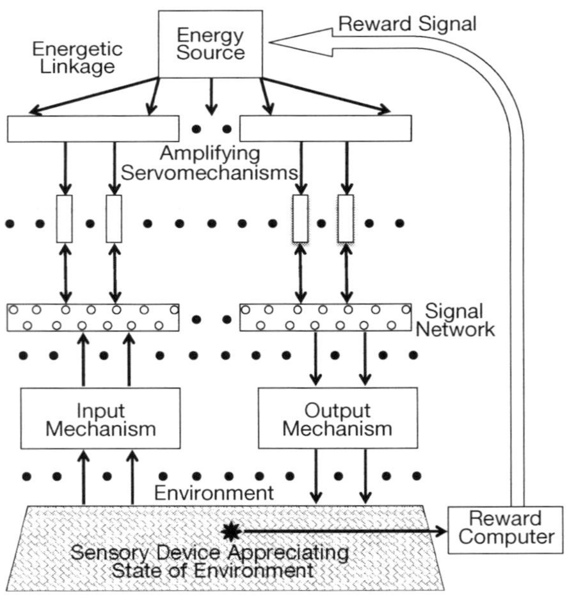

Figure 19.6 See text for details.

(From Figure 6, Pask, 1960, adapted with permission, Elsevier.)

The development and asymptotic state of Pask's electrochemical system are analogous to those of the Bénard convection instability depicted in Figure 19.2. Pask's electrochemical system has the character of a dissipative structure. Now the questions: How to tinker? How to craft conditions that could provide an opportunity for the system to relate to its embedding context, to reveal its "relevance criteria"? By monitoring a few electrodes through output devices, the tinker might be able to detect local changes in conductance. Such changes could be indices of the system reacting to one or more environmental events, one or more $E(s)$. The changes could serve as a basis for tinkering with the electrochemical system. For example, when a conductance change is detected, increase the growing capacity of the system as a whole by amplifying the current to the system. The tinker's intuition was that "rewarding" the entire electrochemical system for a conductance change putatively associated with a particular $E(s)$ might result in the system becoming attuned to that $E(s)$. To facilitate inquiry, the tinker defined instances of $E(s)$, for example, sounds differing in frequency. Pask (1960, p. 261), the tinker, summarized his tinkering thusly:

> We have made an ear and we have made a magnetic receptor. The ear can discriminate two frequencies, one of the order of fifty cycles per second and the other on the order of one hundred cycles per second. The 'training' procedure takes approximately half a day and once having got the ability to recognize sound at all, the ability to recognize and discriminate two sounds comes more rapidly . . . The ear, incidentally, looks rather like an ear. It is a gap in the thread structure in which you have fibrils which resonate at the excitation frequency.

In addition to acoustic and magnetic distinctions, attunement to distinctions of temperature, pH level, and vibrations were also found. In each case, what was being registered was a stable (one might say invariant) feature of the environment embedding the system of cooperative metallic threads. Contemporary investigations by Bird and colleagues (2003) have revealed an analogous phenomenon in the domain of unconstrained intrinsic hardware evolution. They observed a network of transistors self-organize into a primitive radio—specifically, a system that sensed and used radio waves emanating from a nearby personal computer. The notion of *nonobvious variables* introduced in Lecture 12 comes to mind together with a sense of how they might have entered into the governance of organisms.

19.4 Connectionism and Subsymbolism

PSSH is coordinate with a seemingly straightforward inference from the thesis implicit in Lecture 18: that a (universal) Turing machine can implement all possible computations. If one's predilection is to attribute computation to the brain, then the coordination of PSSH and Turing's thesis forewarns that the brain's physical structure will prove irrelevant to this attribution. The brain's formal properties are what matter, not its physical properties.

The typical anatomical image of the brain's microstructure is that of association or interconnectivity of cells. A scientific intuition of considerable historical appeal (touched upon in Lectures 13 and 14) is that fundamental mental capabilities such as perception are to be understood in terms of this connectivity. If the brain is to be understood through its connections (its *connectionism*), then mind should be understood in like fashion. It is a connectivity of mental entities befitting the scale of the individual cell and/or multiple cells functioning as a unitary collective. These mental entities can be viewed as abstract neurons—processing units that implement computation through (simple) interaction—and networks of abstract neurons. Appreciating how that could be the case requires conceptualizing an interaction as "sending numbers" (Rumelhart, 1986, p. 135) from any one abstract neuron to other abstract neurons over the links that connect them.[10] Pursuing this connectionist perspective with an eye on the reality of neurons imposes a priori constraints on how this species of computation behaves. Notably, neuronal-like entities should behave in the time scale of neurons (i.e., magnitudes of time slower than the functional entities in computers) and they should, like neurons, interact cooperatively and in parallel. Here's the bare-bones definition of a connectionist computer alias parallel distributed processing system (Ellis & Humphreys, 1999): "A connectionist computer consists of a set of simple, but richly connected processing units. Each unit receives a number of inputs which it sums. A single outcome is derived from the latter sum and broadcast to other units" (p. 4).

In systems satisfying PSSH, the entities over which computations are conducted have two defining properties: They refer to other things and they participate in operations governed by syntax. They are properly described as symbols. They denote concepts (entities that can be interpreted semantically) and they are governed by formal rules (the laws that define the computational system to which they belong). It can be argued that neither of the preceding holds for connectionist systems (Smolensky, 1986, 1987). For them, semantic interpretations are of activity patterns defined over ensembles of multiple abstract neurons. For them, manipulations by formal rules of passing activation are conducted on the individual activations of the abstract neurons. Entities properly describable as symbols are not part and parcel of connectionist systems.

If connectionism does not deal in symbols denoting concepts, what does it deal with? For want of a word, it can be said that connectionism deals with *subsymbols* (Smolensky, 1987). Clark (1989, p. 113) tells the tale of subsymbols in terms of "The ball broke the window," a variant of which we can tell here. The sentence invokes an activity pattern of abstract neurons with a potentially isolable subpattern that could be said to stand for "ball." The same subpattern, however, would not occur for "ball"—could not stand for "ball"—in the phrase "the baby lifted the ball." The subpattern in the first case is inclusive of hardness-related microfeatures. The subpattern in the second case is inclusive of heaviness-related microfeatures. The two different contexts for "ball" alter its subsymbols (Smolensky, 1988). Implicit in these remarks is the hypothesized highly distributed nature of connectionist systems. It can be expressed as follows: "In the symbolic paradigm the context of a symbol is manifest *around* it and consists of other symbols; in the subsymbolic paradigm the context of a symbol is manifest *inside* it and consists of subsymbols" (Smolensky, 1988, p. 17).

19.5 Population Thinking

Conversationally, one can refer to brain as a symbol-manipulating system—that is, conforming to PSSH—on the seemingly reasonable claim that brain (yours, mine) does computation. So, brains are something like computers, functionally speaking. But are computers like brains? This question does not invoke an immediate "yes." The hesitation arises, in part, because of the self-evident material difference and, in part, because of an obvious difference in origin—that a brain assembles itself and a computer does not. Brain and nervous system emerge from a succession of developmental events, obvious and nonobvious, internal and external (Lecture 12).[11] Edelman (1988, 1992) identifies the cellular level of this developmental process with a form of recognition. By use of the term "recognition," Edelman intends something eccentric relative to common understanding (but not, as we shall see, relative to scientific understanding).

> I mean the continual adaptive mapping or fitting of elements in one physical domain to novelty occurring in elements of another more or less independent physical domain, a matching that occurs without prior instruction.
>
> (Edelman, 1992, p. 74)

His exemplar of recognition is evolution, a non-teleological process—without purpose, without final cause. His explanatory vehicle is the immune system.

Theories of immunity have essentially been theories of antibody production in relation to foreign molecules or *antigens*.[12] Their concern has been the origin of the specificity of antibody production. In 1930, Breinl and Haurowitz expressed the challenge in these terms (Hodgkin, Heath & Baxter, 2007):

> We can now generate an almost infinite number of artificial antigens which cannot be found in nature. It is not feasible that the organism is constantly producing antibodies for thousands of artificially generated antigens.
>
> (p. 1019)

Proposed models of antibody specificity have taken one of two forms, either *instructional* or *selective*. In the instructional variant, a foreign molecule leaves an imprint of itself on the combining site of the antibody in a manner analogous to casting a mold "much as a cookie is impressed in dough by a cookie cutter" (Edelman, 1988, p. 186). The immune system therefore has a template of, or an instruction for, that which is to be recognized. In the selective variant, antigen exposure induces the elaboration of a sample of antibodies from a range of preexisting specificities. The selective variant functions like evolution—without purpose, without final cause, without representations of what it should beget.

We can benefit from making an acquaintance with population thinking. One reason is that it bears on the contrast introduced in Lecture 3 between indirect perception and direct perception. Whereas indirect perception is typically couched in instruction-like terms, apposite PSSH, direct perception is not.

19.5.1 Species

At the core of population thinking is the emphasis on the uniqueness of each member of a species. What is referred to colloquially as a "class" of organisms is more properly appreciated as a population of unique individuals. As Mayr (1975, 1982) stresses, prior to Darwin the theory of species was essentialism, a philosophical stance that all objects (e.g., organisms) and classes of objects (e.g., species) have essential characteristics, not accidental characteristics. Individual variation was dismissed as noise. Darwin saw individual variation as the basis of change—a realization that he came to slowly (Mayr, 1975, 1982). The planet's multiple classes of organisms, past and present, arose in a bottom up fashion *by means of natural selection acting upon the multiplicity of unique individuals in each of the multiple populations.*

19.5.2 Antigen–Antibody Relation

An analogue of population thinking about evolutionary time can be advanced for somatic time (the lifetime of an individual organism). Variety in the DNA of an organism's antibody-producing cells (*lymphocytes*) results in an enormous variety (10^6–10^7) of cell types, each distinguished from the other by one or more antibody molecules attached to its surface. To be emphasized are the facts that antibodies and lymphocytes are unique to the individual and have myriad specificities prior to any contact with any foreign body (Benjami & Leskowitz, 1991; Edelman, 1992).

Any antigen (e.g., virus, bacterium) entering the body will encounter a population of antibodies. The antigen binds to those cells in the population that are sufficiently approximate to the shape of its antibodies. That is, *the antigen selects from among all of the specificities in the population those specificities that enable the antigen-antibody binding to occur*. Each of these matching cells in the population of antibodies then divides repeatedly, to yield more cells of the same kind with antibodies of the same kind. In brief, by deploying a strategy akin to natural selection the immune system selects a cell line adept at dealing with a specific pathogen threat to the body at large. Selective adaptation—in the sense of attunement-to-antigens—self-assembles.

The description just given amounts to the thesis that prior to any encounter with any foreign molecule, the body possesses the capability of manufacturing an indefinitely large number of different antibodies, each uniquely distinguished by the shape of the site at which it binds with an antigen. Edelman (1988) celebrates this somatic ability to classify novelty with the words, "an adaptation so refined that the initial idea used to explain it was instructionist" (p. 190).

19.5.3 *Implications for Brain*

Among the many implications of population thinking—of outcomes following from evolution-like selection and not from instruction—is that uniquely specified connections within brain cannot exist. As Edelman (1988, 1992) takes pains to point out, the variation implied by evolution-like selection is of such a magnitude that precise point-to-point wiring, as in an electronic device, cannot occur. We should not expect brains and nervous systems within the species of any phylum of the Kingdom Animalia to be identical in connectivity from one species member to another.[13] This expectation holds at the microscopic scale of individual neurons and at the relatively molar scale of the cortical regions, the so-called maps, of the sensory and motor systems. In respect to the maps, evidence suggests that not only do they differ from individual to individual (e.g., Hutsler, Loftus, & Gazzaniga, 1998; Mueller, Wang, Fox, Yeo et al., 2013) but that, within the individual, they can undergo time variations in their boundaries and structural organization (e.g., Feldman & Brecht, 2005; Merzernich, Nelson, Stryker et al., 1984). Edelman (1992, p. 28) opines that "the variance of neural maps is not discrete or two-valued but rather continuous, fine-grained, and extensive."

19.5.4 *Invariance over Heterogeneity*

Recognition that individuality is synonymous with uniqueness (no extant duplicates) means that each individual part and whole of any given organism of any given species differs (e.g., anatomically, biochemically) from the parts and wholes of all of its conspecifics past, present and future (cf. Bergman, Afifi, & Miyauchi, 2012; Williams, 1956). Above this heterogeneity, however, sits invariance (Elsasser, 1998)—that is, any part or any whole is functionally the same (within normal bounds) in each of its indefinitely many within-species instantiations.

19.5.5 Instructional and Selective, Indirect and Direct

As anticipated, a parallelism can be drawn between the two theoretical perspectives on the immune response, instructional and selective, and the two theoretical perspectives on perception, indirect and direct, respectively. We can do so in terms of the fundamental claim developed in Lecture 3: What makes a perceptual theory a theory of direct perception is the assertion of specificity.

If we are permitted some small liberty with the perception-related term *sense* then we can cast the defining properties of the immune[14] system as follows:

1 It can sense non-self (antigens) separately from self (antibodies). It is exteroceptive and proprioceptive.
2 It can sense existing antigens never encountered previously and antigens that do not yet exist but could exist. It is infinitely perceptive.
3 Its sensing of any antigen benefits from having sensed that antigen previously. It is tunable and educable.

This casting allows us to recognize the immune system as kindred to a perceptual system in Gibson's (1966, 1979/1986) sense. Let antibodies be agency A and antigens be A's environment (niche) E. Then we can say that A neither constructs E nor infers E. *And, most significantly, we can say that at every instant, whether E's state is a repetition or a novelty, the state of* A *is specific to the state of* E.

As we did at the end of Lecture 18, we recall Figures 3.1 and 3.2 so as to highlight that the two figures contrast in respect to "selective" and "instructional," respectively (terms synonymous with non-inferential and inferential, respectively). The implied commonality between systems characterized by Figure 3.1 and immune systems is the grounding of their functionality in specificity. Whatever the organism in Figure 3.1, its perceiving, like the immune system's sensing, can encompass all of the indefinitely many varied encounters it has in its niche, whether those encounters be habitual or once only.

19.6 The Top–Down Fallacy

Top–down knowledge is often touted as a prima facie requirement of perception. Fowler (1990) rebuffs this tout in the strongest of terms. The rebuff provides an appropriate conclusion to the lecture. First, if top–down knowledge is absent at birth, then the only means by which it can be acquired is perceptual. Second, any top–down knowledge acquired by means of perceiving can be no more meaningful and accurate than the perceiving by which it was acquired. If it were the case that perception is ineffectual in the absence of top–down knowledge, then top–down knowledge acquired perceptually would likewise be ineffectual. To cut to the chase, acquiring useful top–down knowledge requires acquiring true knowledge by means of perceiving. Only perceiving *directly* can ensure that.

Notes

1 A "to" phrase can do the same job. For example, "Fred hopes to drive his dad's new car." for "Fred hopes that he can drive his dad's new car." And "that" can be omitted—that is, merely implied.

2 There are approximately 20 chemically different kinds of amino acids composing proteins with string lengths between 50 and 2000 in number (Alberts, Johnson, Lewis, et al., 2002).

3 It should be noted that in repetitions of the experimental induction of the convection instability, the fact that each cell arises from fluctuations means that the first emerging cells are most unlikely to repeat in location and order from one induction to the next, which is the case (Swenson, 1989).

4 Difficulties should be noted. Given each layer is a goal-directed behavior the more layers there are the greater the likelihood of interference among goals. Implementing a distributed system of inhibition and suppression to select and coordinate some layers (hence, goals) rather than others is complicated.

5 That nature's systems are frequently imperfect (as might be expected from tinkering) is a theme in Darwin's (1859) *On the origin of species*.

6 For Darwin, parts variation (the organism) came first, followed by transmission to the offspring. Modern theory reverses the argument. Alterations in the DNA precede their manifestation in the organism.

7 A gene is composed of DNA. The absence of a universally valid definition of gene encouraged a temporary focus upon the genome, easily defined as the totality of DNA transmitted across generations. The focus was temporary because gene proved more helpful than genome for understanding development and illnesses (Morange, 2001).

8 $E(s)$ is a continuum and as such can be partitioned in mutually incompatible ways (e.g., like a cheese round that can be sliced into triangles, rectangles, columns, etc., but not simultaneously). These ways could, however, be compatible if they could be interpreted as distinct partitions of the same reality on different levels of granularity (Smith, 2009; for details, see Bittner & Smith, 2003).

9 The dimensional form of force is ML/T^2 for grams × (centimeters/seconds squared).

10 Long-term consequences of processing in connectionist systems are manifest as weights assigned to connections. Temporary consequences of processing are manifest as activation patterns.

11 The specification of protein shape by genes does not suffice. The real determinant is the behavior during epigenesis of individual cells, the unpredictable paths traveled and the unpredictable moment and place of dying.

12 Derived from "antibody-generator."

13 The term *connectome* has been suggested (Seung, 2012) for an individual's connectivity, uniquely defined by the reweighting, reconnecting, rewiring and regenerating that is incident to individualized experiences.

14 There are, in fact, two immune systems—innate and adaptive. Discussion here is in respect to the latter.

References

Alberts, B., Johnson, A., Lewis, J., Raff, M., Roberts, K., & Walter, P. (2002). *Molecular biology of the cell* (4th ed.). New York: Garland Science.

Baliga, N. S. (2008). The scale of prediction. *Science, 320*, 1297–1298.

Barwise, J., & Perry, J. (1983). *Situations and attitudes*. Cambridge, MA: MIT Press.

Benjami, E., & Leskowitz, S. (1991). *Immunology: A short course*. New York: Wiley.

Bergman, R. A., Afifi, A. K., & Miyauchi, R. (2012). *Illustrated encyclopedia of human anatomic variation*. Retrieved from: www.anatomyatlases.org/AnatomicVariants/AnatomyHP. shtml.

Bird, J., & Layzell, P. (2002). The evolved radio and its implication for modeling the evolution of novel sensors. *Evolutionary Computation* (*CEC02 Proceedings*), *2*, 1836–1841.

Bird, J., Layzell, P., Webster, A., & Husbands, P. (2003), Towards epistemically autonomous robots: Exploiting the potential of physical systems. *Leonardo, 36*, 109–114.

Bittner, T., & Smith, B. (2003). A theory of granular partitions. In M. Duckham, M. F. Goodchild, & M. F. Worboys (Eds.), *Foundations of geographic information science* (pp. 117–151). London: Taylor & Francis.

Brooks, R. (1991). Intelligence without representation. *Artificial Intelligence, 47*, 139–159.

Brooks, R. (1999). *Cambrian intelligence: The early history of the new AI*. Cambridge, MA: MIT Press.

Carello, C., Turvey, M. T., Kugler, P. N., & Shaw, R. (1984). Inadequacies of the computer metaphor. In M. Gazzaniga (Ed.), *Handbook of cognitive neuroscience* (pp. 229–248). New York: Plenum Press.

Cariani, P. (1992). Emergence and artificial life. In C. G. Langton, C. Taylor, J. D. Farmer, S. Rasmussen (Eds.), *Artificial life II* (pp. 775–797). Reading, MA: Addison-Wesley.

Cariani, P. (1993). To evolve an ear: Epistemological implications of Gordon Pask's electrochemical devices. *Systems Research, 10*, 19–33.

Chomsky, N. (1958). Linguistics, logic, psychology, and computers. In J. W. Carr (Ed.), *Computer programming and artificial intelligence, an intensive course for practicing scientists and engineers: Lectures given at the university of Michigan, Summer 1958* (pp. 429–456). Ann Arbor: University of Michigan College of Engineering.

Clark, A. (1989). *Microcognition: philosophy, cognitive science, and parallel distributed processing*. Cambridge, MA: MIT Press.

Coen, E. (1999). *The art of genes*. Oxford, UK: Oxford University Press.

Darwin, C. (1859). *On the origin of species*. London: Murray.

Dawkins, R. (2006). *The selfish gene*. NewYork: Oxford University Press (original work published 1976).

Edelman, G. M. (1988). *Topobiology: An introduction to molecular embryology*. New York: Basic Books.

Edelman, G. M. (1992). *Bright air, brilliant fire: On the matter of mind*. New York: Basic Books.

Ellis, R., & Humphreys, G. (1999). *Connectionist psychology*. Hove, UK: Psychology Press.

Elsasser, W. M. (1998). *Reflections on a theory of organisms*. Baltimore, MD: Johns Hopkins University Press.

Feldman, D. R., & Brecht, M. (2005). Map plasticity in somatosensory cortex. *Science, 310*, 810–815.

Fowler, C. A. (1990). Calling a mirage a mirage Direct perception of speech produced without a tongue. *Journal of Phonetics, 18*, 529–541.

Gibson, J. J. (1966). *The senses considered as perceptual systems*. Boston, MA: Houghton-Mifflin.

Gibson, J. J. (1986). *The ecological approach to visual perception*. Mahwah, NJ: Erlbaum (original work published 1979).

Hodgkin, P. D., Heath, W. R., & Baxter, A. G. (2007). The clonal selection theory: 50 years since the revolution. *Nature Immunology, 8*, 1019–1026.

Hutsler, J. J., Loftus, W. C., & Michael S., & Gazzaniga, M. S. (1998). Individual variation of cortical surface area asymmetries. *Cerebral Cortex, 8*, 11–17.

Jacob, F. (1977). Evolution and tinkering. *Science, 196*, 1161–1166.

Jacob, F. (1982). *The possible and the actual*. New York: Pantheon.

Kugler, P. N., & Turvey, M. T. (1987). *Information, natural law, and the self-assembly of rhythmic movement*. Hillsdale, NJ: Erlbaum.

Kugler, P. N., & Turvey, M. T. (1988). Self-organization, flow fields, and information. *Human Movement Science, 7*, 97–129.

Lewontin, R. C. (1982). Organism and environment. In H. C. Plotkin (Ed.), *Learning, development and culture* (pp. 151–170). New York: Wiley.

Mahner, M., & Bunge, M. (1997). *Foundations of biophilosophy*. New York: Springer.

Mayr, E. (1975). *Evolution and the diversity of life*. Cambridge, MA: Harvard University Press.

Mayr, E. (1982). *The growth of biological thought: Diversity of evolution and inheritance*. Cambridge, MA: Harvard University Press.

Merzenich, M. M., Nelson, R. J., Stryker, M. P , Cynader, M. S., Schoppmann, A., & Zook, J. M. (1984). Somatosensory cortical map changes following digit amputation in adult monkeys. *Journal of Comparative Neurology, 224*, 591–605.

Morange, M. (2001). *The misunderstood gene*. Boston, MA: Harvard University Press.

Moravec, H. (1988). *Mind children: The future of human and robot intelligence*. Cambridge, MA: Harvard University Press.

Mueller, S., Wang, D., Fox, M. D., Yeo, T. et al. (2013). Individual variability in functional connectivity architecture of the human brain. *Neuron, 77*, 586–595.

Newell, A., & Simon, H. A. (1976). Computer science as empirical inquiry: symbols and search. *Communications of the Association for Computing Machinery, 19*, 113–126.

Nilson, N. J. (2007). The physical symbol system hypothesis: status and prospects. In M. Lungarella, F. Iida, J. Bongard, & R. Pfeifer (Eds.). *50 Years of artificial intelligence* (pp. 9–17). Berlin, Germany: Springer.

Noble, D. (2006). *The music of life: Biology beyond the genome*. Oxford, UK: Oxford University Press.

Noble, D. (2013). Physiology is rocking the foundations of evolutionary biology. *Experimental Physiology, 98*, 1235–1243.

Pask, G. (1958). Physical analogues to the growth of a concept. *Mechanization of thought processes. National Physical Laboratory*. HMSO, 2, 879–928.

Pask, G. (1960). The natural history of networks. In M. C. Yovits & S. Cameron (Eds.), *Self-organizing systems* (pp. 232–261). New York: Pergamon Press.

Pattee, H. H. (1977). Dynamic and linguistic modes of complex systems. *International Journal of General Systems, 3*, 259–266.

Pattee, H. H. (1987). Instabilities and information in biological self-organization. In F. E., Yates (Ed.), *Self-organizing systems: The emergence of order* (pp. 325–338). New York: Plenum Press.

Pattee, H. H. (1989). Simulations, realizations, and theories of life. In C. Langton (Ed.), *Artificial life* (pp. 63–77). New York: Addison-Wesley.

Pattee, H. H. (2001). The physics of symbols: Bridging the epistemic cut. *BioSystems*, 60, 5–21.

Petrusz, S., & Turvey, M. T. (2010). On the distinctive features of ecological laws. *Ecological Psychology*, *22*, 44–68.

Rumelhart, D. F. (1986). The architecture of mind: A connectionist approach. In M. I. Posner (Ed.), *Foundations of cognitive science* (pp. 133–160). Boston, MA: MIT Press.

Seung, S. (2012). *Connectome: How the brain's wiring makes us who we are*. New York: Houghton Mifflin Harcourt.

Shapiro J. A. (2009). Revisiting the central dogma in the 21st century. *Annals of the New York Academy of Sciences*, *1178*, 6–28.

Shapiro J. A. (2011). *Evolution: A view from the 21st century*. Upper Saddle River, NJ: Pearson Education.

Smith, B. (2009). Towards a realistic science of environments. *Ecological Psychology*, *21*, 121–130.

Smolensky, P. (1986). Information processing in dynamical systems: Foundations in harmony theory. In D. Rumelhart, J. McClelland, and the PDP Research Group. *Parallel distributed processing: Explorations in the microstructure of cognition, Vol. 1* (pp. 194–281). Cambridge, MA: MIT Press.

Smolensky, P. (1987). Connectionism, AI, and the brain. *Artificial Intelligence Review*, *1*, 95–109.

Smolensky, P. (1988). On the proper treatment of connectionism. *Behavioral and Brain Sciences*, *11*, 1–74.

Swenson, R. (1989). Emergent attractors and the law of maximum entropy production: Foundations to a theory of general evolution. *Systems Research*, 6, 187–197.

Tagkopoulos, I., Liu, Y-C., & Tavazoie, S. (2008). Predictive behavior within microbial genetic networks. *Science*, *320*, 1313–1317.

Touretzky, D. S., & Pomerleau, D. A. (1994). Reconstructing physical symbol systems. *Cognitive Science*, *18*, 345–353.

Turvey, M. T. (2013). Ecological perspective on perception-action: What kind of science does it entail? In W. Prinz, M. Beisert, & A. Herwig (Eds.), *Action science: Foundations of an emerging discipline* (pp. 139–170). Cambridge, MA: MIT Press.

Turvey, M. T., & Carello, C. (1985). The equation of information and meaning from the perspectives of situation semantics and Gibson's ecological realism. *Linguistics and Philosophy*, 8, 81–90.

Williams, R. J. (1956). *Biochemical individuality*. New York: Wiley.

Part 3

Ecological Perspective

Lecture 20

Ecology: The Science that Reasons Why

A theory of perception ought to be a theory for all organisms. The theorizing spelled out in the lectures so far has focused mainly on one phylum (humans) of one kingdom (Animalia). In this lecture, we will begin to consider reasons for widening our focus. The immediately following remarks provide perspective on how wide the focus can be. Although 1.2 million eukaryotic species have been catalogued to date (those of the Kingdoms Animalia, Plantae, Protoctista, and Fungi), there are reasons to believe that 86% of those existing on land and 91% of those existing in the ocean are yet to be identified (Mora et al., 2011). In respect to the Kingdom Bacteria, the number of different species in a single ton of soil may be of the order of 4×10^6 (Curtis, Sloane, & Scannell, 2002). Complicating estimates of the number of species of bacteria worldwide is the absence of a principled basis for deciding what counts (e.g., Doolittle & Zhaxybayeva, 2009).

There is more that should be said about the Kingdom Bacteria and it is of some import that it should be said earlier rather than later. The Kingdom Bacteria has long been recognized as life's dominant form. It originated 3.5 billion years ago, it exists now, and is expected to exist long into the future. It has long been considered as the most abundant and biochemically diverse form of life, the most resistant to eradication, and the most varied in habitat, functioning in more regions of the planet than the four eukaryotic kingdoms combined. On this matter, Stephen Jay Gould (1982/1998) comments:

> But we cannot grasp this fundamental fact, and so much else about evolution, until we abandon our biased view of life as a linear chain leading to human complexity at a pinnacle, and focus instead upon the rich range of diversity as the primary phenomenon of life's spread and meaning.
>
> (p. xiv)

The dominance of bacteria and Gould's dictum notwithstanding, it has become evident that the governing conjecture formulated in the 19th century, that eukaryotic species are derivative of bacteria, is in need of revision. The

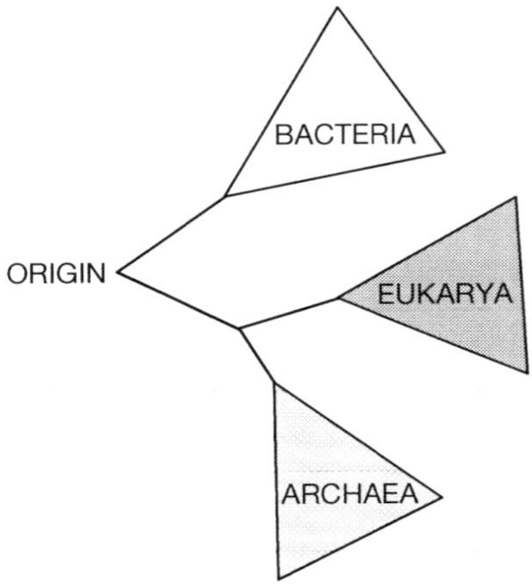

Figure 20.1 Tree of life's three domains according to ribosomal RNA sequences. Lines indicate sequence change.

(From Pace, 2006, adapted with permission, *Nature*.)

relatively recent discovery (Woese & Fox, 1977) of another class of organisms at the nanometer scale of bacteria, referred to as archaea,[1] has revolutionized thinking (e.g, Woese, Kandler & Wheelis, 1990). While archaea are similar to bacteria in size and simplicity of structure, their molecular organization[2] may relate more closely to that of eukaryotes than to that of bacteria. Our present but rapidly complexifying[3] understanding of the relation among bacteria, archaea, and eukaryotes—a current depiction of the tree of life—is shown in Figure 20.1 (Pace, 2006; Woese, 2004).

20.1 Thermodynamics and Living Things

It has been remarked that ecology is "the science that reasons why" (Colinvaux, 1978). For an ecologist, living things have traditionally invited questions of the following sort: Why are some living things common and others rare? Why are some large and others small? Why are they so curious in their ways? Elton's (1927/2001) two original questions of "Why should large animals be so remarkably rare?" and "Why should living things come in discrete sizes?" were answered by Lindeman's (1942) theory of trophic (nutritional) transactions within an ecosystem: Rarity and discreteness are the direct consequences of the 2nd law of thermodynamics. All natural processes (such as the nutritional flows of an ecosystem) increase universal entropy.[4] They degrade the quality of energy—its availability to do work. It was a revolutionary answer, confirmed by modern systems analysis (Ulanowicz, 1995), but one whose significance has yet to be fully appreciated.

20.1.1 Species Membership is a Profession and Earning a Living Implies Agency

Gibson (1977) and Colinvaux (1978) phrase matters nicely. Every organism has to earn its living. *Habitat* is where it does so. *Niche* is how it does so. Gibson (1977) considers niche to be a set of possibilities or opportunities for action. He refers to them as *affordances*. On Lindeman's theory, the numbers of organisms able to earn a living at each distinguishable range of sizes is set by the opportunities for the individual organism's way of life. For each range, only some fraction of the kilocalories/m^2/year of the size range below is food. Relatively discrete sizes of organisms arise because, on average, each kind of living thing must be bigger than the things it feeds on.

All organisms, in all kingdoms (Margulis & Schwartz, 1982/1998), manifest some degree of autonomy and control, *however minimal*, in their encounters. Agency encompasses (a) variation of means to bring about an end (flexibility), (b) coordinating current control with upcoming states of affairs (prospectivity), and (c) coordinating current control with preceding states of affairs (retrospectivity) (cf. E. Gibson, 1994; Reed, 1996). The agency of earthworms (animals with limited sensory organs and no discernible brain) provides a historically apposite example (Darwin, 1881; Turner, 2000). Their job description includes the plugging and lining of their burrows. In doing this job, earthworms select leaves for substance and size, pulling each leaf into the burrow in ways specific to its shape. When the air is warm and moist, an earthworm's leaf choices are less selective. A persistent constraint on selection, however, is the size of the leaf relative to the size of the burrow's exit. When leaves are not available, then small stones are used for the same purpose (or pieces of paper as Darwin showed experimentally). Earthworms are *aware of* their situation in this definitional sense: They perceive meaningful distinctions, befitting their job description, and organize their actions accordingly (J. Gibson, 1979/1986; Reed, 1996; Turvey, 2013). Similar claims can be made for the Kingdoms Plantae (e.g., Carello, Vaz, Blau, & Petrusz, 2012), Protoctista (e.g., Latty & Beekman, 2010), and Fungi (Rayner, 1997; Rayner, Watkins, & Beeching, 1999).

The contention that agency and what it encompasses is *necessarily the case* for all species in all kingdoms would seemingly face its strongest test in respect to the microbial kingdoms of Bacteria and Archaea. It is therefore of some significance that for both there is evidence of prospective behavior. Most notable are the behavioral changes anticipatory of the day-to-night and night-to-day transitions. The evidence is well established and plentiful for individual bacteria (e.g., Bell-Pedersen, Cassone, Earnest et al., 2005) and similarly available, but in lesser degree, for individuals of the recently discovered archaea (e.g., Whitehead, Pan, Masumura et al., 2009). More pertinent are experiments and simulations showing that bacteria can attune to new temporal interrelationships among changes in environmental factors, suggesting that they can learn to be anticipatory and preparatory in regard to relatively novel contexts for the plying of their trades (Baliga, 2008; Tagkopoulos, Liu & Tavazoie, 2008). In this most basic sense of expressing prospectivity and retrospectivity, microbial life is of like kind with Animalia.

20.1.2 Agency Must Follow from First Principles

Kauffman (2000, p. 8) defines an autonomous agent as "a physical system, such as a bacterium, that can act on its own behalf in an environment."[5] The definition presumes a specific functional order. It is of singular import to highlight that natural selection presupposes agency—that is, it presumes the aforementioned specific functional order. If such is indeed the case, then the primary source of agency cannot be natural selection (e.g., Barham, 1996). Consider the neo-Darwinian notion of "fitness." It presupposes either (a) differential reproduction (*what survives, survives*) or (b) adapted-ness (*what is well designed survives*). Under presumption (a) natural selection reduces to a tautology. Under presumption (b) natural selection begs the question of the origin of design, the question of functional order. It would seem that the question to be raised must be of a more fundamental nature: How is agency emergent from first principles? For reasons that follow, we will phrase the question as that of how agency is emergent from the laws of thermodynamics.

20.1.3 Why So Much Variety?

As the ecologist Colinvaux observed, "There is really nothing else so odd about life as its variety (Colinvaux, 1978, p. 6)." Why should living things be so varied? That is, why is there so much variety of perception–action, so many job descriptions, and so many kinds of agents? This Elton-type question seems to require an answer beyond the scope of the 2nd law of thermodynamics. And it seems to require an answer in terms of a directed single evolutionary process at the scale of the planet. That such an answer might be the case has been broached (Swenson, 1997, 2010; Swenson & Turvey, 1991). Its cornerstones are as follows: (1) maximum entropy production, alias energy quality reduction, as a physical selection principle (thermodynamic fields will behave in such a fashion as to get to the final state—minimize the field potential or maximize the entropy—at the fastest possible rate given the constraints); (2) the inexorability of order production (order production is inexorable because order produces entropy faster than disorder); (3) evolution as a global phenomenon (the earth system at its highest level evolves as a single global entity); and (4) informationL. In the coordination of self-organizing dynamics with informationL, access is provided to otherwise inaccessible opportunities to produce ordered flow and to dissipate, thereby, the geo-cosmic potential at faster rates.

Earth's history has continually reworked free energy[6] into increasing numbers of different configurations and conformations. No single class of intentional systems, no single species, has all the perception–action capabilities needed to degrade all forms of free energy (Annila & Salthe, 2010). The multiple kinds of ways of earning a living are what they are, one might argue, because they extend the means for dissipating the planet's free energy resources, for enhancing the rate of its entropy production (cf. Michaelian, 2012). Figure 20.2 reflects the foregoing argument and gives expression to the consequences of the four cornerstones identified above. Of special note is Cornerstone (1). It has been advanced as a 4th law[7] of thermodynamics.

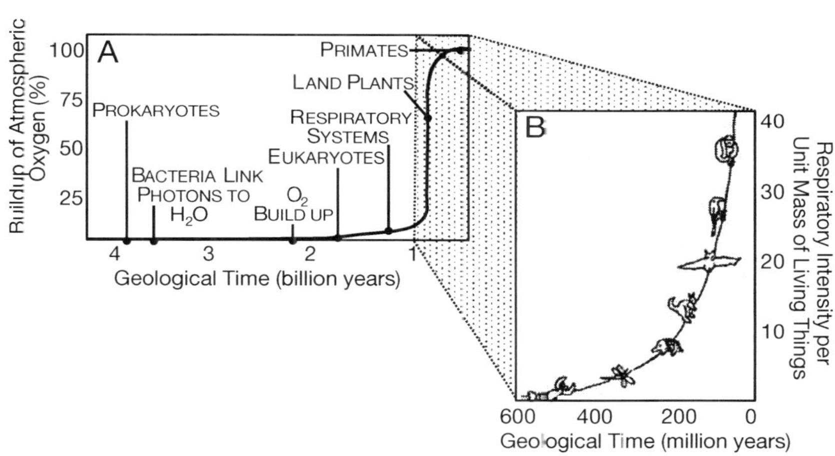

Figure 20.2 Over geological time, measured in billions of years, atmospheric oxygen (O_2) incremented gradually at first and then at a (comparatively) rapid pace with increasing numbers and varieties of life forms until it reached its current level of 21% of the atmospheric gases (100% on the vertical axis of A). The accumulation began about 2 billion years ago when the earth's O_2-binding chemicals became saturated and the O_2 released by bacteria during photosynthesis was free to enter the atmosphere. The O_2 accumulation is a measure of a progressive ordering or internal entropy production of the planetary system as a whole. What panel B shows is that within the last billion years the rate at which the planet's chemical energy was "burned up" through O_2 use increased coordinate with the rate at which the respiration per unit mass of living things increased. The latter did so as the numbers and kinds of organisms increased. Together, A and B suggest that organisms and planet constitute a unitary system under a principle of maximizing the rate of entropy production (Swenson & Turvey, 1991).

(From Figure 11.2, Turvey & Shaw, 1995, Toward an ecological physics and a physical psychology. In Solso & Massaro (Eds.), *The science of the mind: 2001 and beyond*. Adapted with permission of Oxford University Press, USA.)

20.1.4 Order Produces Entropy Faster than Disorder and Some Kinds of Order Produce it Faster than Other Kinds of Order

We can return to Figure 19.2 depicting the surface-tension-driven (STD) Bénard convection instability,[8] a prime example of a self-organizing fluid system. Figure 19.2's lower panel shows a transition, with increasing temperature, from no planforms[9] to hexagonals. Physically, the transition is one between conduction and convection. Conduction is local random interactions among molecules[10] that are manifest macroscopically as a motionless fluid. Convection is a matter of molecules moving in collectives. An impression can be gleaned from the two middle panels of Figure 19.2. The depicted fluid flows act much like conveyer belts transporting energy, that is, transporting molecules interacting randomly (Bejan, 2000, p. 160).

Figure 20.3 schematizes the self-organization of a variant of the STD Bénard convection instability experiment (Eckert, Besterhorn & Thess, 1998). The self-organization proceeds from Region I of no planforms, to Region II primarily of hexagons, to Region III primarily of squares.[11] As can be seen, the heat flux increases across the three regions. Any increase in the heat flux transferred by the cellular pattern slows down the increase of the temperature difference between bottom and surface in the upstream regions. Hexagon cells slow down this increase at a higher rate than no cells, and square cells do so at a higher rate than hexagon cells. Behind this rate increase is a cell's perimeter-area ratio.[12] This ratio for a square Bénard cell exceeds that of a hexagonal Bénard cell by approximately 25% (Eckert & Thess, 2006).

The foregoing is consonant with the hypothesized 4th law: For a given system and a given condition of thermal flow, that organization that can produce the maximal rate of entropy production (energy quality reduction) for the given circumstances will self-assemble. Figure 20.4 provides a glimpse

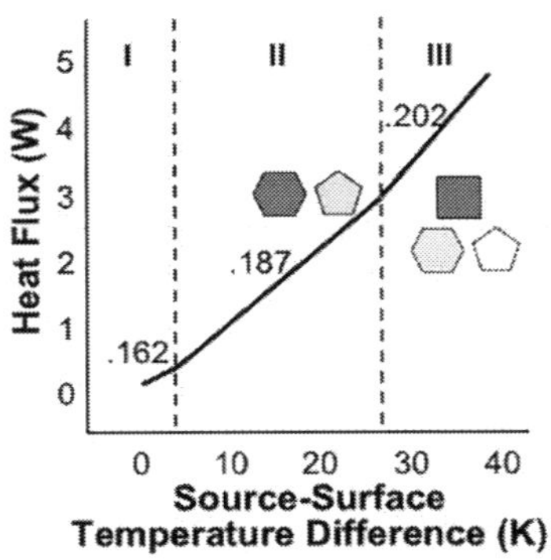

Figure 20.3 Depiction of results of Eckert, Besterhorn, & Thess (1998). See text for details.

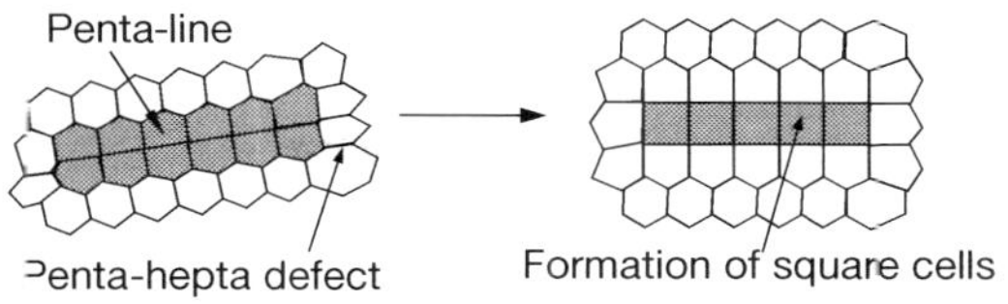

Figure 20.4 Transformation process from hexagons to squares. (*Left*) Formation of a double line of pentagons ("penta-line") which has its origin at the pentagon of the penta-hepta defect. (*Right*) Undoing of the penta-line and spreading of two fronts of pentagons into hexagonal areas. In the interior of the original penta-line square cells are formed.

(From Figure 6 in Eckert, Besterhorn, & Thess, Square cells in surface-tension-driven Bénard convection: experiment and theory. *Journal of Fluid Mechanics*, 356, 155–197, 1998, adapted with permission, Cambridge University Press.)

into how such can be the case. Pentagon cells mediate the transition from hexagons to squares.

20.2 Tinkering Again

We can take the opportunity of our deepening appreciation of the STD Bénard convection instability to enhance intuitions about tinkering (Lecture 19). In the examples that follow, tinkering amounts to manipulations of boundary or auxiliary conditions. Although they are human manipulations in the capacity of experimentation, it is not too difficult to view them as fortuitous natural occurrences. From a 4th law perspective they could be viewed as cases of opportunism, that is, taking immediate advantage of any circumstance of possible benefit. Here are two examples. The tinkering in one case (the ratchet) is with the form of the substrate to which heat is applied (Figure 20.5a). The tinkering in the other case (the clock) is with the surface of the oil that is being heated (Figure 20.5b). Ratchets (e.g., Hoffman, 2012) and clocks (e.g., Kugler & Turvey, 1987/2016) are desiderata for living things.

Figure 20.5a shows a layer of fluid exhibiting STD Bénard convection over a heated substrate with either symmetrical grooves or grooves with right-left asymmetry, the latter in two sizes. In the symmetrical case the fluid flow is strictly that of recirculation. In the asymmetrical cases, there is in addition a lateral flow at a considerably slower pace. Its direction depends on the depth of the fluid (additional to the temperature difference across the fluid). This system acts as a ratchet—a mechanical device that allows movement in only one direction. Specifically, it is a fluidic ratchet: The local structure of the thermally driven convection interacts with the asymmetry of the local topographical pattern and causes a net global fluid flow in only one direction (Strook et al., 2003). Figure 20.5b shows a layer of fluid exhibiting STD Bénard convection with an object (e.g., a flat acrylic rectangle) afloat on the

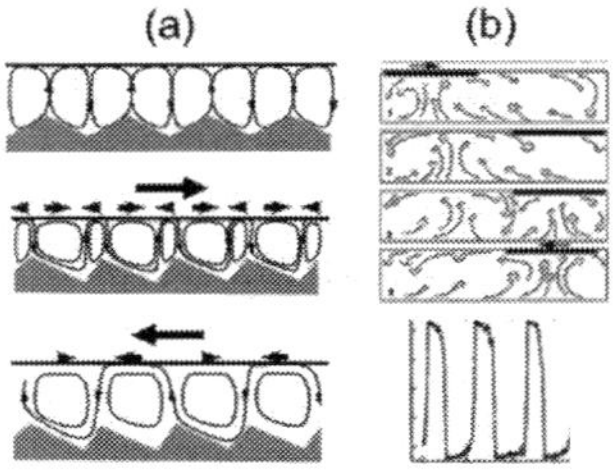

Figure 20.5 (a) Tinkering with the substrate of a STD Bénard convection instability produces ratchets (b) Tinkering with the free surface of a STD Bénard convection instability produces clocks

a: (from Strook, Ismagilov, Stone, & Whitesides, Fluidic ratchet based on Marangoni-Bénard convection, *Langmuir, 19*, 4358-4362. © 2003, American Chemical Society, reprinted with permission).
b: (from Zhang & Libchaber, Periodic boundary motion in thermal turbulence. *Physical Review Letters*, *84*, 4361–4364, 2000, reprinted with permission, American Physical Society).

surface acting as a special boundary condition. Oscillation arises from (a) the floating boundary perturbing and changing the convection flow pattern, and (b) the convection flow pattern repositioning the floating boundary (Zhang & Libchaber, 2000). Tinkering with the size of the floater changes the period of oscillation. From this one self-organizing system, a full spectrum of periodicities or clocks can be made manifest via a change in one boundary condition.

20.3 Ecological Realism

The answer given to the Elton-type question of why living things should be so varied was in terms of the variety of earth's sources of free energy. Under the aegis of a 4th law, gene tinkering is formative of biological entities that are specific to the free energy sources they degrade. The specificity is in respect to metabolism (how a source is harnessed) and behavior (how a source is obtained). It is best expressed as niche specificity. Species co-existing in the same habitat do so on the basis of niche differences supporting metabolic and behavioral differences, no matter how subtle the niche differences might be. In brief, ecological realism is realism defined at nature's ecological scale in a niche-specific way.

The foregoing definition elaborates earlier deliberations in the present lecture (Section 20.1.2). It holds for all Six Kingdoms regardless of whether their members stay in place (are sessile) or change place (are motile). Across the manifold of instances, foraging for energy sources varies in behavioral type (running, swimming, flying, drifting, slithering, spreading, burrowing, ramifying, growing), in the energy cost of the behavioral type, in the range of energy sources, and in the energy cost of handling an obtained energy source. In the circumstance of predating in the phylum Craniata they would be the costs of chasing, subduing, opening, ingesting, etc. a preyed upon animal (W. Bell, 1991).

For all organisms, "foraging is answerable to the empirical world, that is, answerable to how things are in so far as how things are is empirically accessible." The statement is McDowell's (1996, xii) with *foraging* substituting for McDowell's *thought*. McDowell's version expresses the thesis that experience plays the leading role in determining what one knows and believes and, perforce, how one thinks. Unsurprisingly, it gives undue emphasis to one species of one phylum in one kingdom—namely, *Homo sapiens* in the phylum Craniata in the kingdom Animalia. Likewise, unsurprisingly it gives undue emphasis to one dimension of that species, namely, *that it has thoughts*. It should be emphasized, however, that the statement in question heralds a sincere attempt to dispel the radical division between mind and world or, more appositely, in an ecological realism sense, between a living thing and the how and the where (the niche and the habitat) of its existence. As foreshadowed in Lecture 2, this radical division—this dualism of organism and environment and its conceptual entailments—would be a persistent feature of the lectures that followed. In Lectures 3–5 and the present lecture, however, we have caught glimpses of how the conventional division can

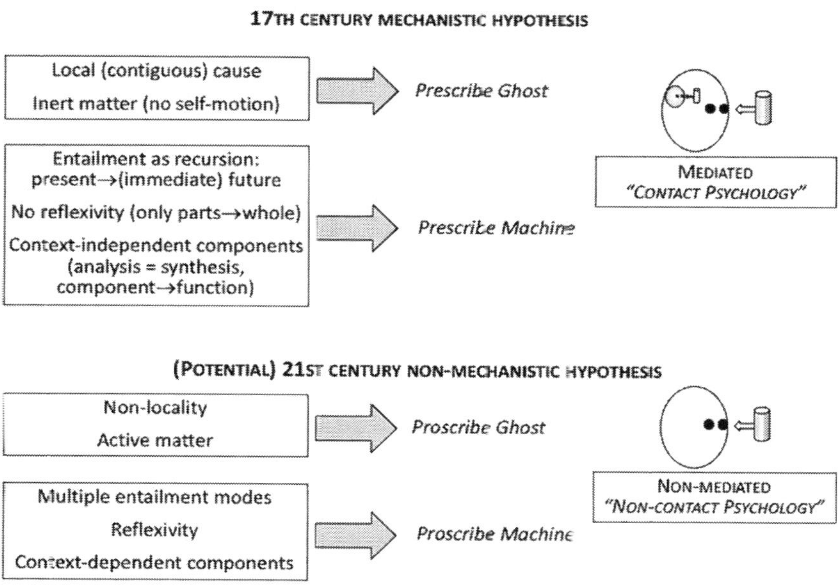

Figure 20.6 The contrast between the historical stance of perception as mediated and the evolving stance of perception as non-mediated.

metamorphose to an unconventional union. Figure 20.6 provides a synopsis of the contrast between the theoretical bedrock from the 17th century to the present and what could be the theoretical bedrock for the future. Dispelling the radical division requires a radical revision.

Notes

1 Derived from the Greek word for ancient. Archaea are often found in extreme environmental conditions, of the kind that would have typified the early development of the planet.
2 That is, their ribosomal RNA molecular sequence.
3 For example, Hug, Baker, Anantharaman, et al. (2016).
4 Entropy can be said to label the manner in which energy is stored (Atkins, 1984/1994). Energy E of amount X stored at a high temperature will be of relatively low entropy and high quality. Energy E of amount X stored at a low temperature will be of relatively high entropy and low quality. Quality refers to E's availability for doing work.
5 See also Kauffman (2003).
6 Roughly, the amount of internal energy of a physical (solid, liquid or gas) system that is available to perform work.
7 The 3rd law of thermodynamics is long established. As temperature approaches absolute zero, the entropy of a system approaches a constant.
8 Often referred to as the Marangoni–Bénard Convection.
9 Planform is an object's contour viewed from above.
10 The motion of atoms and molecules creates heat or thermal energy.
11 This evolution to squares (in a horizontal layer of fluid with a free upper surface heated from below) can take weeks.
12 In respect to the practical matter of heating buildings, the significance of the perimeter/area ratio as opposed to perimeter alone has been recently recognized (Rees, Thomas & Zhou, 2000).

References

Annila, A., & Salthe, S. (2010). Physical foundations of evolutionary theory. *Journal of Non-Equilibrium Thermodynamics*, *35*, 301–321.

Atkins, P. W. (1994). *The 2nd law: Energy, chaos and form*. New York: Scientific American Books (original work published 1984).

Baliga, N. S. (2008). The scale of prediction. *Science*, *320*, 1297–1298.

Barham, J. (1996). A dynamical model of the meaning of information. *BioSystems*, *38*, 235–241.

Bejan, A. (2000). *Shape and structure from engineering to nature*. New York: Cambridge University Press.

Bell, W. J. (1991). *Searching behavior: The behavioural ecology of finding resources*. London: Chapman & Hall.

Bell-Pedersen, D., Cassone, V. M., Earnest, D. J., et al. (2005). Circadian rhythms from multiple oscillators: Lessons from diverse organisms. *Nature Reviews Genetics*, *6*, 544–556.

Carello, C., Vaz, D., Blau, J. J. C., & Petrusz, S. (2012). Unnerving intelligence. *Ecological Psychology*, *24*, 241–264.

Colinvaux, P. (1978). *Why big fierce animals are rare*. Princeton, NJ: Princeton University Press.

Curtis, T. P., Sloane, W. T., & Scannell, J. W. (2002). Estimating prokaryotic diversity and its limits. *Proceedings of the National Academy of Sciences*, 99, 10494–10499.

Darwin, C. (1881). *The formation of vegetable mould through the action of worms, with observations of their habits*. London: Murray.

Doolittle, W. F., & Zhaxybayeva, O. (2009). On the origin of prokaryotic species. *Genome Research*, *19*, 744–756.

Eckert, K., & Thess, A. (2006). Secondary instabilities in surface-tension-driven Bénard-Marangoni convection. In I. Mutabazi, J. E. Wesfreid, E. Guyon (Eds.) *Dynamics of spatio-temporal cellular structures: Springer tracts in modern physics* (pp. 163–176). Berlin, Germany: Springer.

Eckert, K., Besterhorn, M., & Thess, A. (1998). Square cells in surface-tension-driven Bénard convection: experiment and theory. *Journal of Fluid Mechanics*, *356*, 155–197.

Elton, C. (2001). *Animal ecology*. Chicago, IL: University of Chicago Press (original work published 1927).

Gibson, E. J. (1994). Has psychology a future? *Psychological Science*, *5*, 69–76.

Gibson, J. J. (1977). The theory of affordances. In R. Shaw & J. Bransford (Eds.), *Perceiving, acting, and knowing: Toward an ecological psychology* (pp. 67–82). Hillsdale, NJ: Erlbaum.

Gibson, J. J. (1986). *The ecological approach to visual perception*. Mahwah, NJ: Erlbaum (original work published 1979).

Gould, S. J. (1998). Foreword. In L. Margulis & K. V. Schwartz, *Five kingdoms*. New York: W. H. Freeman (original work published 1982).

Hoffman, P. M. (2012). *Life's ratchet*. New York: Basic Books.

Hug, L. A., Baker, B. J., Anantharaman, K., et al. (2016). A new view of the tree of life. *Nature Microbiology*, *1*, 1–6.

Kauffman, S. (2000). *Investigations*. New York: Oxford University Press.

Kauffman, S. (2003). The emergence of autonomous agents. In N. H. Gregersen (Ed.), *From complexity to life* (pp. 47–71). New York: Oxford University Press.

Kugler, P. N., & Turvey, M. T. (1987). *Information, natural law, and the self-assembly of rhythmic movement*. Hillsdale, NJ: Erlbaum.

Latty, T., & Beekman, M. (2010). Food quality and the risk of light exposure affect patch-choice decisions in the slime mold Physarum polycephalum. *Ecology*, *91*, 22–27.

Lindeman, R. L. (1942). The trophic-dynamic aspect of ecology. *Ecology*, *23*, 399–418.

Margulis, L., & Schwartz, K. V. (1998). *Five kingdoms*. New York: Freeman (original work published 1982).

McDowell, J. H. (1996). *Mind and world*. Cambridge, MA: Harvard University Press.

Michaelian, K. (2012). Biological catalysis of the hydrological cycle: Life's thermodynamic function. *Hydrology and Earth Systems Science*, *16*, 2629–2645.

Mora, C., Tittensor, D. P., Sina, A., et al. (2011). How many species are there on earth and in the ocean? *PLoS Biology*, 9, e1001127.

Pace, N. R. (2006). Time for a change. *Nature*, *441*, 289.

Rayner, A. D. M. (1997). *Degrees of freedom: Living in dynamic boundaries*. London: Imperial College Press.

Rayner, A. D. M., Watkins, Z. R., & Beeching, J. R. (1999). Self integration—an emerging concept from the fungal mycelium. In N. A. R Gow, G. D. Robson & G. M. Gadd (Eds.), *The fungal colony*. Cambridge, UK: Cambridge University Press.

Reed, E. S. (1996). *Encountering the world.* Oxford, UK: Oxford University Press.

Rees, S. W., Thomas, H. R., & Zhou, Z. (2000). Ground heat transfer: Some further insights into the influence of three-dimensional effects. *Building Services Engineering Research Technology*, *21*, 233–239.

Strook, A. D., Ismagilov, R. F., Stone, H., & Whitesides, G. M. (2003). Fluidic ratchet based on Marangoni-Bénard convection. *Langmuir*, *19*, 4358–4362.

Swenson, R. (1997). Autocatakinetics, evolution, and the law of maximum entropy production: A principled foundation toward the study of human ecology. *Advances in Human Ecology*, 6, 1–46.

Swenson, R. (2010). Selection is entailed by self-organization and natural selection is a special case. *Biological Theory*, *5*, 67–181.

Swenson, R., & Turvey, M. T. (1991). Thermodynamic reasons for perception-action cycles. *Ecological Psychology*, *3*, 317–348.

Tagkopoulos, I., Liu, Y-C., & Tavazoie, S. (2008). Predictive behavior within microbial genetic networks. *Science*, *320*, 1313–1317.

Turner, J. S. (2000). *The extended organism: The physiology of animal-built structures.* Cambridge, MA: Harvard University Press.

Turvey, M. T. (2013). Ecological perspective on perception-action: What kind of science does it entail? In W. Prinz, M. Beisert, & A. Herwig (Eds.), *Action science: Foundations of an emerging discipline* (pp. 139–170). Cambridge, MA: MIT Press.

Turvey, M. T., & Shaw, R. E. (1995). Toward an ecological physics and a physical psychology. In R. Solso & D. Massaro (Eds.), *The science of the mind: 2001 and beyond* (pp. 144–169). Oxford, UK: Oxford University Press.

Ulanowicz, R. E. (1995). Ecosystem trophic foundations: Lindeman exonerata. In B. C. Patten & S. E. Jorgensen (Eds.) *Complex ecology: The part-whole relation in ecosystems* (pp. 549–560). Englewood Cliffs, NJ: Prentice Hall.

Whitehead, K., Pan, M., Masumura, K-i., Bonneau, R., & Baliga, N.S. (2009). Diurnally entrained anticipatory behavior in Archaea. *PLoS ONE*, *4*, e5485.

Woese, C. R. (2004). A new biology for a new century. *Microbiology and Molecular Biology Reviews*, 68, 173–186.

Woese, C. R., & Fox, G. (1977). Phylogenetic structure of the prokaryotic domain: The primary kingdoms. *Proceedings of the National Academy of Sciences*, *74*, 5088–5090.

Woese, C. R., Kandler, O., & Wheelis, M. L. (1990). Towards a natural system for organisms: Proposal for the domains Archea, Bacteria and Eucarya. *Proceedings of the National Academy of Sciences*, *87*, 4576–4579.

Zhang, J., & Libchaber, A. (2000). Periodic boundary motion in thermal turbulence. *Physical Review Letters*, *84*, 4361–4364.

Lecture 21

Barriers to Ecological Realism

In Lecture 20 we reached what can only be called a radical conclusion: Realism takes as many forms as there are species. Realism is an ecological concept. At various places in the earlier lectures we discussed barriers to ecological realism as thwarts to the understanding of perception, with some barriers discussed more explicitly than others. Figure 21.1 portrays several of the more prominent barriers as an arch of interlocking stones with the keystone being organism-environment dualism (Lecture 2). The pillars of Figure 21.1, one should note, are dualisms that have come to prominence in the modern era with advances in the biological sciences—dualisms that have been questioned, most notably by Weiss (1973) and Gottlieb (1997). We encountered the "pillars" in Lecture 12.

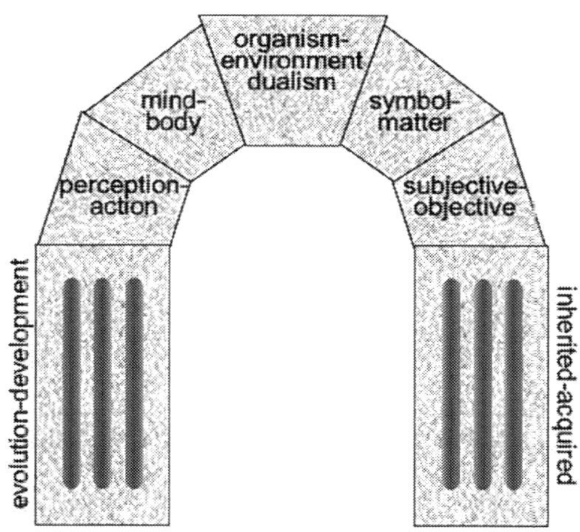

Figure 21.1 Barriers to realism. The primary barrier, the keystone, is organism–environment dualism.

(From Figure 11.1, Turvey & Shaw, 1995, Toward an ecological physics and a physical psychology, in Solso & Massaro (Eds.), *The science of the mind: 2001 and beyond*. Adapted with permission of Oxford University Press, USA.)

The primary goal of the present lecture is to underscore that the radical division (mind–body dualism) as crafted by Descartes and caricatured by the man-in-the-inner-room is merely one of several significant manifestations of organism–environment dualism. The historical tendencies, whether mentalist (pro the radical division) or behaviorist (contra the radical division), have been to construe organisms in their roles of perceivers and actors as logically separable from the environments that they perceive, learn about, and behave with respect to (Turvey & Shaw, 1979). The present lecture supplements Lectures 2 and 3.

There is an organizational wholeness or systemism of organism and environment that tends to go unrecognized, even denied (cf. Bunge, 2000). We can turn to the seemingly lowly earthworm to provide us with an example of this systemism and, simultaneously, to broaden our conceptions of "environment" and "tinkering."

21.1 Recognizing the Systemism of Organism and Environment: The Earthworm's Functional Kidney

In *The Formation of Vegetable Mold through the Action of Worms*, Darwin (1881) presented himself as a *uniformitarian*. The term is taken from geology. It relates to the thesis that processes in operation in the remote geological past are not different from processes in operation now. For Turner (2000), Darwin's uniformitarianism is evidenced by Darwin's belief that

> small, seemingly insignificant processes could be enormously powerful agents for change if they were allowed to operate over a sufficiently long time.
>
> (p. 116)

The common earthworm, as we know it, is physiologically unsuited for terrestrial life. Its organs for balancing water support high rates of filtration and selective reabsorption of salts but not water. Its water losses (urine production) are 60–90% a day. It is like a freshwater animal. The evolutionary course of this ocean-originating organism becoming a landlubber has not been a matter of organism-to-terrestrial environment adaptation. To the contrary, *it seems to have been more a matter of the terrestrial environment, specifically soil, being changed by the earthworm to suit the earthworm.* The earthworm's organs for balancing water together with the soil changes engineered by the earthworm provide the functional equivalent of a kidney. A précis of Turner's (2000) exposition follows.

Soils are commonly divided into three horizontal layers ("horizons") with different features at different depths. The top layer, referred to as aerial, is subject to atmospheric influences. In the aerial layer worms are in danger of drying out. The bottom layer, referred to as aquatic, is subject to water influences. In the aquatic layer worms are in danger of suffocating. The middle layer, referred to as edaphic,[1] is subject to soil conditions such as drainage and coarseness, conditions influenced significantly by earthworms. In respect to drainage, earthworms construct enduring, mucus-coated tunnels through which they can crawl and water can percolate downward. In respect to the reducing of soil coarseness by the disordering process of weathering, earthworms counter in two primary ways. First, their secreted mucus leads to aggregations of soil particles. Second, their ingesting of soil, digesting of organic matter and bacteria, and provisioning of mucus and calcite, mixed and churned, culminate in *casts*—comparatively large, fecal pellets that are fertile and erosion resistant (see also Edwards & Lofty, 1972; Lunt & Jacobson, 1944). In the edaphic layer, earthworms can live and thrive.

Darwin's uniformitarianism is in the gradualness of the "seemingly insignificant processes" of mixing and churning, crawling and tunneling. Locally, at the scale of the earthworm, they yield a coordination of organism and environment with the functionality of a kidney. Globally, at the scale of soil's edaphic horizon worldwide, they yield a foundation for furthering the planet's rate of entropy production (Lecture 20, Figure 20.2) through the multitude of living things supportable by fertile soil (Addiscott, 2010). In sum, we have given ourselves a further reason for appreciating the interactive process *sans* plans that is evolution, a further example of Nature's tinkering (Coen, 1999; Jacob, 1977, 1982).

21.2 Seven Doctrines Prescribed by Organism–Environment Dualism

The theoretical stance of organism–environment dualism, whether it is taken explicitly or implicitly, licenses companion theoretical positions or doctrines that serve to crystalize the dualism. They are identified in the left column of Table 21.1. We encountered the doctrines of intractable non-specificity and incommensurability of natural kinds in Lecture 15 and the doctrine of perception as proposition making and fallible in Lectures 16 and 18.

Companion to intractable non-specificity is the doctrine of the independence of perception from stimulation. The often-cited evidence for the independence doctrine is that where the proximal stimulation is fixed, perception may vary (e.g., the Necker cube); and where proximal stimulation is variable, perception may be unchanged (e.g., the retinal orientation of an object in the frontal plane varies with head movement, but the perceived orientation does not). In accepting these companion doctrines as identifying the initial conditions for perception, it follows that insofar as perception is veridical, insofar as any member of Animalia relates to its environment adaptively, *the animal as perceiver must embody a theory of its niche and habitat and a theory of how niche[2] and habitat structure energy distributions*. Whatever epistemic mediators are proposed, if they are to be taken seriously, they must

Table 21.1 Thwarts to Realism and Direct Perception (*left*) and (Potential) Abettors of Realism and Direct Perception (right)

Doctrine of intractable non-specificity	Doctrine of necessary specificity
Doctrine of perception as independent of stimulation	Doctrine of perception as specific to information
Doctrine of incommensurability of natural kinds	Doctrine of commensurability of natural kinds
Doctrine of reality as predicative	Doctrine of reality as impredicative
Doctrine of perception as intellectual (proposition making) activity	Doctrine of perception as a state of affairs ("perceiving a place to sit" is comparable to "*sitting on* a sitting place")
Doctrine of physics as complete	Doctrine of physics as incomplete

subsume as a minimum requirement both theories. Nothing less will suffice as a basis for discerning the meaning of reflected light to the eye. For any epistemic mediator advanced as an answer to the *mechanism question* of "How does it work?" one must advance an accompanying answer to the *origin question* of "How did it arise?" (cf. Pattee, 1977).

Closely related to the doctrine of the independence of perception from stimulation are the parallel doctrines of defining reality in an absolute sense or, correspondingly, defining the environment in a strictly predicative manner. Both cleave organism and environment. Both require that organism, whatever the phylum, must *construct* (in some sense of the word) a representation of environment.

The remaining doctrine is that of physics as complete. The doctrine was broached in Lectures 1–3 in respect to organism and in respect to environment, and articulated in various forms and in different degrees in the lectures that followed. On this doctrine we must dwell. In the forging of a theory of direct perception, it is perhaps the doctrine of greatest practical significance.

Viewed in a historical context it is self-evidently the case that physics-the-discipline at any given point in time is not complete. There is always more to come, where more is often something different and, occasionally, something radically different. Physics-the-discipline evolves quantitatively and qualitatively. The physics-as-complete doctrine is (a) the acceptance of the current state of physics-the-discipline as fact and (b) the adoption of physics-the-discipline in its current state as the basis for explanation. Although the doctrine is fully understandable and rational, abiding it without some circumspection can lead to complications. Consider, for example, light as radiant energy in the form of rays. From the perspective of the retinal mosaic, light rays are distinguished only by intensity and wavelength giving rise to the puzzle of how the indefinite number of visual perception's descriptors is induced from the paucity of light's descriptors. As the previous lectures have made clear, science has been comfortable with the strategy of resolving this discrepancy through the ascription of inferential prowess brought to bear on a fully articulated image not on a mosaic of colored points.

21.3 Reflected Light

In Lecture 11 we encountered the non-intuitive notion that illuminated surfaces and luminous bodies are visible but light itself is not. Here we encounter the non-intuitive characteristics of light multiply reflected from non-planar surfaces.

Light from a source (such as the sun, or a light bulb) is scatter-reflected or diffused by the faces and facets of surfaces. In the case of a layout of facing surfaces—consider for simplicity, a furnished room with planar walls, ceiling, and floor as depicted in Figure 21.2—the consequence of scattering is multiple-reflection or reverberation, an endless bouncing of light from surface to surface, a network of convergence and divergence that is indefinitely dense. *Multiple-reflection (including inter-reflection and mutual-reflection[3]) endows the light in the room with uniqueness*—that is, it renders the light in the room *specific to the room*. In Gibson's (1966) terminology, the uniqueness exists at the level of each pencil of light (a point in the room), at the level of the set of all pencils (the room itself), and at the level of each series of adjacent pencils (point-to-point translation within the room).

The first true theoretical efforts to address reflection from natural surfaces—that is, surfaces that are rough (technically, not planar at all length scales)—began in the 1980s. As highlighted by Maradudin and Méndez (2007):

> just over 20 years ago, it was recognized that the introduction of multiple scattering into the theory of the scattering of light from randomly rough surfaces yields a variety of effects that have no counterparts in the results obtained on the basis of single scattering theories.
>
> (p. 162)

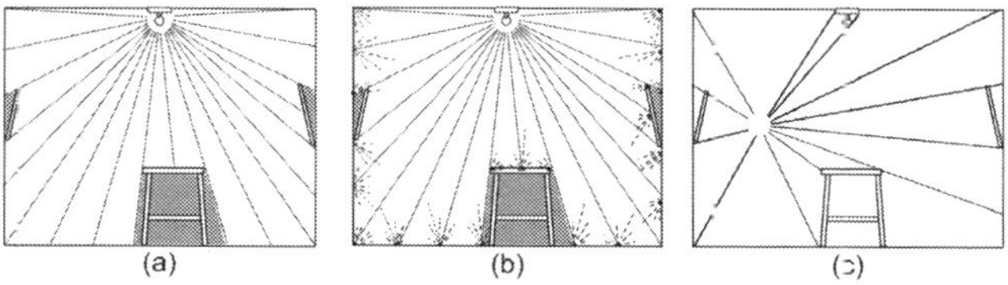

Figure 21.2 Toward Gibson's optic array. (a) Radiant light illuminating an enclosure; (b) scatter reflection; (c) light ambient to a stationary point of convergence with lines depicting borders arising from optical differences due to surface inclination and reflectance.

(From Figures 10.1, 10.2, and 10.4, Gibson, 1966, adapted with permission.)

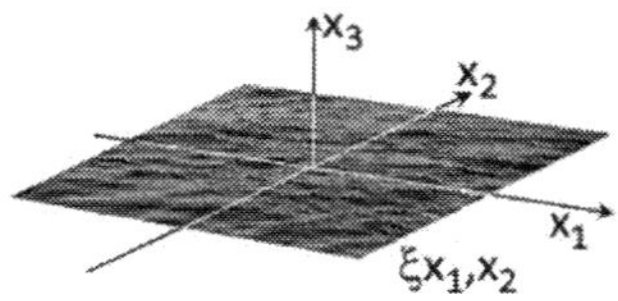

Figure 21.3 Two-dimensional irregular surface. $\xi(x_1, x_2)$ is a surface profile function.

Single scattering is the historical, textbook depiction of light reflected from a planar surface absent any irregularities. In the developing enterprise, multiple reflection or scattering is the structure of light induced by irregularity in one dimension (departure from the plane in the x_1 direction) and by irregularity in two dimensions (departure from the plane in both the x_1 and x_2 directions, Figure 21.3). The structure arises from the presence of many light "scatterers" or "diffusers"—the nooks and crannies, the hills and dales, of an isolable surface. Theoretical studies of such (non-Gaussian random) surfaces are hamstrung by the lack of random functions for which the characteristic functional is known (Maradudin & Méndez, 2007). Nonetheless, insights are accumulating about the form the new optical quantities should take (e.g., Simonsen, Maradudin & Leskova, 2010). Intuitions about the gross variations of structure manifest by reflected light as a function of irregularity of surface texture are obtainable from Figure 21.4.

The foregoing provides the opportunity to underscore the magnitude of the challenge posed by ecological optics: The foundation for optical information in the specificational sense is the physics of multiple reflection by, and multiple reflection among, indefinitely many reflecting surfaces, each of non-Gaussian randomness that is different from surface to surface. These physics and its

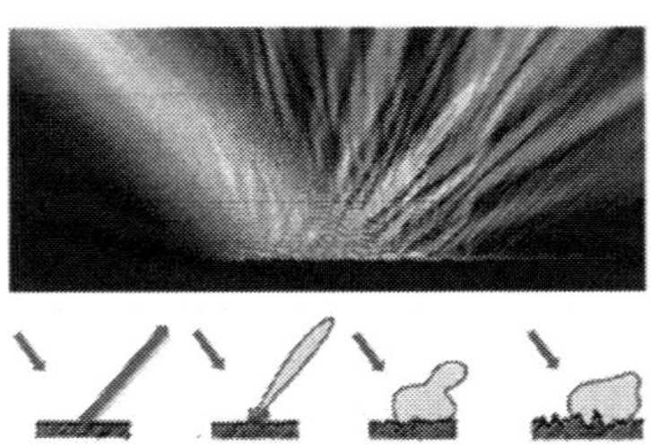

Figure 21.4 (*Top*) Distribution of reflected light (*rightward*) from a rough surface illuminated from a light source (*leftward*). (*Bottom*) Schematics of the reflection of light from the leftward light source. (*From left to right*) A planar surface and three surfaces of increasing irregularity.

(From Figures 1 and 2, I. Simonsen. Optics of surface disordered systems: A random walk through rough surface scattering phenomena, *European Physical Journal: Special Topics*, *81*, 1–103, 2010. With kind permission of *The European Physical Journal* (*EPJ*).

allied mathematics are embryonic. The embryonic evaluation applies equally to ecological acoustics, ecological mechanics, and ecological chemistry—to the patterned energy dispersals that make possible perceiving by listening, touching, smelling and tasting in all their manifest forms within the Six Kingdoms (Turvey, 2013).[4]

21.4 On "Physics of Reflection as an Endowment"

The fact that inter- and mutual reflection of light by a room's surfaces renders the light in the room specific to the room (Figure 21.2) is grounding for hypotheses of the following kind: (a) that perception from any vantage point and any sequence of vantage points is specific to the room and (b) that perception of the room is not a matter of abductive inference but a matter of invariance-detection or resonance (of, as yet, some undetermined kind). The optical support for visual perception is necessarily a matter of the physical principles of inter- and mutual reflection, but the visual system's mode of response to the optical support (the act of visually perceiving) is not.

As we came to appreciate in Lectures 11 and 12, experiments within the framework of unconscious inference, historical and contemporary, are framed in terms of the abductive inference rejected in (b). Their focus is whether the principles of light reflection can be shown to inhere in the act of visually perceiving—unconsciously inferring—one's illuminated spatial surroundings. That is, does the endowment of the visual system include the principles of light reflection? The question was identified in Lecture 12 as a paradox: The third grade of sense in vision must be endowed with knowledge of the connection between visual sensations and spatial reality prior to knowing about that reality through unconscious inference.

21.4.1 Implicit Comprehension of the Laws of Reflection

A typical layout of surfaces illuminated from above will, as noted earlier, necessarily entail the illumination of one or more surfaces by light reflected from one or more neighboring surfaces. Multiple reflection is a physical consequence of surface illumination, one that is obviously conditional on the particulars of the surface layout. A change in the layout of a given set of surfaces for the same source of illumination will entail lawfully a change in the pattern of multiple reflections. Suppose, however, that one could fix both surface layout and illumination, and arrange matters such that the surface layout *as perceived* is not that *as presented*. Would the surface layout *as perceived* express different multiple reflections?

Surprisingly, perhaps, one can in fact address this seemingly anomalous question (Bloj, Kersten & Hurlbert, 1999; see also Gergenfurtner, 1999). For example, a participant views the surface layout through a pseudoscope, a device that swaps the view of the left (right) eye with that of the right (left) eye. The barebones of such a device is shown in Figure 21.5 (right column). It is shown in the context of viewing a variant of the so-called Mach card (lower row, Figure 21.5), an arrangement of two surfaces that when viewed from above have the form ʌ or v. In the experiment of Bloj et al., participants viewed the ʌ form with magenta paper on the left and white paper on the right. In Figure 21.5 magenta is represented by dark grey.

There were two conditions of viewing. In Condition 1 participants viewed ʌ through a fake pseudoscope (no lenses). They saw the white paper of the Mach card as faintly pink (represented as off-white in Figure 21.5 middle).[5] The latter effect was expected on the hypothesis that the visual system, under conditions of normal viewing, discounts the effects of multiple reflections. On this hypothesis, the light reflected from the magenta (m) surface onto the white (w) surface would be basically ignored. In Condition 2, participants viewed the special Mach card through a legitimate pseudoscope. The consequence is depicted in Figure 21.5 (middle and bottom rows). The Mach card was seen as inverted—ʌ became v—and the white paper on the left was seen as strongly magenta (represented in Figure 21.5 bottom right by the left panel's increased grayness).

What would account for this non-intuitive change in color? Suppose that, absent a change in light, the visual system infers, in the abduction sense of infers, that the change in color was most likely the effect of the change in shape (from ʌ or v, Bloj et al., 1999). This inference from effect to cause implies, at a minimum, that the visual system instantiates an understanding

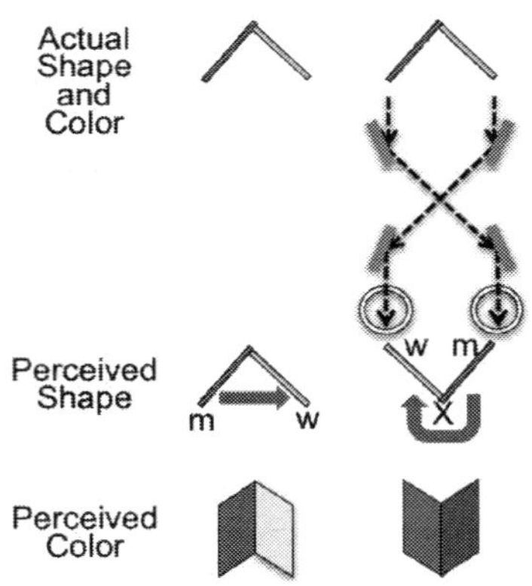

Figure 21.5 Experiment of Bloj et al. (*Left column*) Actual shape (bird's-eye view), perceived shape of Mach card with inter-reflection of magenta (m) side on white (w) side, and perceived color (m on left, "pink" on right). (*Right column*) Actual shape, pseudoscope, perceived shape with impossibility of inter-reflection, and perceived color (near-m on left, m on right).

(From Figure 2, Gergenfurtner, 1999, adapted with permission, *Nature*.)

of the physics of light reflection, most particularly, multiple reflection, and specific knowledge of the reflectance function of colored surfaces (in the present case, magenta).

Gibson's (1979/1986) view on conjectures such as the preceding is worth noting. For him, they all come down to the following:

> In order to perceive the world one must already have ideas about it. Knowledge of the world is explained by assuming that knowledge of the world exists. Whether the ideas are learned or innate makes no difference; the fallacy lies in the circular reasoning.
>
> (p. 304)

21.4.2 Principal of Generic Views

The foregoing case for abduction was articulated with the viewer at one station point. How would abduction fare if the station point were free to vary? For example, if the viewer's relation to the Mach card was oblique (e.g., off to the side or looking down from above) rather than facing? In some quarters of computational vision/Artificial Intelligence a necessary criterion is that successful "perception" should not require the "viewer" to be in a specific relation to the distal surface layout. This is referred to as the *principle of generic views* (e.g., Freeman, 1994). Its violation is cause for rejecting a candidate abduction hypothesis. For any given animal, the relations of distance and orientation to surface layouts will, by and large, be indefinitely many and at the choosing of the animal. In ecological settings, visual perception of *x* is broadly invariant over the multiplicity of a mobile animal's distance and orientation relations to *x*.

21.5 Three Difficulties of the Bayesian Formalism *qua* Abduction

We can conclude this lecture with a few brief remarks on the potential of the Bayesian formalism (recall Lecture 12)—the formalism commonly used for expressing abduction. Arguably, the appeal of the formalism is its *normative* nature, meaning that it is based on what is considered to be the usual or correct way of doing something (such as judging the color of an illuminated Mach card). That usual or correct way is presumed to be rational—that is, it involves a number of self-consistent beliefs with prescribed probabilities and a selective updating of those probabilities by evidence (e.g., additional facts, more data).[6]

Three difficulties are worth noting (Glymour, 2001). First, the belief updating is often assumed within the formalism to be indifferent to the order in which new facts are incorporated. For biological phenomena, however, such as adapting and learning, the sequential order of the formative experiences tends to matter. Second, the formalism is computationally intractable. In the absence of being foretold, the number of possible hypotheses that can be entertained is so large ("astronomical") that heuristics are required to protect against having to evaluate all the possibilities. Third, there is a disarming problem with novelty. A consistent Bayesian method for introducing new, unobserved causes is lacking, a situation worsened by the fact that significant causes reside in the class of nonobvious independent variables (as discussed in Lecture 12). In Glymour's (2001) words:

> [N]o correct, feasible, general Bayesian procedure is known that provides correct information—in the large sample limit—about the existence of unobserved common causes of observed variables.
>
> (p. 97)

Affirmation of the qualms surrounding the aforementioned difficulties[7] is to be found in a re-examination by Marcus and Davis (2015) of a study on infant learning by Gweon, Tenenbaum and Schulz (2010). Whereas Gweon et al.'s original assumption was that the infants had to consider implicitly four hypotheses of equal a priori plausibility, the re-examination revealed that the number was closer to four dozen, engendering more than 7,500 equally well-motivated Bayesian models.

Notes

1 A term meaning resulting from or influenced by the soil as contrasted with influenced by the climate.
2 To reiterate, niche refers to how an organism earns its living. The earning is a variety of behaviors befitting a variety of life's circumstances. The organism must perceive the behaviors and their adequacy so they might be controlled. For that to be the case, the organism must have a theory about how what it does to earn its living structures energy distributions.
3 Light reflected from surfaces illuminated by a light source can illuminate areas that are not illuminated by the light source. Further, two or more surfaces illuminated by a common source can illuminate each other.
4 Returning to the man-in-the-inner-room perspective, the perceiving of any surface layout would involve determining the statistics of the surface and/or inferring through abduction the topography of the surface from the local intensity values at the retina.
5 Participants matched Munsell chips to the perceived color of the white paper.
6 Roughly, Bayesian updating is changing an initial or *prior* probability estimate e.g., P(A) on the basis of one or more new facts, e.g., B and C, with associated probabilities P(B) and P(C), to produce a *posterior* probability estimate.
7 For an overview, see Marcus & Davis (2013, 2015).

References

Addiscott, T. M. (2010). Entropy, non-linearity and hierarchy in ecosystems. *Geoderma*, *160*, 57–63.

Bloj, M., Kersten, D., & Hurlbert, A. (1999). Perception of three-dimensional shape influences colour perception though mutual illumination. *Nature*, *402*, 877–879.

Bunge, M. (2000). Systemism: The alternative to individualism and holism. *Journal of Socio-Economics*, *29*, 147–157.

Coen, E. (1999). *The art of genes*. Oxford, UK: Oxford University Press.

Darwin, C. (1881). *The formation of vegetable mould through the action of worms, with observations of their habits*. London: Murray.

Edwards, C.A., & Lofty, J.R. (1972). *Biology of earthworms*. London: Chapman & Hall.

Freeman, W. T. (1994). The generic viewpoint assumption in a framework for visual perception. *Nature*, *368*, 542–545.

Gergenfurtner, K. R. (1999). Reflection on color constancy. *Nature*, *402*, 855–856.

Gibson, J. J. (1966). *The senses considered as perceptual systems*. Boston, MA: Houghton Mifflin.

Gibson, J. J. (1986). *The ecological approach to visual perception*. Mahwah, NJ: Erlbaum (original work published 1979).

Glymour, C. (2001). *The mind's arrows: Bayes nets and graphical causal models in psychology*. Cambridge, MA: MIT Press.

Gottlieb, G. (1997). *Synthesizing nature and nurture: Prenatal roots of instinctive behavior*. Mahwah, NJ: Erlbaum.

Gweon, H., Tenenbaum, J. B., & Schulz, L. E. (2010). Infants consider both the sample and the sampling process in inductive generalization. *Proceedings of the National Academy of Sciences*, *107*, 9066–9071.

Jacob, F. (1977). Evolution and tinkering. *Science*, *196*, 1161–1166.

Jacob, F. (1982). *The possible and the actual*. New York: Pantheon.

Lunt, H. A., Jacobson, G.M. (1944). The chemical composition of earthworm casts. *Soil Science*, 58, 367–374.

Maradudin, A. A., & Méndez, E. R. (2007). Light scattering from randomly rough surfaces. *Science Progress*, *90*, 161–221.

Marcus, G. F., & Davis, E. (2013). How robust are probabilistic models of higher-level cognition? *Psychological Science*, *24*, 2351–2360.

Marcus, G. F., & Davis, E. (2015). Still searching for principles: A response to Goodman et al. (2015). *Psychological Science*, *4*, 542–544.

Pattee, H. H. (1977). Dynamic and linguistic modes of complex systems. *International Journal of General Systems*, *3*, 259–266.

Simonsen, I. (2010). Optics of surface disordered systems: A random walk through rough surface scattering phenomena. *European Physical Journal: Special Topics*, *81*, 1–103.

Simonsen, I., Maradudin, A. A., Leskova, T. A. (2010). Scattering of electromagnetic waves from two-dimensional randomly rough perfectly conducting surfaces: The full angular intensity distribution. *Physical Review A*, *81*, 013806.

Turner, J. S. (2000). *The extended organism The physiology of animal-built structures*. Cambridge, MA: Harvard University Press.

Turvey, M. T. (2013). Ecological perspective on perception-action: What kind of science does it entail? In W. Prinz, M. Bessard, & A. Herwig (Eds.), *Action science: Foundations of an emerging discipline* (pp. 139–170). Cambridge, MA: MIT Press.

Turvey, M. T., & Shaw, R. E. (1979). The primacy of perceiving: An ecological reformulation of perception for understanding memory. In L.-G. Nilssen (Ed.),

Perspectives on memory research: In honor of Uppsala University's 500th anniversary. Hillsdale, NJ: Erlbaum.

Turvey, M. T., & Shaw, R. E. (1995). Toward an ecological physics and a physical psychology. In R. Solso & D. Massaro (Eds.), *The science of the mind: 2001 and beyond* (pp. 144–169). Oxford, UK: Oxford University Press.

Weiss, P. A. (1973). *The science of life: The living system—a system for living*. New York: Futura.

Lecture 22

Ontology at the Ecological Scale

The lecture's point of departure is J. J. Gibson's (1979/1986) assertion: "If what we perceived were the entities of physics and mathematics, meanings would have to be imposed on them. But if what we perceive are the entities of environmental science, their meanings can be *discovered*" (p. 33). The word "entities" in this quotation situates our present enterprise within ontology. Dictionary definitions[1] of ontology allow (a) a branch of metaphysics concerned with the nature and relations of being and (b) a particular theory about the nature of being or the kinds of things that have existence. Definition (b) is slightly more preferable. We are in pursuit of a theory and the dictionary definition of "entity" is that which has a real and independent existence.

As we shall come to see, the present lecture initiates consideration of the following ontological strategy: supplant the historical and commonplace *mind–body dualism* (more broadly, *mind–matter dualism*) by *organism–environment duality* as the framework for inquiry into issues of perception and action in particular and matters of psychology and its related philosophy in general (Turvey & Shaw, 1995). *Dualism* is the quality or state of having two incommensurate (different or opposite) aspects. *Duality* is the quality or state of having two commensurate (mutual and reciprocal) aspects.

Whereas mind–body dualism has focused ontological inquiry on one species (human) of one phylum (craniata) of one kingdom (Animalia), the warrant of organism–environment duality is an ontology that encompasses all species of all phyla of all Six Kingdoms. Further, whereas mind–body dualism has focused ontological inquiry on the special qualities of human mental states (e.g., thought, ideas), the warrant of organism–environment duality is an ontology befitting prospective control as manifest, in greater or lesser degree, by each and every organism (e.g., Reed, 1996; Turvey, 1992; Turvey & Shaw, 1995). Prospective control is concerned with future events, typically, goals to be realized. It is founded on an ecological-scale desideratum of the following kind (cf. Gibson, 1979/1986, p. 223): *To perceive things is to perceive how to get about among them and what to do or not to do with them.*

22.1 Prospective Control: Fibroblast as Exemplar

To gain appreciation of the possible universality of prospective control and of the aforementioned desideratum, we can hardly do better than to examine the behavior of fibroblasts. These are cells that both construct and maintain the extracellular matrix (ECM) of the mammalian body and, additionally, travel within it. The ultimate significance of fibroblasts is that ECM is the mechanically supportive and regulatory framework for all of the mammalian body's cells.

In exhibiting directionally controlled crawling, a fibroblast expresses forms of mechanosensitivity that are analogues of animal exteroperceptive and exproprioperceptive capabilities (Turvey & Fonseca, 2014). These capabilities are manifest by the cell as a forceful probing of the ECM by means of its lamellipodia and filopodia.[2] They have been revealed, for the most part, by experiments on prepared two-dimensional substrates. In respect to a substrate's ability to support the cell's locomotion, the probing can be said to comprise: (a) anchoring to and pulling on the substrate, and (b) organizational changes in the cell's cytoskeleton[3] in response to the detected rigidity (stiffness) of the substrate (e.g., Discher, Janmey, & Wang, 2005). We assume that cell locomotion, paralleling animal locomotion, can be reliably successful only if "perception" ensures contact with the facts of ECM, facts of the cell ecology. Registering the disposition[4] of one ECM region's ability to support locomotion as better than another ECM region's ability requires detecting ECM stiffness as an invariant measure over variations in (a) tension at the cell's focal (integrin) attachments to the ECM, and (b) the cell's cytoskeletal organization.

A further highlighting of fibroblast selectivity with respect to surface rigidity is warranted. A substrate is divided by the experimenter so as to have a sharp border between two levels of stiffness designated "firm" and "soft." A fibroblast approaching the transition from the soft side proceeds readily to the firm side. It does so with an increase in its traction forces and in its body area, and with the lamellipodia that initiated the firm contact assuming the leading probing role. In contrast, approaching the transition from the firm side is marked by (a) arresting forward crawling and (b) either rotating so as to crawl parallel to the transition or retracting the contacting lamellipodia (Lo, Wang, Dembo & Wang, 2000).

In sum, it would seem that the perceiving of ECM regions by a fibroblast is the perceiving of "how to get about among them and what to do or not to do with them." Fibroblast behavior is prospective. It is in respect to possibilities for action.

22.2 Rejecting the Classical Dichotomies

The foregoing anticipates that our concern is an ontology befitting the ecological scale, an ontology that bears on the organisms composing the Six Kingdoms, particularly, the "how" of their living (their niches) and the "where" of their living (their habitats). We should expect this ecological ontology to differ substantially from the ontologies that shaped the thinking of the likes of Descartes, Locke, Berkeley, Hume, and Kant and their contemporary adherents. In Lecture 5 we confronted appearance versus reality, pragmatic truth versus absolute truth, in the context of a vine (*Monstera gigantea*). It was our introduction to ecological ontology. Although not referred to as such, Mario Bunge's (1977) *Treatise on Basic Philosophy: Volume 3*, entitled *The Furniture of the World*, is an implicit ecological ontology that has been deployed as such and explicitly developed as such (Turvey, Shaw, Reed & Mace, 1981; Turvey, 1992).

Consider, for example, the classical dichotomy of Being versus Becoming. In our consideration, we will use the term *thing* for an entity or substantial individual endowed with all of its (substantial) properties (Bunge, 1977, p. 110). We can then say, in respect to the being–becoming dichotomy, that it is a distinction drawn between things that do not change and changes that transpire without things—changeless things versus thingless changes. Ecological ontology holds that at the scale of living things and their environments there is no such dichotomy. There are only *changing things*, where thing is an entity defined as a substantial, propertied individual (think of an individual fibroblast, think of a river bank). Consider, as a further example, the classical dichotomy of Substance and Form alias propertyless things and thingless properties, respectively. Ecological ontology holds that there are only propertied things. It also holds that intrinsic properties and mutual (relational) properties are equally substantial properties. Both are real.[5]

What of space and time? In ecological ontology, space and time are relations involving things. In respect to space, there is no absolute thing-free space and there is no space-free thing (no thingless spaces, no spaceless things). Ecologically, *space* refers to the mutual separations among things. The separation between two things can be defined as the set of things lying or interposed between them. Given that there are only changing things, none of the multiple kinds of separation are fixed. All undergo change, however plodding that change might be. At the ecological scale, space is dynamic. The bottom line is that, ecologically, neither space nor things exist by themselves; only mutually spaced things exist.

Analogous arguments can be made for time. There is no absolute thing-free time and there is no time-free thing (no thingless times, no timeless things[6]). Ecologically, *time* refers to the mutual sequencing of, and mutual nesting of, things. An unchanging thing would be timeless, but there are no timeless things—that is, neither time nor things exist by themselves. There are no durationless things, no thingless durations.

22.3 Action Possibilities: The Concept of Affordance

Our fundamental premise will be this: All organisms of all Six Kingdoms exhibit "awareness of" defined as the perceiving of possibilities for action and organizing behavior accordingly.[7] Gibson (1977, 1979/1986) introduced the term *affordance* for an action possibility. Lombardo (1987) expresses the significance of affordances thusly:

> Affordances provide the "connection" between perception and behavior, for it is affordances which are perceived and it is affordances that are used and adjusted to vis-à-vis behavior. Gibson's concept of affordances was developed to provide a description of the environment relevant to ways of life.
>
> (p. 355)

The necessary complement of affordance has been termed *effectivity* (Turvey & Shaw, 1979).[8] Affordance and effectivity can be expressed in the following manner (after Shaw, Turvey, & Mace, 1982):

> Situation X *affords* activity Y for organism Z on occasion O if and only if X and Z are mutually compatible on dimensions of relevance to Y.
>
> Organism Z *effects* activity Y in situation X on occasion O if and only if Z and X are mutually compatible on dimensions of relevance to Y.

Figure 22.1 provides an appreciation of the occasion variable O and the functionally specific variability of Y. It is modeled after von Uexküll's (1934/2010, p. 93) classical analysis. On the occasion of lacking the protection of its shell that is provided by sea anemones (a protection against squids), the hermit crab perceives a sea anemone as something to put on its shell and does so. On the occasion of lacking the dwelling provided by its shell, the hermit crab perceives a sea anemone as a possible enclosure and tries to crawl into it. On the occasion of lacking food, but having both protection against squid and a dwelling, the hermit crab perceives a sea anemone as a possible food item and tries to eat it.

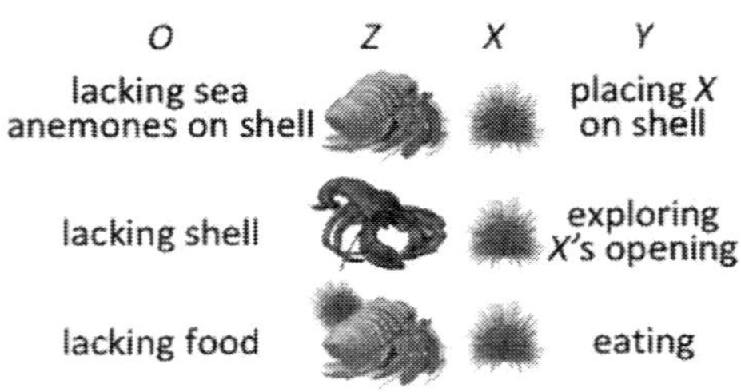

Figure 22.1 The occasion variable O of the affordance formulation expressed in von Uexküll's (1934/2010) study of the sea anemone where Z is organism, X is situation and Y is activity.

(From Figure 12, Turvey, 2015, adapted with permission, Imprint Academic.)

It is of some note that history seems to have missed von Uexküll's (1934/2010, p. 117) insistence that search is first and foremost in respect to "tone" not "image"—that is, to a prevailing character or quality rather than to a specific thing. For the crab of Figure 22.1, the three distinct tones are, respectively, that the thing in question affords temporary protection, that the thing in question affords dwelling within, and that the thing in question affords eating.

A guiding conjecture (Turvey & Shaw, 1979; see also Petrusz & Turvey, 2010) is that, in perceiving, an organism perceives the coordination of *X*, *Y*, *Z*, and *O* as a *single complex particular* (cf. Kripke, 1980).[9] Consider what counts for a branch to be a lizard's perch (*X*) for predating (*Y*). For the lizard *Anolis*, behavioral ecology identifies it as a place that is view from-able, jump from-able with accuracy, and sprint upon-able with maximal speed. It is a function of the lizard's leg length, the branch's breadth, and the branch's texture (Irschick & Losos, 1999; Moermond, 1979). We have no single word that conjoins all these properties. We have no single word, or even a simple combination of words, to define this particular, but representative, affordance.

22.4 Action Possibilities: The Dynamics of Affordance Perception

In everyday activity, a person will commonly perceive whether a visible object affords grasping with one hand or with both hands. In experiments in which wooden blocks of different widths are presented in orderly fashion from one width size to the next, a transition occurs from using one of the aforementioned manual modes to the other (Lopresti-Goodman, Turvey, & Frank, 2011). The transition depends on the ratio of the object's width to the span of the hand. It also depends on the *presentation sequence* of size (increasing versus decreasing). It is of some significance that the observed conventional positive hysteresis (i.e., a larger transition ratio for the increasing sequence) is accommodated by dynamical principles (e.g., Haken, 1991, 1996) that typify self-organizing systems (Frank, Richardson, Lopresti-Goodman, & Turvey, 2009).

Subsequent research by Lopresti-Goodman and colleagues (Lopresti-Goodman, Turvey & Frank, 2013) has taken the dynamical principles inhering in affordance perception a step further. Their research identified and addressed conditions of unconventional negative hysteresis (i.e., a larger transition ratio for the decreasing sequence). Of significance is the implication that a second control parameter is at play in the self-organization of affordance perception—a parameter seemingly regulated by the dynamics (referred to, conventionally, as inhibitory) of agent–task–environment qua system.

22.5 Generalizing from Animalia to (Single Cell) Protoctista

The descriptors "awareness of," "functionally specific variability," and "affordance/effectivity" used in Section 22.3 for *Anolis* (a species in the Kingdom Animalia) apply equally to single cell organisms in the Kingdom Protoctista, for example, those belonging to the genus *Difflugia*. For present purposes, the significant effectivity of *Difflugia* is the construction of a shell (also referred to as a test) by some members of the genus. Figure 22.2a shows a representative *Difflugia*'s fit to its self-assembled shell. Figure 22.2b–d shows three kinds of *Difflugia* distinguished and defined primarily by the forms of their shells.

The genus *Difflugia* seemingly satisfies the dictionary definition of the ability "to build." Its members construct their homes by first selecting materials, then ordering and uniting materials by gradual means into a composite whole. Different actions are afforded at different phases of home building by particles differing in size and mineral properties. For *Difflugia coronata*, the shell comprises 200–300 "stones" cemented together. Seven to eight spikes adorn the top and the opening is ornamental with a pleated collar. Shell size is about 150 micrometers in diameter. Although less complicated than *D. coronata*, the gradations of "stones" in the shell of *D. accuminata* should be appreciated: largest near the middle, smaller towards the apices.

Selection of materials reveals the sensitivity of the genus to the affordances related to grain size. The size distribution and mineral composition of the grains selected by *D. oblonga* for building differ from the size distribution and mineralogical composition of the sediment from which *D. oblonga* selects its grains (Armynot du Châtelet, Noiriel & Delaine, 2013). *D. oblonga* selects

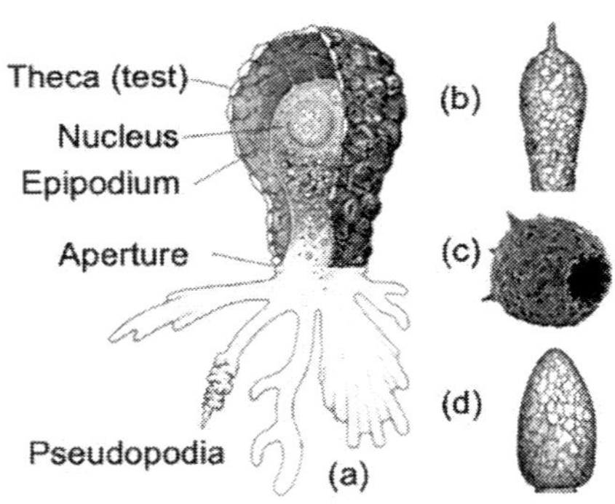

Figure 22.2 (a) A representative *Difflugia*'s fit to its self-assembled shell; (b) *D. accuminata*; (c) *D. coronata*; and (d) *D. oblonga*.

(Adapted with permission: (a–c) from Ferry Siemensma, www.arcella.nl/difflugia; and (d) Ralf Meisterfeld, Tree of Life Web Project.)

from the small-size fraction of the sediment with a preference for low-density silicates close to quartz density. A constraint on grain selection is the size of the eventual shell aperture and, perforce, the eventual size of the inhabitant (Figure 22.2a provides perspective).

As with animal species, members of *Difflugia* may engage in behaviors that make available a specific affordance of a particular thing. An example has been reported for the genus *D. tuberspinifera*, a genus very similar in shell design to *D. coronata* (Figure 22.2c). It is with respect to the undulations of the pseudostome (see the pleated opening of *D. coronata*). *D. tuberspinifera*'s pseudopodia manipulate a rotifer (an animal prey item) covered with a thick, shell-like cuticle so as to situate the pseudostome "teeth" between the animal's cuticle and the animal's body (Han, Wang, Xu et al., 2011). In this situation, the pseudostome of *D. tuberspinifera*'s shell (akin to an inverted bottle top) affords the activity of prying apart the hard and soft tissues of rotifer making the rotifer available for ingesting.

D. tuberspinifera's catching and consuming express a "remarkable agility" (Han et al., 2008, p. 198). It must first perceive that the catch is rotifer, that is, it is a thing X_i that affords ingesting in a particular way Y_i. In so perceiving, *D. tuberspinifera* assembles pseudopods that permit investigating the rotifer's covering cuticle and assessing the rotifer's size. *D. tuberspinifera* then orients to the bottom of the rotifer—that is, away from the mouth end—perforating the cuticle near the rotifer's foot. It does so deploying the "teeth" in coordination with temporarily assembled pseudopods that help provide the necessary leverage. Finally, it ingests the rotifer foot-first. In sum, *D. tuberspinifera* (and, patently, *Difflugia* in general) create, monitor and control action degrees of freedom and do so without a nervous system. As Han et al. (2008) comment respectfully: "Predatory amoebae may thus be single-celled, but are in no way behaviorally primitive" (p. 200).

22.6 Is Affordance a New Kind of *Primary* Quality?

This is an apposite occasion to revisit notions introduced in Lecture 5. Given a grey stone, one can predicate "length" of the stone in relation to a ruler and "weight" of the stone in relation to a balance. Both the ruler and the balance are like the grey stone—they are also objects of some kind. Length and weight are said to be primary qualities. Although length and weight are expressed in relation to another object, each quality is deemed to be an inherent property of the grey stone. We can define a primary quality *P* such as length or weight as follows: Predication relative to some other thing (such as a ruler or a balance) is *P* if and only if the predicated property is *expressed by* its relation to the other thing but does not *inhere in* the other thing or in the relation.

Classically, the quality *P* does not apply to the stone's color. The conventional understanding is that color *inheres in an observer*, an animal endowed with color vision. Classically, grey is a dimension of consciousness.

It is classified as a secondary quality. Historically, a secondary quality *S* such as color or taste has been defined as follows: Predication relative to some other thing (such as an animal endowed with color vision) is *S* if and only if the predicated property is *expressed by* its relation to the other thing and *inheres in* the other thing.

The development of the physics of non-sentient macroscopic objects over the centuries has been tethered to *P*. The development of the psychology of sentient macroscopic objects over the centuries has been tethered (primarily) to *S*. Conventional understanding is that neither *P* nor *S* applies to objects at the quantum scale. Arguably, what marks the quantum scale is the relation between the studied object and the means—another object, a scientific instrument—by which it is studied. A manifest property or quality of a quantum object is *expressed by* and *actualized by* (or, *inheres in*) the relation with this other object. It can be termed a relational property or quality *R* that exists potentially in the studied object as a disposition regardless of whether an object/instrument exists that can actualize it (Gomatam, 1999). Of the three properties or qualities *P*, *S* and *R*, only *R* can be predicated of an affordance. This conclusion echoes the preceding argument and accords with a definition of affordance as a disposition tantamount to an actual state of affairs *minus* particular conditions (Turvey, 1992). On provision of the conditions, actuality ensues—the affordance is realized as shown in Figure 22.1. The realization is as a particular relation, R_i. However, as Figure 22.1 makes evident, one cannot equate a thing's affordance (the sea urchin's affordance for the hermit crab) with any single R_i. For an *R* to be manifest, and in what form, depends on O (the occasion).

A significant conjecture follows from Gomatam's reasoning (see especially pp. 185–186) that, ontologically, *R* complements *P*: *Affordance realized as a relation, is not so much a third ontological quality as it is a new kind of primary quality.*[10] Echoing this conjecture, Fajen and Phillips (2013) ask whether affordances are so fundamental that judgments of conventional metrical properties are necessarily constrained by them, and Lee, Lee, Carello and Turvey (2014) opine that estimates of conventional physical dimensions may be elliptical reports of affordances.

We would do well at this juncture to remind ourselves of the historical or received view of perception's nature. We need to do so in a manner that befits the themes of the present lecture. We can do so through the following two assertions (see Fodor & Pylyshyn, 1981; Turvey et al., 1981):

Assertion 1. By virtue of its physical makeup, a perceiver is linked lawfully to the conventional physical properties of light, sound, molecular distributions in the air, etc.

Assertion 2. By virtue of its intellectual makeup, a perceiver is linked non-lawfully to the behaviorally significant properties (i.e., affordances) of the surrounding surfaces and substances.

Ideally, the juxtaposition of (a) the affordance-based behavioral achievements of *D. tuberspinifera*, and (b) the implication of affordance as a primary quality, can be appreciated as an essential counter to Assertions 1 and 2.

22.7 The Dispositional and the Relational

The use of relation in respect to the use of disposition in defining affordance requires elaboration. Terms used in philosophy to describe what is meant by disposition include power, ability, potency, capability, tendency, potentiality, proclivity, and capacity, among others.[11] We can use these terms to gain a purchase on the notion of affordance as interpreted by Reed (1996).

> An affordance is only a relation when used. Affordances are not relations. They are resources for obtaining value from the environment through regulated action. Affordances are available to come into relationships with organisms, *but this need not happen*.
>
> (pp. 26–27)

Of particular significance in the foregoing quotation is the term "resources." The words power, potency, potentiality, and capacity in the list of disposition's descriptors are close relatives of resource. Reed's separation is seemingly recognition of affordance as a *disposition* of situation or thing X that transforms on occasion O to affordance as a *relation* R.[12]

Allow that dispositions are causally relevant (Harré, 1970; McKitrick, 2005). Then, taking advantage of Heil's (2005) thematic enumeration of disposition, we can say the following of any given thing X in the environment of any given organism Z: (a) X's dispositions are actual, not merely possible; (b) X's dispositions are properties intrinsic to it (they are neither relations nor "relational properties"); (c) X's dispositional nature is not wholly revealed via a reductive conditional analysis;[13] (d) X's being dispositional is not a contingent feature; (e) X's dispositions are not "higher level" properties (i.e., not grounded in "lower level" non-dispositional properties; (f) X's manifestation of dispositions is a manifestation of reciprocal disposition partners (recall any panel of Figure 22.1); (g) X's dispositions can manifest themselves differently with different reciprocal disposition partners (recall all three panels of Figure 22.1).

Returning to Reed's perspective above, affordances are dispositions of environmental layout that can be made manifest by reciprocal dispositions of organisms. Relation *R* between organism Z and situation X is afforded, on the occasion O, when Z uses X in the course of implementing activity Y.

22.8 Affordances: A Lawfully Benign Relativism

Pursuant to Gomatam (1999), we can ask whether *R* is what Bohr and Einstein sought as a basis for interpreting quantum mechanics consistently at micro and macro scales. Inconsistency was worrying insofar as it suggested a malign relativism: different scales, different experimental contexts, expressing different phenomena, implying different natures. Harré (1997) summarizes Bohr's position as follows. An apparatus (A) is not in general a transparent medium on the world (W). To the contrary, phenomena are made manifest by A–W complexes. As we noted in Lecture 7, the concept of complementarity was inspired by the so-called duality paradox: Radiation as W is a wave when A is a receiving antenna and a particle when A is a photomultiplier. The dispositions that phenomena (such as radiation) reveal are dispositions of A–W complexes.

Casting the matter in the language of affordances, Harré (1997) contends that an A-W complex affords a phenomenon Π if and only if W has the power to engender Π. Thus, one kind of A–W complex engenders electrons and another kind of A–W complex engenders waves (with engender understood as "cause to make manifest"). Harré presents the case where W is a garden and A is either a human or a bee. By virtue of the difference in their lifestyles, the affordances of a garden for human and bee differ, as do the spectral distributions within which the affordances for human and bee are optically specified: A_{HUMAN}–W engenders light that is VIBGYOR; A_{BEE}–W engenders light that is UVVIBG.[14] The affordances of the garden for a bee are different from those for a human. But the garden, *independent of bees and people*, affords one activity-relevant color layout for bees and another for people. And this, as Harré underscores, *is a property of the garden.*

Consider Figure 22.3. The affordance of a brink in a surface (as the world W) is a case in point. The affordance differs for animals of different sizes (as apparatus A): A_{LARGE}–W engenders the activity of stepping down; A_{MEDIUM}–W engenders the activity of jumping down, and A_{SMALL}–W engenders the activity of crawling down. This threesome of affordances is a property of the brink. Likewise, for W as a gap in a surface and A as a human either walking

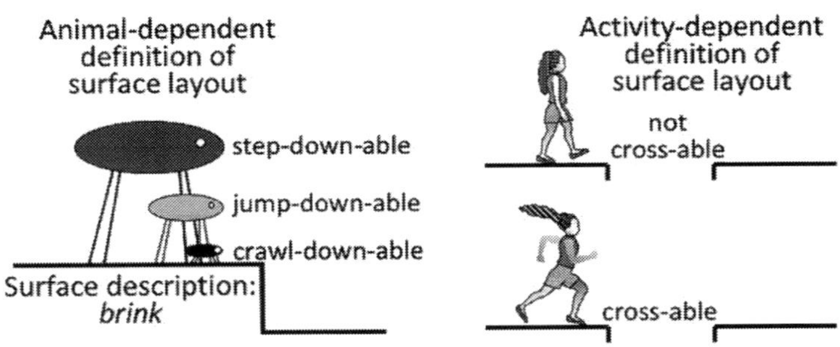

Figure 22.3 (*Left*) Affordance of brink is relative size (animal/depth) dependent. (*Right*) Affordance of gap for a given animal is speed-dependent.

(From Figure 10, Chemero & Turvey, 2007, adapted with permission, Springer.)

slowly or running quickly: $A_{WALKING}$–W engenders not crossable and $A_{RUNNING}$–W engenders crossable. This twosome of affordances is a property of the gap. The bottom line is that affordance allows science to say that "there are properties of the world such that their empirical content is always given by their mode of manifestation" (Harré, 1997, p. 28).

To reiterate, an A–W complex affords a specific phenomenon only if W has the power to generate such a phenomenon when intimately interconnected with the relevant A. In the terms of the affordance formulation used above, Harré's position is that a quantum experimental situation *X* affords a mode of manifestation alias activity *Y* for world *W* on occasion *O* if and only if *X* and *W* are mutually compatible on dimensions of relevance to *Y*. The upshot at quantum and ecological levels is a lawfully benign relativism.

22.9 Intensional Description and Conceptual Ascription

In Figure 22.1, we cast the hermit crab as perceiving a particular thing (a sea urchin) as a "cover shell with-able thing," or a "crawl into-able thing," or an "eat-able thing," depending on the occasion.[15] For the particular occasions identified in Figure 22.1, we assigned to the hermit crab the properties "can perceive cover shell with-able things," "can perceive crawl into-able things," and "can perceive edible things," respectively. Each of the preceding involves a borrowing of a property of the environment to predicate a property of the hermit crab. In each case of "can perceive," a property of one kind of thing—namely, the sea urchin—is borrowed and applied to another kind of thing—namely, the hermit crab. Thus, we have the notion of a property—for example "cover shell with-able"—of a sea urchin (a perceivable thing) and a property of the hermit crab (a perceiver thing) which disposes the hermit crab to perceiving "cover shell with-able." In attaching the property "cover shell with-able" to the property "can perceive," we have concocted what can be referred to as an intensional[16] context (cf. Turvey et al., 1981).

Intension is the meaning or connotation of an expression (as opposed to its extension or denotation). The intension of a predicate expression (a common noun or an adjective) is often taken to be a concept (Audi, 1999). In consequence, it is historically and typically the case that in giving an organism an intensional description, a perceptual theorist's intent is to ascribe to the organism the concept of one or more properties of the embedding environment. It mandates that to perceive property *x* of *X*, *Z* must have a concept of property *x* of *X*. This mandate is the "intellectual makeup" in Assertion 2 above. It was the implicit core of the lectures in Parts 1 and 2. It is founded primarily on the assumption that no energy medium singly or in conjunction with other energy media is structured by property *x* of *X* in a way that is specific to property *x* of *X*. Property *x* of *X* has to be borrowed by the theorist in the form of a concept deemed innate or acquired. It is the familiar perspective of the man-in-the-inner-room. It runs counter to ecological realism.

An ecological understanding of intensional description looks as follows (after Turvey et al. 1981, Section 11):

1 To describe one thing Z (organism) in terms of the properties of another thing X (environment), properties to which Z is sensitive, is not to ascribe to Z concepts of the properties of X.[17]
2 An intensional context of the kind "Z can perceive property *x* of X" or "Z perceives property *x* of X and acts accordingly" is merely an indirect way of referring to a lawful relation of properties.

Together, 1 and 2 inform us that when the expression "organism Z perceives the affordance *a* of a thing X" designates an actual state of affairs it *does not* mean that Z has a concept of *a* that mediates the perception of *a* and *does* mean that there is a lawful basis to the perception of *a* by Z. This, in a nutshell, is the thesis of direct perception. Its exposition and proof rests on the development of a perspective-dependent ecological physics (e.g., Shaw, 2001) or, what might be termed, a semantic physics (Petrusz & Turvey, 2010).

22.10 What Environment Affords is Objective, Real, and Physical (but in a Non-Classical Sense)

Consider two animals, an ant and a cat, in the proximity of a stone (Figure 22.4b). The focal *P* property of the stone is height (Figure 22.4a). It is objective in the conventional sense that it is expressed through its relation to another thing (e.g., a ruler). The *R* properties of the stone in respect to the current states and locations of cat and ant in Figure 22.4b include (1) jump upon-able for the cat but not for the ant, (2) climb up-able for the ant but not for the cat, (3) walk around-able for both cat and ant, and (4) pass through-able for neither cat nor ant. They are real in the impredicative sense.

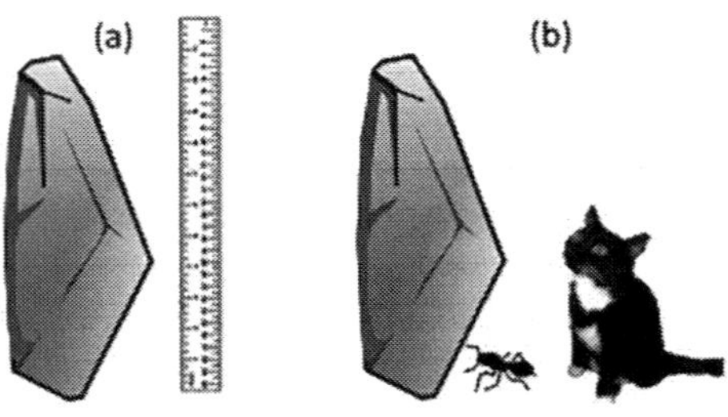

Figure 22.4 (a) Primary/predicative property: Height. (b) Relational/impredicative property: Jump up on-able (not crawl up-able) for cat. Crawl up-able (not jump up on-able) for ant.

(From Figure 16, Turvey, 2015, adapted with permission, Imprint Academic.)

Our introduction to the notion of impredicativity was in Lecture 3 in respect to the two natures of the mathematical notion of set, predicative and impredicative. It was depicted in Figure 3.7. Its role in Lecture 3 was to communicate the conception of self-referencing and the possibility of an alternative to the historical causal chain perspective on the workings of perception. Here we need to emphasize that whereas the conventional predicative version (set theory) has been to date well suited to the modeling of artificial languages and artificial systems, the impredicative version, referred to as hyperset theory and introduced (primarily, and relatively recently) by Aczel (1988), is more accommodating of natural languages and natural systems (e.g., Barwise & Etchemendy, 1987; Barwise & Moss, 1996; Kercel, 2003; Núñez, 2008). It nests the predicative form as a special case. Arguably, it is what is required to formalize affordance (e.g., Chemero & Turvey, 2007, 2008; Turvey, 2004).

Property (i) of Figure 22.4b, for example, is defined impredicatively—that is, in terms of the system of which the stone is a part (the cat-stone system). Property (i) is also physical in the "quantum compatible" superpositional sense—that is, it is in no definite state. Other action possibilities are simultaneously and equally present (e.g., walk round-able, hide behind-able, rest next to-able). Accordingly, in the absence of a stone-related act by the cat one might refer to the cat-stone system as *coherent*. However, given an act by the cat (namely, jumping up on the stone thereby realizing jump up on-able) one might refer to the cat–stone system as *decoherent*, because properties (i) and (iii), *by virtue of the cat's act*, are currently null and void. In the meantime, however, given no act by the ant, the ant–stone system remains superpositional and, perforce, coherent. If the foregoing reasoning passes muster, then one is encouraged to consider the possibility of a deep link between decoherence and ontology grounded in the fundamental link between decoherence and dissipation.

Aside from rare nondissipative systems (e.g., superfluids, superconductors), a macroscopic system will never be found in a quantum superposition of macroscopically different states (Omnès, 1994).[18] From the indefinitely many quantum states, decoherence distills a small number of broadly characterized properties (Lindley, 1996). The primary and secondary qualities comprising the classical ontology are canonical. In common English, they are "Size, position, speed; color, texture, hardness; solidity and fluidity; smell, taste, and sound" (Lindley, 1996, p. 216). This distillation from the vast randomness of quantum states by decoherence is reliable and deterministic. It stands in sharp contrast to the individual quantum states in both number and kind.

Designation of affordances as "new primary qualities" brings the classical ontology into question. Across the individual organisms constituting the Kingdoms of Bacteria, Archaea, Protoctista, Fungi, Plantae, and Animalia, the number of affordances qua new primary qualities is uncountable. Why such is the case might ensue from the fundamental linkage of decoherence to dissipation (Omnès, 1994) joined with the following understanding introduced in Lecture 20, namely, that the perceiving and acting capabilities coordinate with affordances are what they are because they extend the means for dissipating energy resources—for enhancing the rate of environmental entropy production. As noted in Lecture 20, the understanding in question reflects what has come to be labeled in some quarters as the *Law of Maximum Entropy Production* (Mahulikar & Harwig, 2004; Martínez-Kahn & Martínez-Castilla, 2010; Swenson & Turvey, 1991). To reiterate, the proposed law states that a given system will select the path or assemblage of paths out of available paths that minimizes the potential or maximizes the entropy at the fastest rate possible, given the current circumstances or constraints.

If living things are inseparable from their surroundings and both are part of a directed single planetary-scale evolutionary process, then the number and variety of organisms and environments can be said to follow from an opportunistic strategy that produces progressively more ways, and more intense ways, to generate entropy. That is, more organism–environment systems implicates more affordances, higher levels of order, and greater entropy rate (Figure 20.2). To quote Annila and Salthe (2010):

> [E]volution into species richness is no objective as such but is common because generally more diverse sources of free energy are accessed by diverse mechanisms. No single species is equipped with all interaction mechanisms to draw from all sources. This is because history has continually reworked surviving energy gradients into increasing numbers of different configurations and conformations.
>
> (p. 312)

Figure 22.5 adapted from Smith (1996, p. 146) provides us with an apt finish to the present lecture. It expresses the fit or lack thereof between an

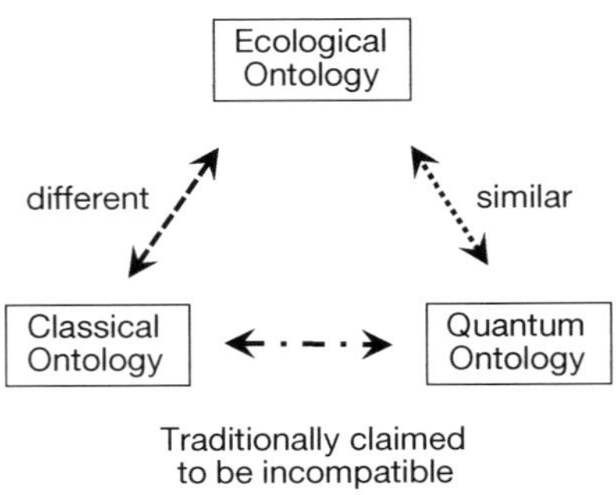

Figure 22.5 Proposed relation among quantum, classical, and ecological ontologies. (From Figure 17, Turvey, 2015, adapted with permission, Imprint Academic.)

ontology motivated by nature's ecological scale and the two ontologies that govern contemporary science, that of Newtonian mechanics and that of quantum mechanics. Ideally, we have come to appreciate that an ecological ontology could be minimally as rich, and maximally more far reaching, than the established ontologies that have thus far given shape to established thinking on perception. And, ideally, we have also given ourselves a sense of what the non-mediated, non-contact theory of perception introduced in Lecture 20, Figure 20.6, might look like.

Notes

1 Definitions are from *Merriam-Webster*.

2 These are, respectively, sheet-like and filament-like extensions of cytoplasm that form transient attachments to the substrate.

3 The cytoskeleton is a network of intra-cell protein filaments and microtubules that contributes to the cell's shape, internal organization and movement.

4 The term "disposition" has been used here and there in the preceding lectures. At this juncture, we need to recognize its use in conventional physical analysis: a property of a thing that is potential, latent, or possible—that is, not occurrent.

5 Whereas a predicate may represent a substantial property, rightly or wrongly, possessing a substantial property is not a matter of true or false.

6 Bunge (1977, p. 303) remarks: "if anything looks timeless then it has been improperly investigated."

7 Within ecological thinking, constructions of the kind "awareness of *x*" are preferred over "awareness" neat. The role of the latter is commonly used in the sense of "aware" to designate a state of mind.

8 The term is owing to von Neumann (1966, p. 78). For him, it meant the potentiality to do things, how involved were the purposive operations.

9 See Fodor (1998) and Millikan (2000) for arguments favoring an atomistic interpretation of concepts.

10 Further, given that *R* is potential in situation X on occasion O whether or not O occurs means that X has the quality of aboutness in respect to Z. The implication is that intentionality is, first and foremost, the mark of the relational. It is not, first and foremost, the mark of the mental, as commonly claimed.

11 See Choi, Sungho and Fara, Michael, "Dispositions," *The Stanford Encyclopedia of Philosophy* (Spring 2014 Edition), Edward N. Zalta (ed.), available at: http://plato.stanford.edu/archives/spr2014/entries/dispositions/

12 In the literature on affordance, some have focused on the dispositional aspect (e.g., Lopresti-Goodman et al. 2013; Turvey et al., 1981; Turvey, 1992) and some have focused on the relational aspect (e.g., Chemero, 2003, 2009).

13 The analysis is a matter of identifying one or more subjunctive conditionals: to say that an object has the disposition to do F is just to say that it does F if the circumstances are such-and-such.

14 Where UV is ultraviolet, V is violet, I is indigo, B is blue, G is green, Y is yellow, O is orange, R is red.

15 We are constructing something similar to what Bell (1993), in the domain of quantum mechanics, has referred to as *be*ables (short for may-*be*ables) and typically written without the italics. In respect to future theoretical physics Bell suggests it should not be fundamentally about "measurements" and "observables" but about *be*ables: objective properties assigned to objects. For Bell, the observables of quantum mechanics are "*made* out of beables" (p.41).

16 It is worth underscoring that intensional is not the same word as intentional. The two words are, however, related (Audi, 1999).

17 Generally speaking, to describe one thing in terms of a property of another thing to which it is sensitive or responsive is not a matter of ascribing a concept. Consider "jellied eels are nauseating." The property "nauseating" is borrowed from humans—namely, the property of making humans retch. In asserting that "jellied eels are nauseating" one is not, of course, ascribing to jellied eels a concept of this human property.

18 Quantum coherence can, in particular biological circumstances (e.g., photosynthetic complexes), be relatively long-lived extending up to the picosecond range (Chin, Huegla, & Plenio, 2012).

References

Aczel, P. (1988). *Non-well-founded sets*. Stanford, CA: CSLI Publications.

Annila, A., & Salthe, S. (2010). Physical foundations of evolutionary theory. *Journal of Non-Equilibrium Thermodynamics*, *35*, 301–321.

Armynot du Châtelet, E., Noiriel, C., & Delaine, M. (2013). Three-dimensional morphological and mineralogical characterization of testate amebae. *Microscopy & Microanalysis*, *19*, 1511–1522.

Audi, R. (1999). *The Cambridge dictionary of philosophy*. Cambridge, UK: Cambridge University Press.

Barwise, J., & Etchemendy, J. (1987). *The liar: An essay on truth and circularity*. New York: Oxford University Press.

Barwise, J., & Moss, L. (1996). *Vicious circles*. Stanford, CA: CSLI Publications.

Bell, J. S. (1993). *Speakable and unspeakable in quantum mechanics*. Cambridge, UK: Cambridge University Press.

Bunge, M. (1977). *Ontology I: The furniture of the world*. Dordrecht, Netherlands: D. Reidel.

Chemero, A. (2003). An outline of a theory of affordances. *Ecological Psychology*, *15*, 181–195.

Chemero, A. (2009). *Radical embodied cognitive science*. Boston, MA: MIT Press.

Chemero, A., & Turvey, M. T. (2007). Complexity, hypersets, and the ecological approach to perception-action. *Biological Theory*, *2*, 23–36.

Chemero, A., & Turvey, M. T. (2008). Autonomy and hypersets. *Biosystems*, *91*, 320–330.

Chin, A. W., Huegla, S. F., & Plenio, M. B. (2012). Coherence and decoherence in biological systems: Principles of noise-assisted transport and the origin of long-lived coherences. *Philosophical Transactions of the Royal Society* A, *370*, 3638–3657.

Discher, D. E., Janmey, P., & Wang, Y. L. (2005). Tissue cells feel and respond to the stiffness of their substrate. *Science*, *310*, 1139–1143.

Fajen, B. R., & Phillips, F. (2013). Spatial perception and action. In D. Wallace & L. Nadel (Eds.). *Handbook of spatial cognition* (pp. 67–80). Washington, DC: APA Books

Fodor, J. A. (1998). *Concepts: Where cognitive science went wrong*. Oxford, UK: Oxford University Press.

Fodor, J. A., & Pylyshyn, Z. W. (1981). How direct is visual perception? Some reflections on Gibson's ecological approach. *Cognition*, 9, 139–196.

Frank, T. D., Richardson, M. J., Lopresti-Goodman, S. M., & Turvey, M. T. (2009). Order parameter dynamics of body-scaled hysteresis and mode transitions in grasping behavior. *Journal of Biological Physics*, *35*, 127–147.

Gibson, J. J. (1977). The theory of affordances. In R. E. Shaw & J. Bransford (Eds.) *Perceiving, acting and knowing* (pp. 67–82). Hillsdale, NJ: Erlbaum.

Gibson, J. J. (1986). *The ecological approach to visual perception*. Mahwah, NJ: Erlbaum (original work published 1979).

Gomatam, R. V. (1999). Quantum theory and the observation problem. In R. Núñez & W. J. Freeman (Eds.), *Reclaiming cognition: The primacy of action, intention and emotion* (pp. 173–190). Thorverton, UK: Imprint Academic.

Haken, H. (1991). *Synergetic computers and cognition*. Berlin, Germany: Springer.

Haken, H. (1996). *Principles of brain functioning*. Berlin, Germany: Springer.

Han, B. P., Wang, T., Lin, Q. Q., Dumont, H. J , (2008). Carnivory and active hunting by the planktonic testate amoeba *Difflugia tuberspinifera*. *Hydrobiologia*, *596*, 197–201.

Han, B-P., Wang, T., Xu, L., Lin, Q. Q., Jinyu, Z., & Dumont, H. J. (2011). Carnivorous planktonic Difflugia (Protista, Amoebina Testacea) and their predators. *European Journal of Protistology*, *47*, 214–223.

Harré, R. (1970). Powers. *British Journal for the Philosophy of Science*, 21, 81–101.

Harré, R. (1997). Is there a basic ontology for the physical sciences? *Dialectica*, *51*, 17–34.

Heil, J. (2005). Dispositions. *Synthese*, *144*, 343–356.

Irschick, D. J., & Losos, J. B. (1999). Do lizards avoid habitats in which their performance is submaximal? The relationship between sprinting capabilities and structural habitat use in Caribbean Anoles. *American Naturalist*, *154*, 293–305.

Kercel, S. W. (2003). Endogenous causes—bizarre effects. *Evolution and Cognition*, *8*, 130–144.

Kripke, S. (1980). *Naming and necessity*. Cambridge, MA: Harvard University Press.

Lee, Y., Lee, S., Carello, C., & Turvey, M. T. (2012). An archer's perceived form scales the "hit-ableness" of archery targets. *Journal of Experimental Psychology: Human Perception and Performance*, *38*, 1132–1143.

Lindley, D. (1996). *Where does the weirdness go?* New York: HarperCollins.

Lo, C. M., Wang, H. B., Dembo, M., & Wang, Y. L. (2000). Cell movement is guided by the rigidity of the substrate. *Biophysical Journal*, *79*, 144–152.

Lombardo, T. J. (1987). *The reciprocity of perceiver and environment: The evolution of James J. Gibson's ecological psychology*. Hillsdale, NJ: Erlbaum.

Lopresti-Goodman, S. M., Turvey, M. T., & Frank, T. D. (2011). Behavioral dynamics of the affordance "graspable" *Attention, Perception, & Psychophysics*, *73*, 1948–1965.

Lopresti-Goodman, S. M., Turvey, M. T., & Frank, T. D. (2013). Negative hysteresis in the behavioral dynamics of the affordance "graspable". *Attention, Perception, & Psychophysics*, *75*, 1075–1091.

Mahulikar, S. P., & Harwig, H. (2004). Conceptual investigation of the entropy principle for identification of directives for creation, existence and total destruction of order. *Physica Scripta*, *70*, 212–221.

Martínez-Kahn, M., & Martínez-Castilla, L. (2010). The fourth law of thermodynamics: The law of maximum entropy production (LMEP). An interview with Rod Swenson. *Ecological Psychology*, *22*, 69–87.

McKitrick, J. (2005). Are dispositions causally relevant? *Synthese*, *144*, 357–371.

Millikan, R. (2000). *On clear and confused ideas*. Cambridge, UK: Cambridge University Press.

Moermond, T. (1979). The influence of habitat structure on *Anolis* foraging behaviour. *Behaviour*, *70*, 147–167.

Núñez, R. E. (2008). Mathematics, the ultimate challenge to embodiment: Truth and the grounding of axiomatic systems. In P. Calvo & A. Gomila (Eds.), *Handbook of cognitive science: An embodied approach* (pp. 333–354). San Diego, CA: Elsevier.

Omnès, R. (1994). *The interpretation of quantum mechanics*. Princeton, NJ: Princeton University Press.

Petrusz, S., & Turvey, M. T. (2010). On the distinctive features of ecological laws. *Ecological Psychology*, *22*, 44–68.

Reed, E. (1996). *Encountering the world: Toward an ecological psychology*. Oxford, UK: Oxford University Press.

Shaw, R. E. (2001). Processes, acts and experiences: Three stances on the problem of intentionality. *Ecological Psychology*, *13*, 275–314.

Shaw, R., Turvey, M. T., & Mace, W. M. (1982). Ecological psychology: The consequence of a commitment to realism. In W. Weimer & D. Palermo (Eds.), *Cognition and the symbolic processes II* (pp. 159–226). Hillsdale, NJ: Erlbaum.

Smith, B. (1996). *On the origin of objects*. Boston, MA: MIT Press.

Swenson, R., & Turvey, M. T. (1991). Thermodynamic reasons for perception-action cycles. *Ecological Psychology*, *3*, 317–348.

Turvey, M. T. (1992). Affordances and prospective control: An outline of the ontology. *Ecological Psychology*, *4*, 173–187.

Turvey, M. T. (2004). Impredicativity, dynamics, and the perception-action divide. In V. K. Jirsa & J. A. S. Kelso (Eds.), *Coordination dynamics: Issues and trends* (pp. 1–20). New York: Springer.

Turvey, M. T. (2015). Quantum-like issues at nature's ecological scale (the scale of organisms and their environments). *Mind & Matter*, *13*, 7–44.

Turvey, M. T., & Fonseca, S. T. (2014). The medium of haptic perception: A tensegrity hypothesis. *Journal of Motor Behavior*, *46*, 143–189.

Turvey, M. T., & Shaw, R. E. (1979). The primacy of perceiving: An ecological reformulation of perception for understanding memory. In L-G Nilssen (Ed.), *Perspectives on memory research: In honor of Uppsala University's 500th anniversary* (pp. 167–222). Hillsdale, NJ: Erlbaum.

Turvey, M. T., & Shaw, R. E. (1995). Toward an ecological physics and a physical psychology. In R. Solso & D. Massaro (Eds.), *The science of the mind: 2001 and beyond* (pp. 144–169). Oxford, UK: Oxford University Press.

Turvey, M. T., Shaw, R. E., Reed, E. S., & Mace, W. M. (1981). Ecological laws of perceiving and acting: In reply to Fodor and Pylyshyn (1981). *Cognition*, *9*, 237–304.

von Neumann, J. (1966). *The theory of self-reproducing automata*. Urbana: University of Illinois Press.

von Uexküll, J. (2010). *A foray into the worlds of animals and humans*. Minneapolis: University of Minnesota Press (original work published 1934).

Lecture 23
Ecological Optics Primer

The barrage of conceptual details that was Lecture 22 was motivated by a very simple activity-oriented characterization of perception: To perceive things is to perceive how to get about among them and what to do or not to do with them.[1] The characterization is given expression in Figure 23.1, which is a portrayal of the ecological theme that began Lecture 3: When we observe a dragonfly steering its way through a thicket, and inquire "To what does its perceiving refer?" we should expect the answer "That to which its activity

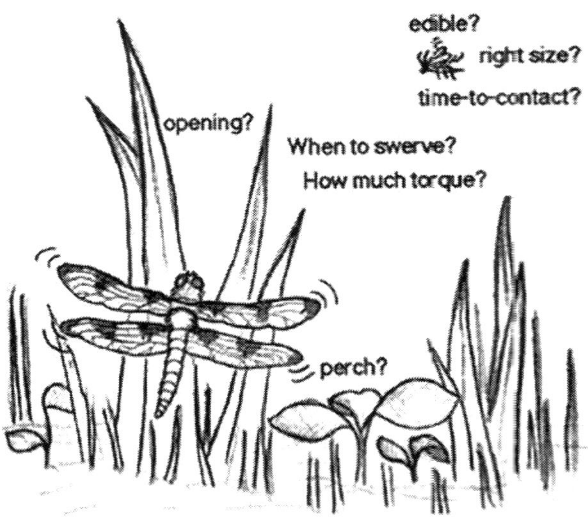

Figure 23.1 A dragonfly in its niche exemplifies the activity-oriented characterization of perception: to perceive things is to perceive how to get about among them and what to do or not to do with them.

(From Figure 11.3, Turvey & Shaw, 1995, Toward an ecological physics and a physical psychology, in Solso & Massaro (Eds.), *The science of the mind: 2001 and beyond*. Adapted with permission of Oxford University Press, USA.)

refers." This is simply to say that the proper "objects" of perceiving are presumed to be the same as those of activity.

Revisiting Lecture 20 (particularly, Figure 20.2), we can note the emergence over the past 550 million years of the Kingdom Animalia and, correspondingly, the diversification of the ability to move in a controlled and directed manner.[2] To have this ability is to be able to perceive what actions the material layout allows with sufficient efficacy to discover energy resources and to implement the circumstances for furthering one's kind. On these considerations, the focus of scientific inquiry into the psychology of perception–action for the Kingdom Animalia is *controlled locomotion*, specifically, visually controlled locomotion (e.g., Fajen & Matthis, 2011; Harrison, Turvey & Frank, 2016; Lee, 1980; Warren, 2009).[3] Unfortunately, the aforementioned focus cannot be the first order of business. Coming fully to terms with visually controlled locomotion requires, at a minimum, dismantling the hegemony of (a) the retinal image, and (b) measures and associated geometries appropriated uncritically from physics. As will become apparent, to pursue requirements (a) and (b) is to question the grounds for calling any instance of perception "illusory."

23.1 Retinal Image is not Axiomatic

The retinal image has been the centerpiece of vision theory for centuries and it has, necessarily, been a prominent feature of the present series of lectures (beginning with Lecture 6).[4] It has been the pre-eminent example of a "third thing" M mediating between animal A and environment *E* (Figure 3.2). In our progression through the historical variants of the man-in-the-inner-room (of a mobile home) it was the second grade of sense. It may be regarded as the primary conceptual barrier to the understanding of visual perception as direct.

Here we entertain the proposition that, despite the hegemony of retinal image in centuries of theorizing about vision, there are substantive reasons to argue that *there is no such entity*—that "retinal image" is a fiction.[5] It fell to the likes of Campbell (1817) and Bentley (1954/1975), more than a century apart, to point out that the celebrated scenario we encountered in Lecture 6 has little if anything to do with the nature of vision in living animals. In respect to the issues posed by the scenario, Campbell and Bentley contended that an image can be located at a translucent screen (the post-surgery state of affairs) *but it cannot be located at a transparent screen* (the pre-surgery state of affairs). When looking through the windshield of one's car, or the windows of one's office, or the lenses of one's eyeglasses, that which one sees is beyond the windshield, the windows, and the lenses, and is responded to behaviorally as such. This fundamental observation assigns the burden of proof for the concept of retinal image to the domain of living vision (i.e., investigation of eyeballs that are alive not dead).

Helmholtz was inclined to believe that the newly invented ophthalmoscope provided such a proof. On the basis of ophthalmoscope observations

(Helmholtz, 1886/2000, p. 92), he described experimental conditions in which a candle positioned off-center would be visible as an inverted image (with identifiable flame and wick at its base) on the inner side of the retina. Helmholtz averred that a view from the front provided by the ophthalmoscope should be inclusive of the retina, the retina's blood vessels, *and the optical images on the retina's surface*. And such, seemingly, was taken to be the case. One says "seemingly" because no further empirical proof via the ophthalmoscope seems to have been forthcoming in the 100-plus years since. What a present-day ophthalmologist sees when using an ophthalmoscope to look into the eye is shown in Figure 23.2 (top). The claim that for any given point of view the environment is imaged on the retina remains a claim seemingly substantiated only for a translucent retina. In reality, one's retinal image is not a thing that can be seen in everyday vision (Gibson, 1979/1986, p. 62), an appreciation reinforced by the retina's multilayered nature and dense

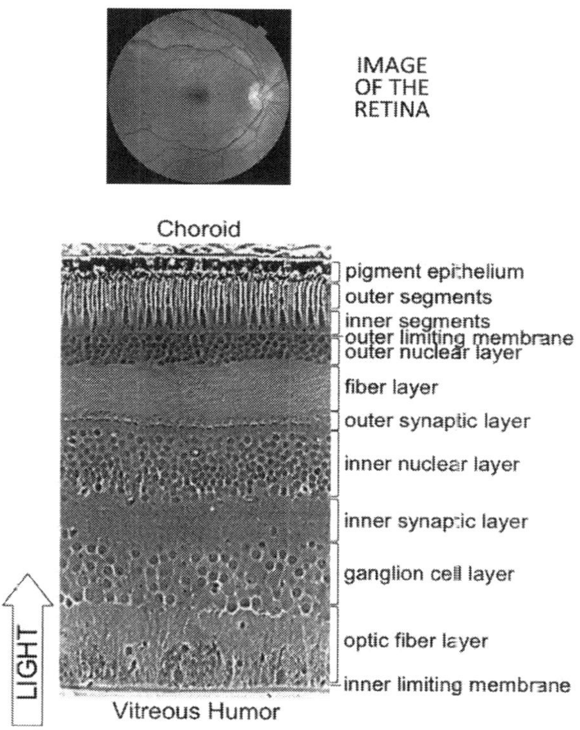

Figure 23.2 (*Top*) Network of blood vessels How does image formation avoid it? (*Bottom*) The layers of the retina; which houses the retinal image?

Top: (by Mikael Häggström, used with permission).
Bottom: (Adapted with permission, Boycott & Dowling, 1969, Royal Society.)

network of blood vessels (Figure 23.2, bottom). Of its 10 layers, which should we interpret as "screen-like"? And given its mish-mash of veins, how could we ever have unencumbered vision?[6]

To summarize the situation in Bentley's careful phrasing (1954/1975),

> retinal image is "just a careless use of words."
>
> (p. 274, Footnote 5)

There is one further observation to be made. It is on the questionable identity, in Bentley's view (1954/1975, p. 279), of retinal image as physical image. It is an observation made in Lecture 11 but one worth repeating here given its deep significance. A stationary layout of surfaces facing an observer can be said to project onto a retinal surface such that there is a point-to-point correspondence between atoms radiating from the facing surfaces and point-coordinates of the retina. This is the retinal image of geometric and physiological optics. Boynton (1974) expressed this conventional understanding thusly by way of dismissing Gibson's (1966) ecological optics:

> We are not in visual contact with objects, or edges, faces, facets, or textures. We are in contact only with photons.
>
> (Boynton, 1974, pp. 300–301)

A lesson from Lecture 11 was that visual experience is what it is not because light emitted from a light source is what it is, but because light reflected from objects, edges, faces, facets, textures, etc., is what it is. Figure 11.7 (upper) made apparent that if light as such were seen, as tables and chairs are seen, then in the course of conversing in a furnished room we would not see the person with whom we are conversing. The light would be in the way. Gibson, it seems, is right. Boynton, it seems, is not.

23.2 The Inverted Retinal Image: Lessons from Prisms

The upper panel of Figure 23.3 conveys a fairly common understanding, historical and contemporary, of the implications of the inverted retinal image—that is, the up-down image reversal at the retina is preserved in the visual cortex[7] but the mental representation is (inexplicably) true to the object's actual orientation relative to the environment. The middle panel of Figure 23.3 communicates the consequence of an inversion prism that orients the retinal image and, perforce, the cortical representation congruent with the object's actual orientation but inverts the mental representation. The bottom panel resurrects our discussion in Lecture 17 of the "in-ness problem" (Figure 17.9). It shows the upshot of adapting to the inversion prism: The mental representation is now also congruent with the object's actual up–down orientation suggesting strongly that neither the inverse projection P1 nor the

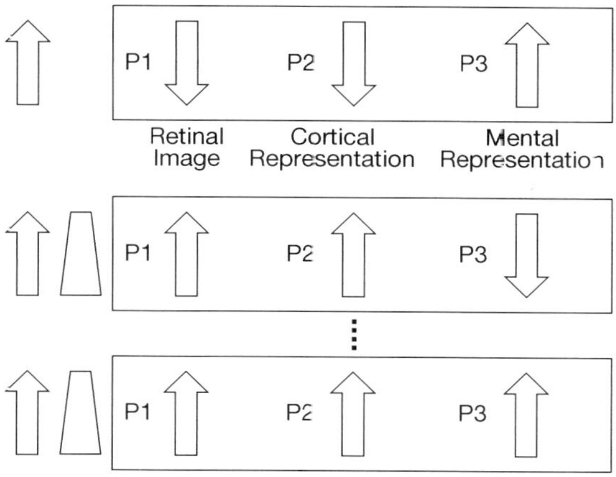

Figure 23.3 Assumption of inverted retinal image in the context of prism adaptation (see text for details).

insensate cortical projection P2, singly or in combination, determine the experiential projection P3 (Shaw & Mace, 2005). Returning to "perception" as opposed to the pedagogically convenient "mental representation," Figure 23.3 concurs with the thesis that the perception of the environmental object is not an effect that "pops out" at the end of a causal chain but rather an experience that longitudinally penetrates all three projections (Shaw & Mace, 2005). The thesis was encountered in its general form in, and given expression through, Figure 3.5. The mixed media of air and tissue are transparent to information about the environmental object.

In respect to generality, however, the conception of prism adaptation portrayed by Figure 23.3 is, in Dolezal's (1982, p. 227) words, "misguided, misleading and linguistically ambiguous." The phenomenon of prism adaptation is not, as the figure might be taken to imply, essentially a matter of retinal image inversion. To reiterate, perceiving things visually is a matter of perceiving how to get about among them, and what to do or not to do with them. *Prism adaptation must be considered in terms of the latter definition.*

What kinds of perceiving would a sighted animal need to meet the definition? The kinds are four in number (Shaw, 2001; Turvey & Fonseca, 2014). They are shown in Figure 23.4 for the particular case of a human climbing a rock face. They are the familiar exteroperceiving (roughly, perceiving the layout of surrounding surfaces) and proprioperceiving (roughly, perceiving the layout of one's body) and the less familiar pro-exteroperceiving (roughly, perceiving the layout of surrounding surfaces relative to the layout of one's body) (Lee, 1978, 1980) and ex-proprioperceiving (roughly, perceiving the layout of one's body relative to the layout of surrounding surfaces). The four kinds of perceiving can be schematized in the manner of Figure 23.5 (Shaw, 2001).

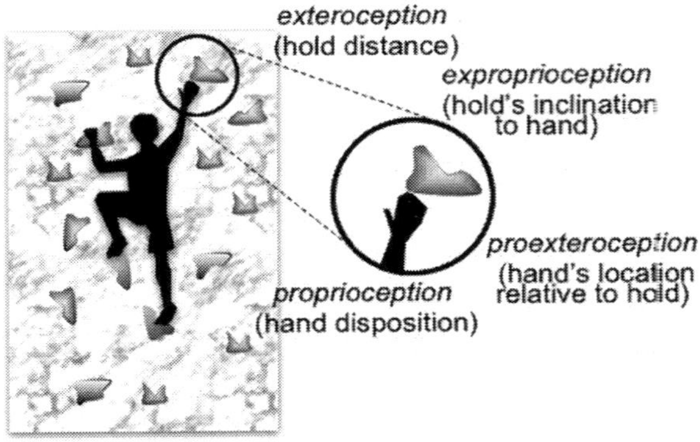

Figure 23.4 The four kinds of perceiving required for everyday perceiving shown in the uncommon context of scaling a rock face arrayed with holds for foot and hand.

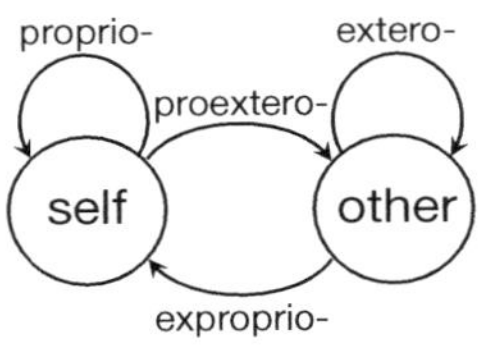

Figure 23.5 Schematic of the four kinds of perceiving.
(From Figure 6, Shaw, 2001, adapted with permission, *Ecological Psychology*.)

Each of the four kinds of visually perceiving is systematically affected by the wearing of prisms. As Dolezal (1982, p. 227) underscores, removing inverting prisms following five weeks of continuous use leads to "massive perceptual confusion" regarding (a) the layout of surrounding surfaces, their clutter, and their motions relative to the perceiver, and (b) the orientations of the perceiver's body segments relative to each other, and to the stationary and moving surroundings. The implication is that adapting to prisms is far more than a matter of the image inversion shown in Figure 23.3 (lower panel). It is a matter of adapting to the prism-induced transformations of the optical information that ordinarily makes possible (one more time with feeling) the getting about among things and doing what one does or does not do with them.

23.3 Preliminary Remarks on Ecological Optics

The seeming paradox of "light itself is not visible" introduced in Lecture 11 and revisited above (Section 23.1) is expressible conventionally and succinctly in the following contrast. Whereas physical optics is in terms of luminous bodies, radiation, and radiant light, ecological optics is in terms of illuminated bodies, illumination and ambient light (Gibson, 1979/1986).

Lecture 11 also introduced us to the illumination of a room by radiant light and the scatter reflection of this radiant light by the variously inclined surfaces of the room (Figures 11.6a and 11.6b, respectively). It also showed an arbitrary location in the room and the arrangement of reflected light that is specific to that location (Figure 11.6c). For any such arbitrary location there will always be a unique arrangement of reflected light specific to it (recall Lecture 21, Section 3). Figure 23.6a shows that same arbitrary location but this time occupied by a viewer. For the viewer, the structure of light at that location is intrinsically informative about the sources of its structure—the layout of the room relative to the viewer's current point of observation. Change that point, as in Figure 23.6b, and the four types of optical information transform systematically.

Although it may not be self-evident, it is the case that we are on the verge of engaging an idea about ambient light that stands in opposition to the historical view that has been the staple of most of the preceding lectures. We are beginning to consider the possibility that, at any vantage point, *the structure of light is intrinsically informative about the sources of its structure, and it is so whether it is time-invariant (observer and environment stationary) or time-variant (observer and/or environment nonstationary)*. The light available to organisms with eyes is not, as tradition would have it, intrinsically mechanical and extrinsically informative (e.g., Lecture 7, Figure 7.1). Gibson's intended understanding of the lines in Figure 23.6 should be noted:

> They are no longer beams of light shrunken to lines; they are boundaries between pencils of rays. They are no longer the paths of photons; they are relations. Hence they no longer represent energy but information.
>
> (Gibson, 1966, p. 193)

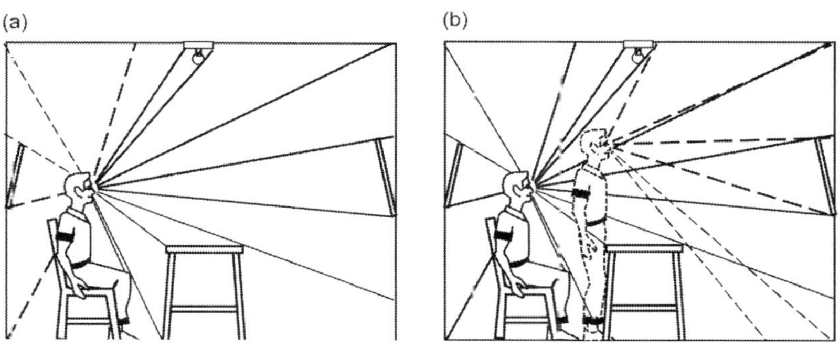

Figure 23.6 (a) Effective optic array (solid lines versus dotted lines) at a person's eye situated at a particular location, and (b) transformation of the optic array by standing up and stepping forward from a seated position.

(From Figures 10.5 and 10.6, Gibson, 1966, adapted with permission)

> The reason for the boundaries in the array is that the faces of the room reflect different amounts and colors of light to a convergent point. No two adjacent faces (or facets) will project the same intensity if they are at different angles of inclination to the source. Moreover, no two adjacent faces (or facets) will project the same intensity if they have a different composition or pigmentation, that is, a different reflectance
>
> (Gibson, 1966, pp. 193–194)

The angles in Figure 23.6 are plane angles. For a depiction of viewing in three-space (the natural circumstance) they would be solid angles—that is, their bases are 2D (areas) not 1D (points). As implied by the preceding quotations, the "lay of the land" for any given terrestrial organism will vary from place to place in elevation and material composition. For the limiting case of a stationary observer, there will be typically very many array boundaries, very many relations due to the nesting of ground regions of multiple sizes and inclinations. Capturing this fact pictorially with plane angles means very many lines. Parallel comments hold for three-space and solid angles, with the "lay of the land" expressed optically in terms of the faces and facets of optical solid angles and their boundaries. Very many boundaries mean very many lines in the depiction. For both the plane and solid angle depictions, the boundaries (i.e., the optical relations) arise from light structuring by surface layout, surface pigmentation, and surface illuminated-ness (see Lecture 11, Section 4).

We should not underestimate the boundaries. They articulate optical solid angles at multiple scales for multiple variations in layout, pigmentation, and illuminatedness. In ordinary, everyday circumstances they are indefinitely many, even for the limiting case of vision from a single station point at a single temporal moment in a frozen (stationary) environment. We are, once again, confronting Malebranche's bold question (Lecture 8, Section 8.1; Lecture 18, Section 5)—a problem that worsens, if that's possible,[8] for the mundane circumstance of time variation in both point of observation and surrounding environment (e.g., a dragonfly hunting in dense foliage on a breezy day, a person walking in a crowded mall or airport). The nested 2D areas of the multiply nested optic solid angles at each station point comprise a multifractal.[9] In the course of locomotion (by fin, wing or limb), this multifractal must transform globally and necessarily in ways specific to the style of locomotion and transform locally in ways specific to the ground and its clutter. Gibson (1966; 1979/1986) hypothesized that under these transformations particular optical variables of higher order would be invariant and specific to the four kinds of facts identified in Figures 23.4 and 23.5.

This preliminary encounter with the conception of information as *information about* is sufficient backdrop for expanding Gibson's foundational hypothesis, that visual perception is specific to optical information. The ecological information hypothesis has three implications.

1 *Incorrigibility*. Optical information is unalterable by psychological and neural factors. Said differently, psychological and neural factors are transparent to optical information. They engage optical information frankly, without pretense.
2 *Nonlocal causality*. Optical information is such that the systematicity of visual perception is coordinate with the systematicity of environment, body, and environment-body relations.
3 *Ontologized epistemology*. Taken together, implications (1) and (2) hold that visually based knowledge of environment, body, and environment–body relations, is grounded in, and acquired through, the specificity of optical information to environment, body, and environment-body relations.

23.4 On Illusions: The Fundamental Issue of Metric

Historically, the information hypothesis, particularly *incorrigibility*, is deemed untenable, primarily on the grounds of visual illusions. As the cornerstone of conventional perception theory, and a staple of academic courses on perception, the class of phenomena tagged as illusions exert a conceptual influence that is broad and persistent. A classical and well-worn instance is a straight stick partially immersed in water. It appears bent. Examining this classical instance will help us to appreciate how misperceptions are misconstrued within mediational (indirect) theories.

Conclusions drawn from bentness of a straight stick in water are typically of the following kind (Turvey et al., 1981). (a) It is an instance of perceptual error. (b) The central nervous system drew an incorrect inference from the play of light at the eyes, namely, that the stick was bent when in fact the stick was straight. (c) This error is a clear denial of direct perception because if perception were direct, then the stick should have been seen as straight, which it is, and not as bent, which it is not.

Hopefully, one's perspective at this stage of this series of lectures inclines one to find such conclusions highly questionable (even doltish). How ought a straight stick look immersed in water if it is really a straight stick? If it looked straight, then it is adamantly clear that perception is a source of deception and error because perception would be letting the straight stick appear as it ought not appear. Patently, a straight-stick-immersed-in-water must structure the light in a way that is true to the laws of light reflection. The differential in refractive indices between the media of air and water cannot be compromised. As clarified more than a century ago by Woodbridge (1913), *there is no intelligible sense in which it can be claimed that the stick ought to appear straight if perception were free of error and if perception were direct.*

Let's consider a different kind of misperception that has the added pedagogical benefits of involving a non-human perceiver and a non-visual perceptual system. Sharks electrically detect things to eat and things that impede locomotion (Kajiura & Fitzgerald, 2009; Kalmijn, 1974). A typical prey item, the flatfish, differs in ionic composition from the surrounding water, producing a bioelectric field partially modulated in the rhythm of the living thing's respiratory movements. A flatfish that has buried itself in the sand will be detectable by a nearby shark. Experiments that simulate the bioelectric field of the flatfish by passing a current between two electrodes buried in the sand reveal the same predatory behavior. The shark digs tenaciously at the source of the field departing from the site when the act fails to reveal an edible thing (Kalmijn, 1971).

Now there is no intelligible sense in which it can be claimed that the source ought to have appeared inedible if the shark's perception were free of error and if the shark's perception of a prey item was direct. In the niche of the shark a lawlike relation exists between an edible thing and an electric field of, say, type F*. To predicate of the shark, (a) "detects electric field of type F*" and (b) "takes to be an edible thing" is not to refer to two different states of affairs, one (namely (b)) that is reached from the other (namely (a)) by an inference. Rather, it is to make reference in two ways to a single state of affairs of the shark-niche system. The linking of (a) and (b) is not something that goes on in the "mind" of the shark, as theories of indirect, mediated perception would have it. The (a)–(b) linkage is in the physics of the ecological system given by the complementation of the shark and its niche.

The pointed question is what should be said of the shark's actions. Aren't they erroneous? Isn't the shark making a mistake? The source of the electric field proved, on investigation, to be an inedible thing. But given the nomic (law-like) relation between "electric field of type F*" and "edible," there is no intelligible sense in which it can be said that the shark's act of investigating the source of the field was wrong. Quite to the contrary, the wrong action for the shark, given its niche and its appetite, would be *not* investigating the source of F* (Turvey et al., 1981).

Attributing to the shark the misperception—the illusion—of perceiving a fish when there is no fish, is clearly a matter of false attribution. An illusion of a very different kind, and far more celebrated, is that experienced when humans and other animals[10] encounter Müller–Lyer figures. Two lines of equal extent are perceived to be unequal in the context of attached angles of different degrees. (The textbook example is Figure 23.7a.) The Müller–Lyer misperception is one of a family of geometric illusions that share in common a disparity between their dimensions as given by standard instruments (e.g., a ruler, a compass) and their dimensions as perceived. Lines that physical measurements reveal as straight, parallel, or intersecting when placed in the context of other lines may be seen as curved (Wundt–Herring illusion), non-parallel (Zollner illusion) or non-intersecting (Poggendorf illusion) (see Lecture 14, Figure 14.3). Is labeling each of these perceptions "illusions" analogous to the case with the shark, a matter of false attribution?

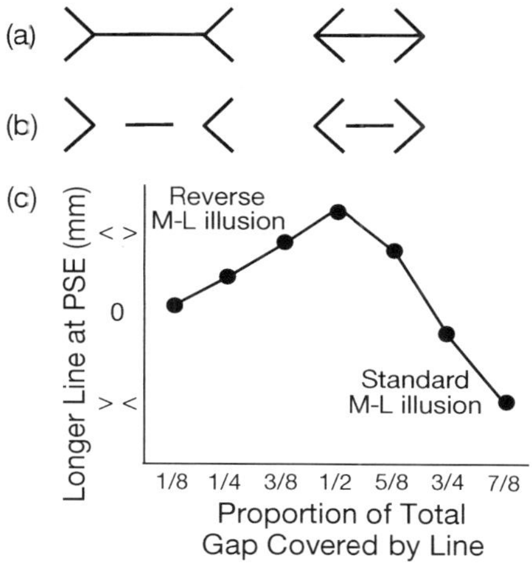

Figure 23.7 (a) Standard Müller–Lyer (M–L) illusion. (b) Reverse M–L illusion. (c) M–L illusion as a function of proportion of total gap covered by line. (PSE: point of subjective equality.)

(From Figure 2, B. J. Fellows, *Quarterly Journal of Experimental Psychology*, *19*, 208–214, 1967, APA, adapted with permission.)

23.4.1 Logic of "Illusion Ascription"

As is evident from the preceding discussion, the label "illusion" is employed when perception of X deviates consistently from the uniformly accepted physical measure of X. Given a mismatch between the psychological and the physical the historical tendency is to ascribe blame to the psychological. Given a measurement disagreement between a natural system, one that has evolved over 3.8 billion years to gauge multivarious (and possibly uncountable) attributes, and a recent human artifact (e.g., a ruler, a compass) that gauges but one attribute, error is attributed to the natural system. This starkly (and sardonically) drawn contrast between a natural system and an artifact inclines one to adopt Shaw and Cutting's (1980, p. 65) perspective on illusions: "There is no 'error,' only a difference to be explained."

A major surmise of Lecture 22 was that the relational quality *R* could be regarded as a new kind of primary quality. It will help to reiterate the details. First, situation X affords activity Y for organism Z on occasion O if and only if X and Z are mutually compatible on dimensions relevant to Y. Second, given satisfaction of the latter conditional, organism Z is afforded relation *R* in respect to situation X on occasion O if and only if Z interacts with X through the mutually compatible dimensions x_i in the course of implementing activity Y. Our goal in this subsection, as odd as it may seem, is to investigate the Müller–Lyer illusion in terms of *R*. We will ask the question of whether an organism's relation to extensions (e.g., a straight edge) is in terms of a metric independent of the organism, the real-number metric, or a metric dependent on the organism, a natural-number metric?

With respect to Figure 23.7a, let the arrow-type (< >) Müller–Lyer figure be X_A and the fin-type (> <) Müller–Lyer figure be X_F. And let the line segment that connects the arrows and the line segment that connects the fins be of equal length L as measured by a ruler. When measured by an organism, L of X_A is less than L of X_F. In using the ruler measure as benchmark one has assumed that Z deploys a real number basis—that is, Z deploys the full array of rational and irrational numbers as shown in Figure 23.8. All points on the number line, all possible distances on the number line, are measurable. An alternative assumption is that Z deploys a natural number basis—that is, the counting numbers or whole numbers when 0 is included. Whereas the geometry underpinning the real numbers is that of infinitesimally small points, the geometry underpinning the natural numbers is that of chords (lines of finite lengths, such as those given by joining any two points on the circumference of a circle). As highlighted in Lecture 9 (Section 3.1), measurement conducted in a chord space is only as precise as the tolerance provided by the shortest chord. It expresses the limited resolving power of natural measuring devices (Shaw & Cutting, 1980).

If perceptual systems are (as it were) natural number systems, then we should expect them to depart systematically from expectations founded on the assumption that they are real number systems. An implementation of pattern determination by computer in a natural number chord space, with chords of equal size, revealed that the endpoints of line segments, vertices, and intersections defined as the centers of chord distributions did not necessarily align with the end-point locations in real number Euclidean space. Specifically, centers of chord distributions were more inward for X_A and more outward for X_F, corresponding to their respective regions of greatest geometric complexity (Parker & Moore, 1972). In brief, in chord space, L of X_A was less than L of X_F.

In Shaw and Cutting's (1980) view, information about the length of the connecting line made available by a pattern's chord density is intrinsic—it is

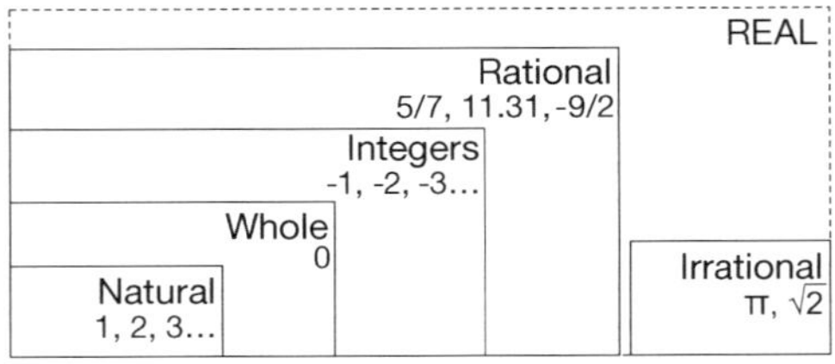

Figure 23.8 The real number system.

a function of the pattern's overall structure. It contrasts with the strictly local provision of information in the real number basis conventionally adopted for the Müller–Lyer figures. Shaw and Cutting's view dovetails with a formal issue in mathematics, that of whether the contrast between natural numbers and real numbers is the contrast between impredicative and predicative, respectively. As you might recall from Lectures 3 and 11 (Section 5), to define something "impredicatively" is to appeal to a totality that includes (or depends upon) the very thing that is to be defined. It is commonly claimed that the characterization of the natural numbers is impredicative (see George, 1987).

In summary, the point being made here by Shaw and Cutting is twofold. First, perception and standard physical measures will sometimes differ because they do not share a common basis of measurement. Perception is impredicative, standard physical measures are predicative. Second, perception of a thing *x* (e.g., —) in one context (e.g., > <) may differ, *on principle*, from its perception in another context (e.g., < >). The principled origin of the difference lies in the impredicative nature of thing-in-context.

Seemingly consonant with the foregoing thesis is the class of observations that define the *reverse Müller–Lyer illusion* (Fellows, 1967) shown in Figure 23.7. In respect to Figure 23.7(b)—the generalized Müller–Lyer display—whether $X_F > X_A$ or not depends on how much of the distance between the fins or arrows is covered by the line between them. If it is outside a particular range of values, then the Müller–Lyer effect is reversed: $X_F < X_A$ (see also Predebon, 1992; Stacy & Pike, 1970).[11] Figure 23.7(c) indicates that the usual Müller–Lyer effect decreases to zero as the line decreases to fill about 70% of the interfins space, and the "reverse" effect (i.e., line between arrows appearing longer) then increases until the line fills about half the interarrows space.

23.4.2 Illusion in the Perspective of Modern-Day Empiricism

At this juncture it would be good to review Lecture 10 (Section 10.6, "Space and its Geometries") and Lecture 12. The latter identified Helmholtz's highly influential thesis that, given current sensations, one sees the spatial properties *that would routinely cause them* (alias, the notion of unconscious inference to the best explanation). Modern-day empiricism (e.g., Howe & Purves, 2005; Purves & Lotto, 2003) has a means of quantifying "routinely." Natural scene geometry (i.e., absent human artifacts) is acquired with a laser range scanner. A database so accumulated allows for the determination of, among other things, the probabilities of everyday encounters with geometric analogues of Müller–Lyer figures. These natural statistics reveal a larger separation for environmental arrangements like X_F (that is, > <) than for environmental arrangements like X_A (that is, < >). They favor Helmholtz's hypothesis to the degree that natural scenes are routinely disposed to X_F. Figure 23.7c suggests, however, that the reverse Müller–Lyer illusion is on a par with the standard Müller–Lyer illusion. Natural scenes are likely inclusive of all variants of

Müller–Lyer figures meaning there is no necessary bias to see X_F arrangements as being wider in span than X_A arrangements.

That probability-based accounts of a perceptual capability will not be very general is underscored by Gilchrist (2006). Consider once again the ostensibly prosaic phenomenon of seeing things as black, grey or white—the innocuous act of perceiving the different degrees of reflectance of surrounding surfaces. The nature of the lightness enigma is that any luminance value of a surface is perceptible as any shade of gray (Lecture 11, Figure 11.8). For a given surface with a given luminance value, a consultation of memories of past encounters will not reveal a typical gray value.

23.4.3 The Ames Room (Its Mischief and Blessings)

Figure 23.9 identifies a very well-known experimental arrangement referred to as an Ames Room that is often taken to be prima facie evidence for (a) the non-specificity of perception, especially under conditions of motionless environment and/or motionless observer, and (b) perception necessarily as a matter of abduction, of inferring from effect to cause (e.g., Ittelson & Kilpatrick, 1961).

The room is constituted primarily by trapezoidal surfaces and viewed through a peephole in one of the walls. Collectively, the optical projection of the walls, floor and ceiling at the designated viewpoint is identical to the optical projection of the walls, floor and ceiling of a conventional rectangular room; the extraordinary Ames Room is perceived as ordinary, as rectangular. The compellingness of the effect is underscored by the viewer's perception of people in the room as either very small or very large depending on their standing location in the room, and by the changes in their sizes (e.g., from "dwarf" to "giant") as they walk or crawl from corner to corner (e.g., Wittreich, 1952/1961).

In the discourse on perception's nature, the Ames Room is promoted as, and taken to be, representative of visual encounters in general (e.g., Gregory,

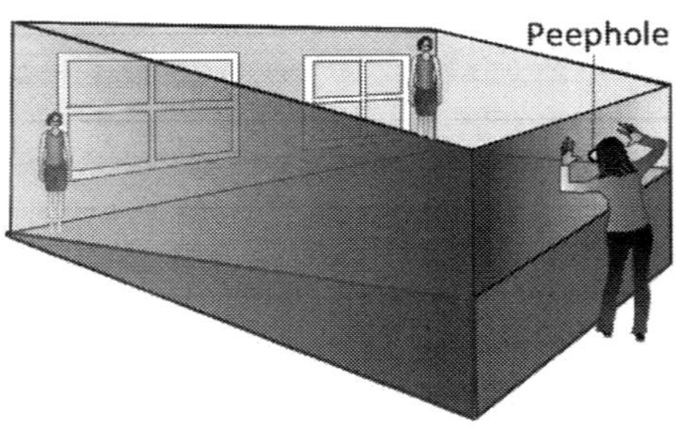

Figure 23.9 People standing inside an Ames Room appear very different in size to an observer at the designated viewpoint.

1978). It has caused much mischief both in the academic study of perception and the layperson's valuation of the fidelity of everyday perception. An important step to countering the mischief is full appreciation of the reasons that an Ames Room cannot occur naturally. As Runeson (1988) cautions:

> [O]nly those equivalent configurations that could actually be encountered present perceptual systems with ambiguity problems they have to deal with.
>
> (p. 298)

An argument can be given that, geometrically, an equivalent configuration such as an Ames Room of restricted size, furnishings, and surface texture, has only a 1 in 100 million chance of occurring randomly. Minus the restrictions, the odds are orders of magnitude smaller. Further, given that the material composing the room and its furnishings cannot be distributed arbitrarily—given gravity and the other laws of solid matter—any chance probability derived from geometric considerations alone is a gross overestimation. The preceding raises a question of considerable import: Are prevailing natural constraints (physical and ecological) of such a kind that they exclude arrangements of surfaces that are only equivalent to a normal room *in a geometric projective sense?* The question's import on the larger theoretical stage is in respect to the historical emphasis (well appreciated in the present course of lectures) on perception's modus operandi as determined by ambiguity rather than by specificity. If the question is answered positively, then perception's modus operandi is not determined by ambiguity; it is determined by specificity. Anomalously, given the original motivation, what the Ames Room inadvertently implies is that the optical structure made available to a single stationary point of observation is specific to the stationary environmental layout that gives rise to that optical structure (Runeson, 1988). This is the Room's primary blessing.

It should be emphasized that reaching this conclusion required invoking constraints beyond those of pure geometry. For Runseson (1988), this latter step is integral to the designating of Gibson's approach as "ecological." It should also be emphasized that the conclusion accords with the contention above that the structure of light (Gibson's optic array) is intrinsically informative about the sources of its structure (environment's material and geometric layout, one's body, one's point of observation), even in the minimal case of sources that are stationary.

23.4.4 *The Lee Room (Optical Information about a Pseudo-Force)*

Other rooms (but of lesser notoriety) are those of the kind introduced by Witkin and Wapner (1950a, b) and Lee and colleagues (Lee & Aaronson,

1974; Lee & Lishman, 1975; Lishman & Lee, 1973). The Lee Room is depicted in Figure 23.10. In its original form, a person stands or walks on an unmoving floor in a movable "room" comprising a ceiling, a wall to the front, and a wall on each side. The room can be swung backward and forward[12] relative to the person. For a person standing still, the optical change so produced is similar in kind to that when the person is moving backward and forward, respectively, about the ankles and/or hips in a stationary surround. When the foregoing room-displacement and optical change are implemented the person, with feet firmly planted on unmoving ground, loses balance, falling backward in the case of the room approaching and forward in the case of the room receding.[13] The backward case is depicted in Figure 23.10. How might this phenomenon be understood?

In the tradition of abduction, the person infers from the increase in the room's retinal image (an effect) that the room is approaching (a probable cause) or that she is leaning/falling forward (another probable cause). From the stationary signals of the vestibular system and muscle proprioceptors (effects), the person infers, to the contrary, that she is standing still (the most probable cause). She concludes that the room is approaching and commands the muscles to bring about a backward lean and/or step.

Shaw and Kinsella-Shaw (2007) offer a contrasting perspective on the phenomenon depicted in Figure 23.10. The destabilization is a consequence of an "optic push," not an inference. The phenomenon reflects a physical principle, not a mental directive. The physical principle is that of the 18th-century scholar D'Alembert. Basically, it is an alternative way of writing

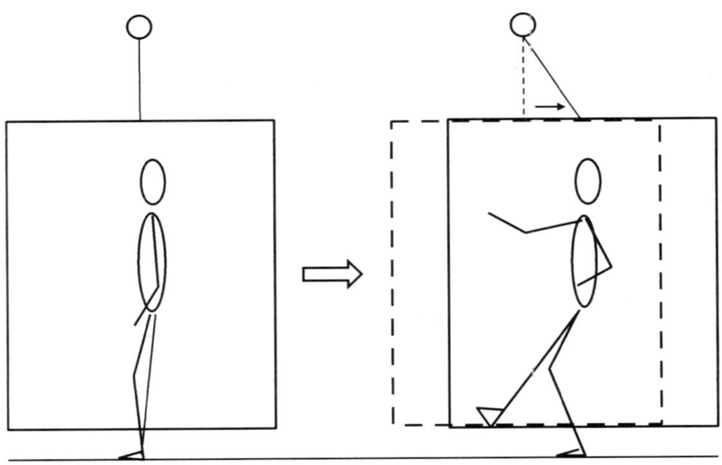

Figure 23.10 The Lee Room.

(From Figure 1, Shaw & Kinsella-Shaw, 2007, with permission, *Ecological Psychology*.)

Newton's 2nd Law. The formulation of inertial force F as equal to mass (m) × acceleration (a) is rewritten as F – ma = 0. The term –ma is then written as I, allowing that the law can be rewritten as F + I = 0—that is, as the zero sum of an inertial force F and a corresponding non-inertial or pseudo force I.

When the person is stationary in the stationary room (Figure 23.10, left), both person and room, physically speaking, are inertial reference frames. Each is in a state of zero rectilinear motion. A mean acceleration of zero would be registered by an accelerometer attached to the person and an accelerometer attached to the room. When the room is moved abruptly with respect to the stationary person (Figure 23.10, right), it does so under an inertial force F = Ma, where M is the mass of the room. Shaw and Kinsella-Shaw hypothesize that the consequent transformation of optical structure specific to the stationary person-in-room system is information about an abrupt change in the person's reference frame from inertial (stationary or uniform velocity) to non-inertial (accelerating). The transformation of the optic array specifies a fictional- or pseudo-force I, where I is incident to the acceleration of the non-inertial reference frame. Succinctly, an optical push is optical information specifying frame discrepancy. Such information is manifest whenever an abrupt change occurs that transforms an observer's inertial reference frame into a non-inertial (accelerating) reference frame (Shaw & Kinsella-Shaw, 2007). The behavior incurred by the push is intentional. It refers beyond itself to something else, namely, attaining upright posture in a detailed manner conditional on the specifics of losing upright posture. For Shaw and Kinsella-Shaw (2007), a chosen response is intentional not because it is chosen but, rather, *because it refers beyond itself.*

23.5 Rethinking the Necker Cube

Conventional visual perception theory has long been inspired by the phenomenon introduced to science by Necker (1832). When viewing a 2D rendition of a rhomboid frame resting on an edge (e.g., Figure 23.11a), one experiences a reversal with "the near becoming far and the far near" (Boring, 1942, p. 268). As is evident from viewing Figure 23.11a, the rhomboid is experienced as an object that vacillates in 3D. In Necker's opinion, the vacillation resulted from involuntary eye adjustments intended to sharpen vision. Wheatstone (1838/1964) contended that the vacillation was strictly a mental matter. Contemporary experiments with the commonplace Necker cube of Figure 23.11b suggest a dynamical coupling of the two hypothesized processes (Einhäuser, Martin, & König, 2004).

The interpretation offered by Wheatstone has been the historically dominant view. We will take it as our focus for the following reason: It is frequently promoted as prima facie evidence for the non-realist nature of perception (e.g., Gregory, 1978)—namely, that what one perceives is mind-dependent.

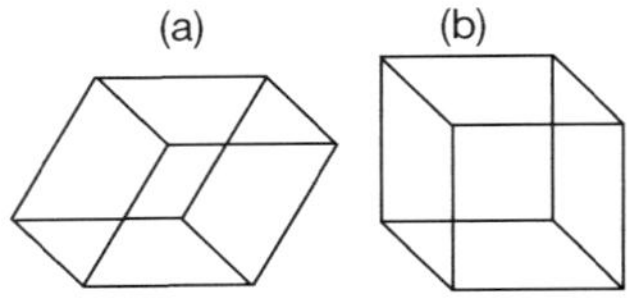

Figure 23.11 The Necker rhomboid and cube.

The "rhomboid" and "cube" in Figure 23.11 are projective mappings from 3D to 2D. Such mappings do not preserve the facts of a rhomboidal or cubical object's orientation. Absent these facts, one cannot make reliable distinctions of the kind (1) clockwise rotation versus counter-clockwise rotation, (2) nearer than versus further than, (3) left of versus right of, and (4) inside of versus outside of (cf. Shaw & Mace, 2005). The *orientability* lost in the 3D to 2D projection is a property intimately linked to *sidedness* as shown in Figure 23.12. Whereas a two-sided surface, depicted by (a), has an orientation (a nearer side and a farther side), the one-sided surfaces, depicted by (b) and (c), do not.

The general significance of the latter fact is in respect to the ecological basis of everyday optical structure (Gibson, 1979/1986). Surfaces are typically opaque and the encountered environment is typically cluttered (see Figures 21.2 and 23.1). With change in the point of observation (envisage such for the dragonfly of Figure 23.1), some previously occluded surfaces become visible and some previously visible surfaces become occluded (Figure 23.6). For any geometry advanced to express the optical information supporting everyday animal locomotion, the facts of occlusion and disocclusion, of deleting and accreting optical solid angles, must be foundational. Accordingly, two-sidedness is the minimal property any candidate geometry (projective or otherwise) must have in order to embrace fully the optical basis of perception by eye (Shaw & Mace, 2005).

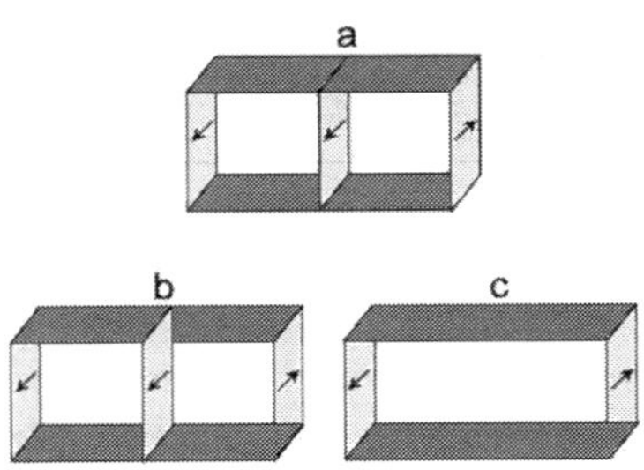

Figure 23.12 Orientability and sidedness: (a) A two-sided surface with orientability; (b and c) one-sided surfaces without orientability.

(From Figure 2.1, Shaw & Mace, 2005, adapted with permission.)

For present purposes, and by way of concluding the present lecture, the upshot of the preceding is that the Necker cube illusion is not an illusion. *It is a geometrically well-motivated perception.* Because the 2D Necker cube is one-sided the optical information about occlusion—what overlapping lines are nearer and what are farther—is necessarily ambiguous. Both orientations are specified. The empirical issue, simply put, is explaining the selection of one of two justified orientations (Shaw & Mace, 2005).

Notes

1 Note that it takes little effort to recognize that the definition applies to the basic orienting system, the auditory system, the haptic system, the haptic-somatic system, and the tasting and smelling system (Gibson, 1966).
2 Figure 20.2 is a sample of Animalia's 37 phyla (Margulis & Schwartz, 1982/1998). The ability includes crawling, walking, running, jumping, flying, gliding, swimming, sliding, burrowing, etc.
3 Arguably, the very human achievements of language, reasoning, and the like, are capabilities that could only arise once controlled bipedal locomotion was firmly in place (see also Brooks, 1991 and Lecture 17).
4 At this juncture retina and/or retinal have appeared in 9 of the preceding 22 lectures and image (in several uses) has appeared in 14 of the preceding 22 lectures.
5 In contemporary usage, "retinal image" as a question to the internet is answered by what should be termed "images of the retina." An example of the latter is Figure 23.3 (*top*).
6 If the eye is a camera, then one might ask whether the final image occurring at death is retained on the retina much like a photograph. The asking was done by Helmholtz's successor in 1871 as Professor at Heidelberg, Willy Kühne. Chemical fixatives could be used to preserve the retinal image for a brief period, a state referred to as an optogram. The latter appeared as a white image on a red or purple background. Unlike a photographic negative, the light and dark areas are not reversed. Kühne (1871) found the optogram to be unstable, fading quickly. It achieved notoriety in its potential use as evidence of the last person seen by a murder victim.
7 For the neuroanatomy, see, for example, Purves, Augustine, Fitzpatrick et al. (1999).
8 As we learned in Lecture 18, the stationary case for an easily countable number of environmental objects is already NP-complete.
9 A multifractal layout of surfaces is a generalization of a fractal system in which a single exponent (the fractal dimension, see Section 9.3.2) is not enough to describe it. A continuous spectrum of exponents (a singularity spectrum) is required.
10 To date, these other animals include fly (Geiger & Poggio, 1975), capuchin monkey (e.g., Suganuma, Pessoa, Monge-Fuentes, Castro & Tavares, 2007), Grey parrot (Pepperberg, Vicinay & Cavanaugh, 2008), and, in a collective nonvisual sense, ant (Sakiyama & Gunji, 2013). It is worthwhile noting that flies also respond to the "waterfall" illusion (Srinivasan & Dvorak, 1979), and that bees respond appositely to the contour illusion of Craik-O'Brien-Cornsweet (Davey, Srinivasan, & Maddess, 1998) and the color illusion of Benham (Srinivasan Lehrer, & Wehner, 1987).
11 Independently discovered by Yanagisawa (cited by Oyama, 1960).

12 The room is attached to a high ceiling by means of a long cable. The room's motion is essentially that of gliding back and forth.

13 A room oscillation as little as 6mm caused adults to sway approximately in-phase with the room. They behaved as if they were hooked to their surroundings unaware of the real cause of their disturbance.

References

Bentley, A. F. (1975). The fiction of "retinal image." In S. Ratner (Ed.), *Inquiry into inquiries: Essays in social theory*. Boston, MA: Beacon Press (original work published 1954).

Boring, E. G. (1942). *Sensation and perception in the history of experimental psychology*. New York: Appleton-Century-Crofts.

Boycott, B. B., & Dowling, G. E. (1969). Organization of the primate retina: light microscopy. *Philosophical Transactions of the Royal Society of London B, 255* (799), 109–184.

Boynton, R. (1974). The visual system: Environmental information. In E. C. Carterette & M. P. Friedman (Eds.), *Handbook of perception, Vol. 1, Historical and philosophical roots of perception* (pp. 285–307). New York: Academic Press.

Brooks, R. (1991). Intelligence without representation. *Artificial Intelligence, 47*, 139–159.

Campbell, J. (1817). On vision. *Annals of Philosophy, 10*, 17–29.

Davey, M. P., Srinivasan, M. V., & Maddess, T. (1998). The Craik-O'Brien-Cornsweet Illusion in Honeybees. *Naturwissenschaften, 85*, 73–75.

Dolezal, H. (1982). *Living in a world transformed*. New York: Academic Press.

Einhäuser, W., Martin, K. A., & König, P. (2004). Are switches in perception of the Necker cube related to eye position? *European Journal of Neuroscience, 20*, 2811–2818.

Fajen, B. R., & Matthis, J. S. (2011). Direct perception of action-scaled affordances: The shrinking gap problem. *Journal of Experimental Psychology: Human Perception and Performance, 37*, 1442–1457.

Fellows, B. J. (1967). Reversal of the Müller-Lyer illusion with changes in the length of the inter-fins line. *Quarterly Journal of Experimental Psychology, 19*, 208–214.

Geiger, G., & Poggio, T. (1975). The Müller-Lyer figure and the fly. *Science, 190*, 479–480.

George, A. (1987). The imprecision of impredicativity. *Mind*, 96, 514–518.

Gibson, J. J. (1966). *The senses considered as perceptual systems*. Boston, MA: Houghton Mifflin.

Gibson, J. J. (1986). *The ecological approach to visual perception*. Mahwah, NJ: Erlbaum Associates. (Original work published 1979)

Gilchrist, A. (2006). Seeing in black and white. *Scientific American Mind, 17*, 42–49.

Gregory, R. L. (1978). *Eye and brain: The psychology of seeing* (3rd ed.). New York: McGraw-Hill.

Harrison, H., Turvey, M.T., & Frank, T. (2016). Affordance-based perception-action dynamics: A model of visually guided braking. *Psychological Review, 123*, 305–323.

Helmholtz, von H. (2000). *Treatise on physiological optics, Vol. III* (J. P. C. Southall, Trans.). Bristol, UK: Thoemmes (original work published 1866).

Howe C. Q., & Purves, D. (2005) The Müller–Lyer illusion explained by the statistics of image-source relationships. *Proceedings of the National Academy of Sciences, 102*, 1234–1239.

Ittelson, W. H., & Kilpatrick, F. P. (1961). The monocular and binocular distorted rooms. In F. P. Kilpatrick (Ed.), *Explorations in transactional psychology* (pp. 154–173). New York: New York University Press.

Kajiura, S. M., & Fitzgerald, T. P. (2009). Response of juvenile scalloped hammerhead sharks to electric stimuli. *Zoology, 112*, 241–250.

Kalmijn, A. J. (1971). Electric sense of sharks and rays. *Journal of Experimental Biology, 55*, 371–383.

Kalmijn, A. J. (1974). The detection of electric fields from inanimate and animate sources other than electric organs. In H. Autrum (Ed.), *Handbook of sensory physiology, Vol. 3* (pp. 149–199). New York: Springer.

Kühne, W. (1871). Nerv- und Muskelfaser. In S. Stricker (Ed.), *Handbuch der Lehre von den Geweben* (pp. 147–169). Leipzig, Germany: Engelmann.

Lee, D. N. (1978). The functions of vision. In H. L. Pick & E. Saltzman (Eds.), *Modes of perceiving and processing information* (pp. 159–170). Hillsdale, NJ: Erlbaum.

Lee, D. N. (1980). The optic flow field: The foundation of vision. *Philosophical Transactions of the Royal Society of London, Series B, 290*, 169–178.

Lee, D. N., & Aronson, E. (1974). Visual proprioceptive control of standing in human infants. *Perception and Psychophysics, 15*, 529–532.

Lee, D. N., & Lishman, J.R. (1975). Visual proprioceptive control of stance. *Journal of Human Movement Studies, 1*, 87–95.

Lishman, J. R., & Lee, D. N. (1973). The autonomy of visual kinaesthesis. *Perception, 2*, 287–294.

Margulis, L., & Schwartz, K. V. (1998). *Five kingdoms*. New York: Freeman (original work published 1982).

Necker, L. A. (1832). Observations on some remarkable optical phaenomena seen in Switzerland; and on an optical phaenomenon which occurs on viewing a figure of a crystal or geometrical solid. *The London & Edinburgh Philosophical Magazine and Journal of Science, 1*, 329–337.

Oyama, T. (1960). Japanese studies on the so-called geometrical optical illusions. *Psychologia, 3*, 7–20.

Parker, D. J., & Moore, D. J. (1972). End points, complexity, and visual illusions. *IEEE Transactions on Systems, Man, and Cybernetics, 2*, 421–429.

Pepperberg, I. M., Vicinay, J., & Cavanaugh, P. (2008). Processing of the Müller-Lyer illusion by a Grey parrot (Psittacus erithacus). *Perception, 37*, 765–781.

Predebon, J. (1992). Framing effects and the reversed Müller-Lyer illusion. *Attention, Perception, & Psychophysics, 52*, 307–314.

Purves, D., Augustine, G. A., Fitzpatrick, D., & Hall, W. C. (2005). *Neurosciences* (Vol. 1). Brussels: De Boeck.

Purves, D., & Lotto, R. B. (2003). *Why we see what we do: An empirical theory of vision*. Sunderland, MA: Sinauer.

Runeson, S. (1988). The distorted room illusion, equivalent configurations, and the specificity of static optic arrays. *Journal of Experimental Psychology: Human Perception and Performance, 14*, 295–304.

Sakiyama T., & Gunji Y-P. (2013). The Müller–Lyer illusion in ant foraging. *PLoS ONE, 8(12)*: e81714.

Shaw, R. E. (2001). Processes, acts, and experiences: Three stances on the problem of intentionality. *Ecological Psychology*, *13*, 275–314.

Shaw, R. E., & Cutting, J. (1980). Biological constraints on linguistic form: Clues from an ecological theory of event perception. In U. Bellugi & M. Studdert-Kennedy (Eds.), *Signed and spoken language: Biological constraints on linguistic form* (pp. 57–84). Weinheim, Germany: Verlag Chemie.

Shaw, R. E., & Kinsella-Shaw, J. (2007). Could optical 'pushes' be inertial forces? A geometro-dynamical hypothesis. *Ecological Psychology*, *19*, 305–320.

Shaw, R. E., & Mace, W. M. (2005). The value of oriented geometry for ecological psychology and moving image art. In J. D. Anderson & B. F. Anderson (Eds.). *Moving image theory: Ecological considerations* (pp. 28–47). Carbondale: Southern Illinois University Press.

Srinivasan, M. V., & Dvorak, D. R. (1979). The waterfall illusion in an insect visual system. *Vision Research*, *19*, 1435–1437.

Srinivasan, M. V., Lehrer, M., & Wehner, R. (1987). Bees perceive illusory colours induced by movement. *Vision Research*, *27*, 1285–1289.

Stacye, B., & Pike, R. (1970). Apparent size, apparent depth and the Müller-Lyer illusion. *Perception & Psychophysics*, *7*, 125–128.

Suganuma, E., Pessoa, V. F., Monge-Fuentes, V., Castro, B. M., & Tavares, M. C. H. (2007). Perception of the Müller–Lyer illusion in capuchin monkeys (Cebus apella). *Behavioral Brain Research*, *182*, 67–72.

Turvey, M. T., & Fonseca, S. T. (2014). The medium of haptic perception: A tensegrity hypothesis. *Journal of Motor Behavior*, *46*, 143–189.

Turvey, M. T., Shaw, R. E., Reed, E. S., & Mace, W. M. (1981). Ecological laws of perceiving and acting: In reply to Fodor and Pylyshyn (1981). *Cognition*, *9*, 237–304.

Warren, W. H. (2009). How do animals get about by vision? Visually controlled locomotion and orientation after 50 years. *British Journal of Psychology*, *100*, 277–281.

Wheatstone, C. (1964). Some remarkable phenomena of binocular vision. In W. N. Dember (Ed.), *Visual perception: The nineteenth century* (pp. 114–129). New York: Wiley (original work published 1838).

Witkin, H. A., & Wapner, S. S. (1950a). Visual factors in the maintenance of upright posture, *American Journal of Psychology*, 63, 31–50.

Witkin, H.A., Wapner, S. S. (1950b). Large oscillating visual displays increase postural instability. *American Journal of Psychology*, 63, 385–392.

Wittreich, W. J. (1961). The Honi phenomenon: A case of selective perceptual distortion. In F. P. Kilpatrick (Ed.), *Explorations in transactional psychology* (pp. 188–202). New York: New York University Press (original work published 1952).

Woodbridge, F. J. (1913). The deception of the senses. *The Journal of Philosophy, Psychology and Scientific Methods*, *10*, 5–15.

Lecture 24

Perceiving "How to Get About Among Things"

In this lecture and the next, we focus on perception in terms of how to get about among things, and we do so in terms of principles common to all organisms. This focus stands in sharp contrast to the historical perspective on space perception/depth perception (Lectures 8–12) as (1) a mental process of interpreting or organizing sensations, and (2) exemplary of the outness problem (Lecture 9). A sentiment expressed by Gibson (1958) serves as a guide:

> If the theories of space perception do not provide an adequate explanation for the visual control of locomotion in animals, let us forget about the former and pay heed to the latter.
>
> (p. 182)

Unsurprisingly, the foundation for addressing this "how" question, whether it be in respect to vision or any other perceptual system, singly or in combination, is the primitive of functional/behavioral ecology: affordance. We can expand its functional/behavioral character as follows (after Turvey et al., 1981):

For all Six Kingdoms, *perception* must be reserved for designating only actual states of affairs: "Z perceives X-affording-*a*" where X is an environmental thing and *a* is an activity performable by Z. Perceiving X-affording-*a* presupposes a law, *L*: An ambient energy property *e* is nomically related to *a* in that it is unique and specific to *a* in Z's niche.

Given *L*, "Z perceives X-affording-*a*" designates an actual state of affairs if:

1 X-affording-*a* is present;
2 the *e* specific to 1 is available to Z;
3 Z detects the *e* defined in 2.

For any organism in any one of the Six Kingdoms, the incorrigible basis for perceiving any given affordance of its environment is the satisfaction of *L* and conditions 1–3.

24.1 "Getting About" by Members of Animalia and Plantae

The dragonfly of interest in Lecture 23 gets about among the things that comprise its surroundings on the basis of information about what things afford, be they fixed (e.g., thing *x* is a barrier to forward locomotion) or variable (e.g., thing *x* is land-on-able, thing *x* is fly-underneath-able). For each and every organism of the Six Kingdoms we can readily entertain the possibility of producing a functional equivalent of Figure 23.1. Consider a member (*Arabidopsis thaliana*) of the Kingdom Plantae. To garner water and nutrients, and to insure anchorage, a plant growing primarily downward must so act as to optimize the architecture of its root system. Doing so requires that a plant "get about among things" co-present in the soil of its habitat, such as rocks, the roots of other plants, and impenetrable soil (Blancaflor & Masson, 2003). It achieves the latter via sensitivity of its roots to gravity, moisture gradients, and barriers to directional growth. On confronting a horizontal barrier (as in Figure 24.1), a root does not buckle as would occur if downward growth persisted, but rather, upon contact, elongates in a direction parallel to the barrier with only its tip in contact with the barrier (Massa & Gilroy, 2003). The root cells behind the tip so organize as to transition collectively from growing parallel to gravity to growing perpendicular to gravity (see Telewski, 2006). On termination of contact with the barrier, root cells return to growing in alignment with gravity.

In both of the preceding examples, getting about among things entails an intimate relation between perception and action. Consider the dragonfly pursuing a mosquito (Turvey & Shaw, 1995). The mosquito's perceptible parameters qua target are direction-to-contact, time-to-contact, and distance-to-contact. The dragonfly's action parameters qua manner of approach to the target are torque-to-contact, impulse-to-contact, and work-to-contact, respectively. Mathematically speaking, the two distinct classes of parameters, those relating to perception and those relating to action, are duals that together form a duality (Shaw & Kinsella-Shaw, 1988). The Möbius band and the relation of cube and octahedron (Figure 24.2) are illuminating. In respect to

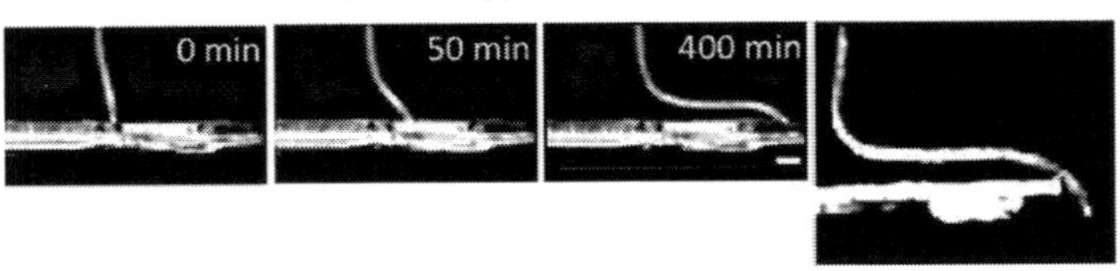

Figure 24.1 The directed root growth of *Arabidopsis thaliana* relative to a barrier. See text for details.

(From Figures 1 and 4, Massa & Gilroy, 2003, adapted with permission, Wiley.)

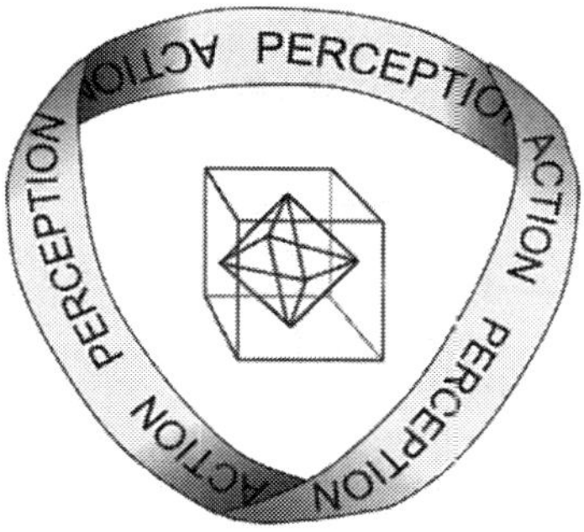

Figure 24.2 See text for details.
(Figure 1, Turvey, 2007, adapted with permission, Elsevier.)

cube and octahedron, although they are pictorially different, they are identical in respect to symmetry operations—intuitively, the ways one can do something to a thing so that having done them the thing looks the same as before. The symmetries of the cube are the symmetries of its dual, the octahedron. Cube and octahedron form a duality.

24.2 Ecological Action Mechanics?

The dragonfly of Lecture 23 (Figure 23.1) expresses the conjoint nature of perception and action: dual processes serving the mutual aim of satisfying a goal in reciprocal ways. The dragonfly's perceiving modulates its acts and its acts modulate its perceiving in a form of causality that is best expressed not as a cycle of separate events but as the co-occurring events of a temporal Möbius Band (Figure 24.2 (*outer*); cf. Turvey, 2007). We will entertain the conjecture of Shaw and Kinsella-Shaw (1988) that this goal-directed behavior of the dragonfly (and of organisms in general) is a kind of action mechanics to be considered on a par ontologically with the action mechanics tied to the speed of light and the action mechanics tied to quanta. This conjecture allows us to catch a further glimpse of what it will mean to comprehend perception as lawful. Figure 24.3 is a necessary pictorial aid to taking that step. It expresses the conceptual charge of formulating at the ecological scale equations of (a) energy conversion and (b) energy distribution. For (a) the challenge is to rescale downwards Einstein's energy conversion equation $E = mc^2$ (where E is energy, m is mass, and c is the speed of light). For (b) the challenge is to rescale upwards Planck's energy distribution equation $E = fh$ (where f is frequency and h is a constant). As they stand, neither (a) nor (b) is suited to the in-between ecological scale. At this in-between ecological scale the analogue of energy conversion cannot be an uncontrolled burst and the analogue of quantum distribution cannot be a random process. In rough and ready terms, Ω_{goal} in

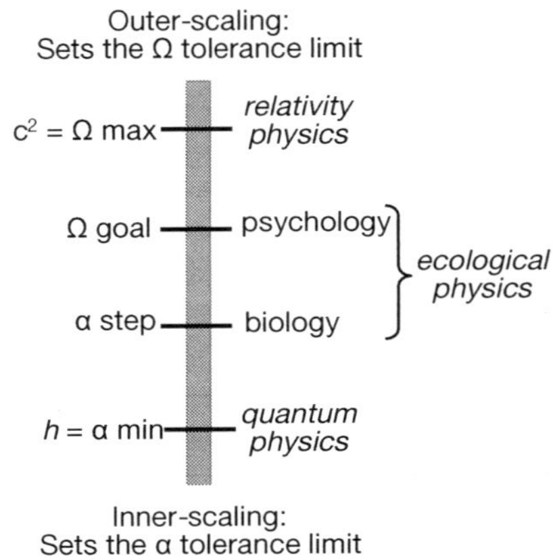

Figure 24.3 The outer and inner scales of an ecological physics. See text for details. (From Figure 1, Shaw & Kinsella-Shaw, 1988, adapted with permission, Elsevier.)

Figure 24.3 is a limit on the controlled conversion of an amount of potential energy (a unit quantity of biomass) into the requisite kinetic energy for achieving a goal. And similarly, in rough and ready terms, the quantity α_{step} is the minimal quantity of metabolic energy needed to move one functionally defined "step" closer to the goal. However Ω_{goal} and α_{step} might be understood eventually, they must necessarily be related to intention and to information about the surrounding states of affairs. "Information about" is our next concern.

24.3 The Optical Basis for Getting About Among Things

As implied by preceding remarks, the function of vision is predominantly in the service of activity, specifically, in the service of getting about (e.g., Gibson, 1966, 1979/1986; Harrison, Turvey & Frank, 2016; Fajen, 2007, 2013; Lee, 1974, 1978, 1980; Warren, 1990, 1998, 2006; Warren, Young & Lee, 1986). The optical basis for this visual service is ecological optics, a point that has been made on several occasions in the preceding lectures. A charge of the present lecture is to elaborate on this point.

24.3.1 Physical Optics, Physiological Optics, Ecological Optics

Merriam-Webster defines optics as the science that studies light and the way it affects and is affected by other things. It defines *physical optics* as a branch of optics that deals with the description and explanation of all optical phenomena in terms of physical theories, namely, wave or undulatory theory, electromagnetic phenomena, or quantum mechanics. Helmholtz (recall

Lectures 10 and 11) introduced the label *physiological optics* for the study of the nervous system's modes of responding to light impressed upon the eye—how light affects the physiology of an animal's visual system. The contemporary journal *Optometry and Vision Science* elaborated physiological optics in these terms: "basic and applied elements of vision research such as adaptive optics and eye dynamics, ocular aberrations and corrections, intraocular scattering, retinal image quality, cornea and lens biomechanics and optics, retina and photoreceptor optics" (Adams, 2012).

In line with the *Merriam-Webster* definition of optics, *ecological optics* is the study of how light is affected by other things. Unsurprisingly, given preceding lectures, these other things are not instances of classically defined primary and secondary qualities, and they are not properties of the visual system's anatomy and physiology. Rather, they are constituents of habitat and niche (the where and how, respectively, of an organism's everyday living) and they are the time-dependent and time-independent relations of organisms to habitat and niche. These other things, and the ways that they affect light, were presaged in Lecture 23. Ecological optics aims to articulate light's extero-, proprio-, expropriо- and proextero-specificity in formal terms. It is an enterprise directed at the nature and status of ambient optical distributions prior to living things and, perforce, independent of the stimulation of receptors (see Gibson 1979/1986; Johansson, 1985; Kugler & Turvey1987; Pepping & Grealy, 2007; Reed 1996; Runeson & Frykholm 1983; Stoffregen & Bardy, 2001). It is an enterprise directed at informationL for vision (as introduced in Lecture 3). In engaging this enterprise, it helps to recall the fact of light's invisibility (Lecture 11, Section 4). The optical basis for visual perception is structured light distributions incident to illuminated surfaces, not light as radiating from a point source.

24.3.2 Optic Flow

Our examination of the Ames Room in Lecture 23 led to the conclusion that the optical structure at a single stationary point of observation is specific to the stationary environmental layout that gives rise to that optical structure. Here we now seek to establish that the transformations of optical structure at a moving point of observation are specific to the environmental layout and to the particular motions of the point of observation. As a first approximation, we seek properties of an optic flow field that inform (a) about the layout of surrounding surfaces relative to an organism, and (b) about an organism's movements relative to the surrounding surfaces. The ultimate goal is properties of the optic flow field that inform about what the surrounding surfaces *afford*—that is, *what they mean for getting about*. Perception as direct dictates that, for an organism to meet the challenges of controlling and coordinating behavior with respect to the surroundings, such optic flow properties must be body- and action-scaled. It also dictates that the optic flow properties must be such as to specify trajectories in terms of "points" in space-time (Lee, 1980). Interceptive behavior in predating or playing (e.g., soccer, tennis) requires being at the right place at the right time. The apposite wording of this conception is Minkowski's, as given in his address in 1908 to the 80th Assembly of German Natural Scientists and Physicians, albeit expressed in a different context (Relativity Theory): "Henceforth space by itself, and time by itself, are doomed to fade away into mere shadows, and only a kind of union of the two will preserve an independent reality."

Figure 24.4 is Lee's (1980) barebones schematic of how rectilinear movement of an organism's point of observation relative to the surroundings generates an optic flow field. Figure 24.4a is a view from the side. Figure 24.4b is a frontal view. For mathematical simplicity, Lee considers a schematic eye—with nodal point O at a height *H* above the ground plane—to be stationary and the environment approaching with velocity *V* in the direction Z to O. Two texture elements *P* and G on surfaces in the environment are identified, G being on the ground surface. Light reflected from *P* and G passes through O giving rise to the moving optic texture elements *P*′ and G′. In the general case, a densely textured environment gives rise to a densely textured optic

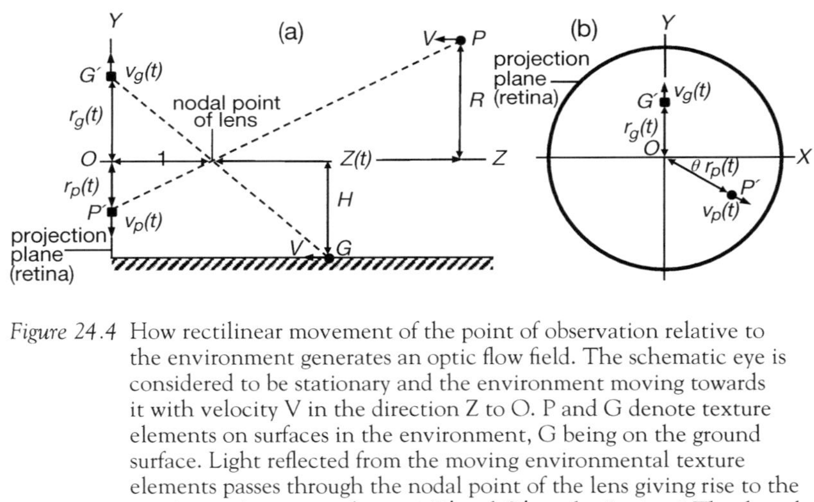

Figure 24.4 How rectilinear movement of the point of observation relative to the environment generates an optic flow field. The schematic eye is considered to be stationary and the environment moving towards it with velocity V in the direction Z to O. P and G denote texture elements on surfaces in the environment, G being on the ground surface. Light reflected from the moving environmental texture elements passes through the nodal point of the lens giving rise to the moving optic texture elements P′ and G′ on the "retina." The densely textured environment gives rise to a densely textured optic flow field wherein all optic texture elements move outwards along radial flow lines emanating from O. How the optic flow field affords information about the environment and about an animal's movement relative to it is explained in the text.

(Adapted from Figure 1, D. N. Lee, The optic flow field: The foundation of vision. *Philosophical Transactions of the Royal Society of London, Series B*, 290, 169–178, 1980. Permission conveyed through Copyright Clearance Center.)

flow field wherein all optic texture elements move outwards along radial flow lines emanating from O.

As will become evident, this simple figure provides enlightenment about a problem that bedeviled the disquisition on space perception encountered in several of the preceding lectures. If the projection plane of Figure 24.4a is interpreted as an image (as a time-independent 2D spatial structure), then the position of an optic texture element, for example, P', relates to the 2D direction *but not the 3D distance* of the environmental texture element P. In the terms of Figure 24.4a, P may be defined relative to the eye by the distance coordinates $Z(t)$ and R together with the angle between the OZP and OZX planes. This angle is given in the optic flow field by the angular coordinate θ of the optic texture element P'. The distance coordinates $Z(t)$ and R, however, are not given optically; from similar triangles in Figure 24.4a:

$$Z(t)/R = 1/r_p(t). \tag{24.1}$$

Wherein lies the missing so-called "depth" dimension? The answer is in the spatio-temporal structure (Gibson, 1966, 1979/1986; Lee, 1980). Differentiating $Z(t)/R = 1/r_p(t)$ with respect to time yields:

$$R/V = r_p(t)^2/v_r(t), \tag{24.2}$$

where V is velocity given by $-dZ(t)/dt$. Eliminating R between Equations 24.1 and 24.2 yields

$$Z(t)/V = r_p(t)/v_r(t). \tag{24.3}$$

That is, the distance coordinates of particular texture elements are optically specified within a scale factor of V. For all visible texture elements in Figure 24.4, the right-hand sides are expressed as $r(t)^2/v(t)$ and $r(t)/v(t)$.

Equations 24.2 and 24.3 are of special value. First, they encrypt information about the relative sizes, distances, and orientations of the surrounding surfaces. Given an appropriate scaling factor, they yield information about an individual organism's surroundings *in terms of the individual organism's size*. Second, they presage understanding of how the relation of an organism to its surroundings can be in terms of the times that getting about in its surroundings will entail if current circumstances persist. In respect to Figure 24.4, $Z(t)/V$ is the time that will elapse for a given V before the point of observation is level with the surface texture element P.[1] Equation 24.3 states that this time, designated τ (or tau) is optically specified by the value of $r(t)/v(t)$. Figure 24.5 elaborates the τ variable. Of special note is the *field of τ values* generated in the act of standing up, and hence moving one's point of observation forward, from a seated position in an object-cluttered enclosure.

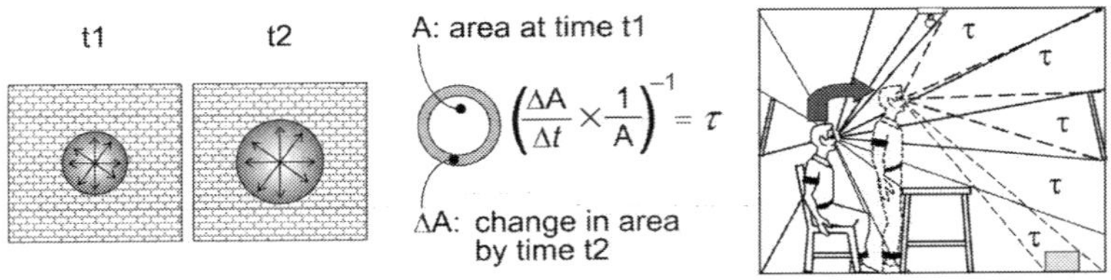

Figure 24.5 The time-to-contact variable. (*Left*) An approaching object generates optical expansion. (*Middle*) How the tau variable (τ) is constructed (Δ stands for change). (*Right*) Standing up from a chair generates a field of τs.

(From Figure 10.6, Gibson, 1966, adapted with permission.)

Taken together, the preceding figures and equations reveal how the optic flow field can be informative about the relative distances, sizes, and orientations of surfaces and objects comprising an organism's surroundings and the times at which contact with them will occur if current conditions persist. We are catching glimpses of the optical foundation for the dragonfly's ability to get about among things. As already alluded to, it must be the case that at any point in its pursuit, an intimate connection holds between seeing direction to contact and seeing torque to contact, and likewise between seeing distance to contact and seeing work to contact (Turvey & Shaw, 1995). Information

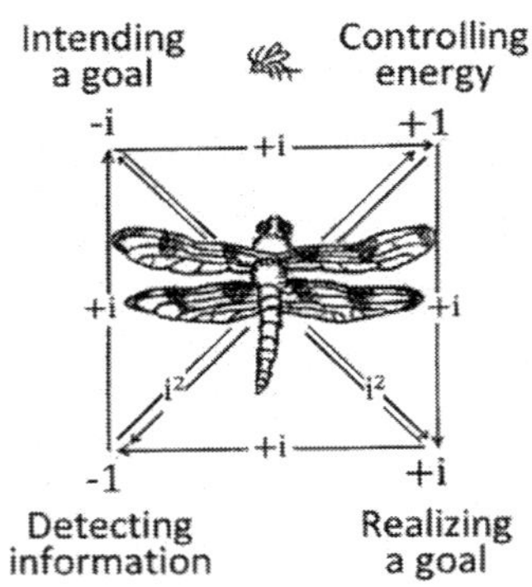

Figure 24.6 The persistence of an intention ("catch that mosquito") over variations in information detection, energy dissipation, and proximity to the "catch"—together with the coherent fitting together of these variations—invites a mathematical group structure analysis. The depicted group is a cyclic group with its four operations linked by the flow operator *i*.

(From Figure 11.3, Turvey & Shaw, 1995, Toward an ecological physics and a physical psychology. In Solso & Massaro (Eds.), *The science of the mind: 2001 and beyond*. Adapted with permission of Oxford University Press, USA.)

that is detected is related to energy that is controlled, but how? It is certainly not in terms of a simple linear chain, first seeing, then doing. In the familiar image of the hunting dragonfly, Figure 24.6 expresses the idea that, in the abstract, the information–energy relation is likely to be in the form of a symmetry group.[2]

24.3.3 Optic Deformation

The base conceptions behind the preceding development of the optic flow field are environment loci, their inclinations to and distances from the observer, and the rates of change in those inclinations and distances. An alternative conception is in terms of kinds of transformations at both global and local scales (e.g., Koenderink, 1986). Figure 24.7 is a depiction of the cardinal forms of these transformations referred to mathematically as divergence, curl, and deformation. Figure 24.8 is a depiction of how the aforementioned transformations apply in respect to a point of observation relative to a stationary layout

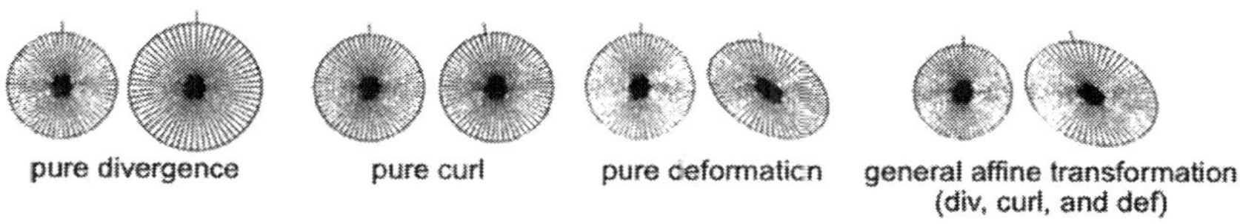

Figure 24.7 Divergence, curl and deformation.
(From Figure 3, Koenderink, 1986, adapted with permission, Elsevier.)

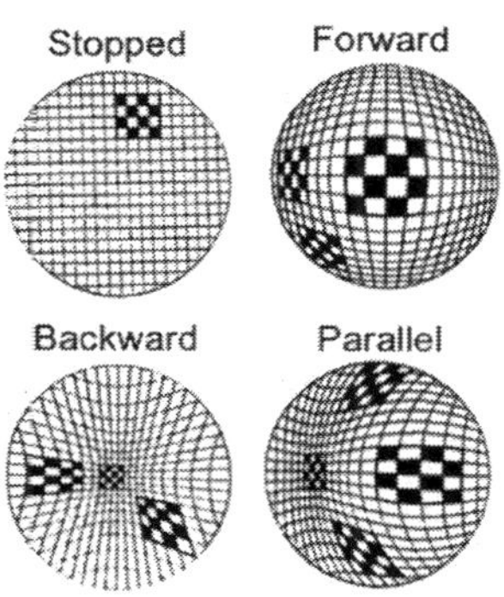

Figure 24.8 Divergence, curl and deformation. The optical deformations due to a translation with respect to a plane surface covered by a grid. (*Left to right*) No movement of point of observation; movement perpendicular toward the plane; perpendicular movement away from the plane; rightward translation parallel to the plane.

(From Figure 5, Koenderink, 1986, adapted with permission, Elsevier).

of environmental surfaces. The point of observation is shown for when it is stationary relative to the layout, when it is moving forward and moving backward relative to the layout, and when it is moving parallel to the layout.

24.3.4 A *Global Array?*

The seemingly obvious thesis that perception is of five types (seeing, hearing, tasting, smelling, and touching) corresponding to five types of energy distributions (optical, acoustical, liquid-borne chemical, air-borne chemical, and mechanical) can be questioned. Stoffregen and Bardy (2001), for example, argue that rather than a unique relation between (a) each energy distribution kind and (b) the affordances of and the behaviors of an organism in its niche, there is a redundancy of specificity, both within any particular energy array and across energy arrays. That is, specification—and hence direct perception—is a fact of the global array, of higher-order relations defined across the different energy forms.

24.4 Specification of What *Will* Occur versus Expectation of What *Might* Occur

It is to our disadvantage to attempt further progress on the topic of optical specification without an acquaintance with history's long-standing perspective on how visually endowed organisms in general accommodate their actions to up-coming circumstances. We can do so through the influential Russian physiologist, Nicolai Bernstein (1967; see Kim & Turvey, 1998).

Unlike his contemporaries, Bernstein's physiology was a physiology of activity, not a physiology of reaction (as prominently represented in the reflex conditioning work of his internationally famous compatriot, Ivan Pavlov). In Bernstein's view, the pertinent issues are those implicated in our earlier (Lecture 23, Figure 23.1) and current depiction of the foraging dragonfly—namely, solving by activity the multiple ever-changing problems posed by niche and habitat. As Bernstein saw matters, the dragonfly and its environment are in a never-ending game. In his words (Bernstein, 1967): "a game where the rules are not defined and the moves planned by the opponent are not known" (p. 173).

In this continuous game, the dragonfly (and the individual organism in general) is not reacting to, not responding reflexively to, the environment and other players. Stated more broadly, the surroundings with respect to which organisms behave are not to be understood as collections of so many triggering stimuli, and the behaving organisms are not to be understood as collections of so many conditioned and unconditioned reflexes. Rather than simply reacting to triggering stimuli, organisms cleverly exploit the information about their surroundings and their movements to control their actions both retrospectively ("after the fact") and prospectively ("before the fact").

In retrospective control, adjustments are made in respect to what has occurred; in prospective control, adjustments are made in respect to what will occur (if current conditions persist).

There are many situations encountered in daily activity for which retrospective control is infeasible. The class of so-called ballistic movements is only controllable prospectively: Throwing at a target, jumping a brink or a barrier, hammering a nail, and so on. Similarly, requiring of prospective control are "movements that forestall others" (Bernstein, 1967, p. 141) such as the predator moving to an extrapolated point in the prey's trajectory and the perceptually analogous achievements of catching a moving object with a hand, passing a ball to a running teammate in basketball or soccer, intercepting the ball with a striking implement in tennis or baseball or cricket, and so on. The following is an apt summary of Bernstein's (1967) stance:

> Each significant act is a solution (or an attempt at one) of a specific problem of action. But the problem of action, in other words the effect which the organism is striving to achieve, is a something which is not yet, but which is due to be brought about. *The problem of action, thus, is the reflection or model of future requirements* (somehow coded in the brain); and a vitally useful or significant action cannot be either programmed or accomplished if the brain has not created a prerequisite directive in the form of the future requirements that we have just mentioned.
>
> (Bernstein, 1967, p. 171, italics added)

Whereas Bernstein saw that retrospective control could be conceptualized through the cybernetic trio of set points, feedback, and corrective signals, he envisaged that conceptualizing prospective control required speculation on the forms of extrapolation by which the future could be anticipated or modeled given present and past conditions. As we will come to appreciate (and, ideally, have already come to appreciate), there are serious limitations, however, to extrapolation as the basis for prospective control.

24.4.1 Modeling the Future and the Problem of Induction[3]

Any form of extrapolation to future states is an induction—that is, it is the determination of some general proposition based on instances.[4] In the prospective control of action, the kinds of general propositions to be reached by induction are of the form "If I keep doing what I am doing, then so-and-so will occur" and "If that thing keeps doing what it is doing, then so-and-so will occur." In formal terms, induction seeks to establish $(\forall x)P(x)$ (in words, "for all x, or for any x, or for every x, x has the property P; $P(x)$ is true") on the basis of particular instances of the set X for which x_i having the property P is known (Rosen, 1991). If the subset of X that is experienced is S, then given the knowledge $(\forall s)P(s)$, do we then have the knowledge that

$(\forall x)P(x)$? It has long been respected that the answer in the general case is "no." With respect to any arbitrary chosen property P, no sample entails anything about an unsampled instance, defining, thereby, the *problem of induction* (e.g., Goodman, 1965) that we encountered in Lecture 4.

The problem of induction can be resolved if the sampled property P manifests a property called *contagion*[5] that is, if the truth of $P(x_i)$ implies the truth of $P(x_j)$ for some other x_js in X. If the sampled property is embodied with a contagious property, induction can be carried out with the value of P with the first element of the set X, $P(1)$, and a rule which embodies an entailment relationship between the value $P(n)$ and its successor $P(n+1)$. A series whose value at n, $P(n)$, entails the next value $P(n+1)$ is called recursive. If a series is recursive, then extrapolation of the entire series from a sample is just a matter of a simple mechanical operation. Hence, through recursion the future can be extrapolated given the knowledge of the present. In mathematics, a device for doing precisely this has been known for some time—Taylor's Theorem, a "magical" device that converts synchrony (what happens at an instant) into diachrony (what happens over a series of instants) (Rosen, 1991, p. 78). Specifically, the conversion of the present to the future is accomplished in Taylor's Theorem through derivatives. Derivatives contain information about the future as well as the past (Rosen, 1991).

Despite the favorable property of contagion, it is nonetheless the case that recursion *tout court* is an unsatisfactory solution to the general problem of modeling the future. Although recursion ensures the entailment relationship between two values at two successive instants of a given series, the initial value out of which a series is generated is completely independent of the recursive rules of the series. Depending on which initial value is chosen, a completely different outcome of a series is obtained. Moreover, the choice of initial value is completely arbitrary. For a mechanical particle on a trajectory solely determined by the force acting upon it, an entailment between two successive states assures a complete description of its behavior. However, as the amount of force varies, the path traveled by the particle similarly varies. At every instant there would be infinitely many different trajectories the particle can traverse given that the range of force values can be infinite. Members of the Six Kingdoms, on the other hand, are capable, in greater and lesser degrees, of aiming themselves toward a target by authoring their own initial conditions (Shaw & Kinsella-Shaw, 1988). This ability to select a path in respect to future goal states is a hallmark of living things. It is why we call them "goal-directed" respectful of the fact that the kinds of goals and the degree of directedness vary with phylum.

Indeed, the recognition that biological movements are goal-directed rather than simple reactions to the environmental stimulus was the rationale behind Bernstein's call for the physiology of activity rather than the physiology of reactions. Specifically, goal-directed movements are movements that are directed to "what must be done" as opposed to reactions that signal "what is"

(Bernstein, 1967, p. 147). To address this problem, Bernstein (1967, p. 161) had to resort to probabilistic extrapolation as the basis for modeling the future. It is highly questionable, however, whether probability estimates based on past experiences can provide sufficient constraint for the prospective control of movements. Patently, experience with a given situation and its contingent events can lead to an expectation of what is likely to occur when the situation reoccurs and such expectations must shape, to an important degree, the selection and conduct of actions. But an *expectation of what might occur* is not the same as *specification of what will occur* and it is the latter that is necessary for the successful prospective control of everyday, commonplace actions in the Six Kingdoms. In the case of a human driving a car, given a stop sign at the junction of two roads, one expects on the basis of very particular experiences that the likely action of approaching cars or trucks will be a slowing, and eventual arresting, of forward motion. Executing the activity of bringing the car to a halt at the stop sign, however, requires specification of the appropriateness of the current deceleration forces brought about by the drivers of their respective vehicles. We ought to suspect that such specification is much more deep-seated and universal. It is grounded in aspects more fundamental than the individual experiences that constitute the basis of probabilistic extrapolation (Kim & Turvey, 1998). A reasonable conjecture is that it is grounded in the lawfulness of optical flow or optical deformation incident to a moving point of observation as briefly considered in Sections 24.1.2 and 24.1.3 (see Harrison, Turvey & Frank, 2016).

24.4.2 The Current Future

The concept of the current future (see Bootsma in Lee, Bootsma, Frost et al., 2009) defines the inquiry initiated by Lee and instantiated in τ and its extensions.[6] The inquiry has been in respect to information about "what leads to what." In terms of the current future, it is *that which will happen if things do not change*.

Consider that which must be done to catch a fly ball in the games of baseball and cricket. How does an outfielder know where to run to make the catch and when to be at the spot where the catch can be made? The outfielder's problem is resolved by abiding a simple behavioral injunction: Synchronize with the ball's optical acceleration and so move as to keep it constant (e.g., Chapman 1968; Fink, Foo, & Warren, 2009; Michaels & Oudejans, 1992). To elaborate, the outfielder steers to the right place to arrive at the right time by a continuous linkage of his or her locomotion to a variable (namely, optical acceleration) of a closed contour in the optic array. The defining experiment (Fink et al., 2009) is distinguished by its manipulation of the ball's trajectory, from parabolic to linear.[7] The "outfielders" in the experiment succeeded in being at the right place at the right time to catch a virtual baseball on a virtual trajectory whether the trajectory was (a) parabolic throughout or (b) parabolic up to the zenith and then linear, with the (a) and (b) trajectories terminating at the same ground plane coordinates (Figure 24.9). The "outfielders" made successful virtual catches by so moving as to keep the rate of the ball's optical expansion constant.

A closely related but more commonplace skill is that of achieving non-injurious contact with the surroundings. Birds alighting on a branch, for example, insure soft contact (minimal momentum exchange) by so moving as to keep the rate of optical expansion of the approached branch at zero (Lee et al., 1992). The solution to the generic problem of visually controlled collisions (e.g., a human catching a ball, a bird landing gently on a branch) is the equating of prospective control with the future that is optically specified at the current agent–environment relation. A change in that relation is a change in the current future.

Prospective control in any case of purposeful movement is realized in General Tau Theory (Lee, 1998, 2009) as the closing of so-called action gaps—the separations between the current states and end states of movement degrees of freedom needed to achieve the action. Figure 24.10 illustrates the kinds of action gaps comprising the case of running over a surface with uneven footing. In each aspect to be controlled—gaze, step distance, and propulsive force—the metric of control is in terms of τ. An unresolved issue inherent to the circumstances depicted in Figure 24.10 and circumstances of like kind is

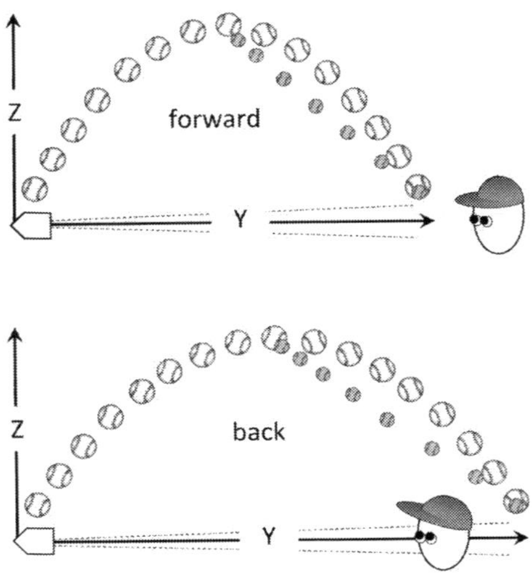

Figure 24.9 Experimental conditions in Fink et al. (2009). Whether the trajectory of the ball was parabolic throughout or linear after the zenith (small baseballs), its landing coordinates were the same: (*top*) 4m in front or (*bottom*) 4m behind the outfielder's starting location (and 4m to the left or right, shown by the dashed lines). Distances are not to scale.

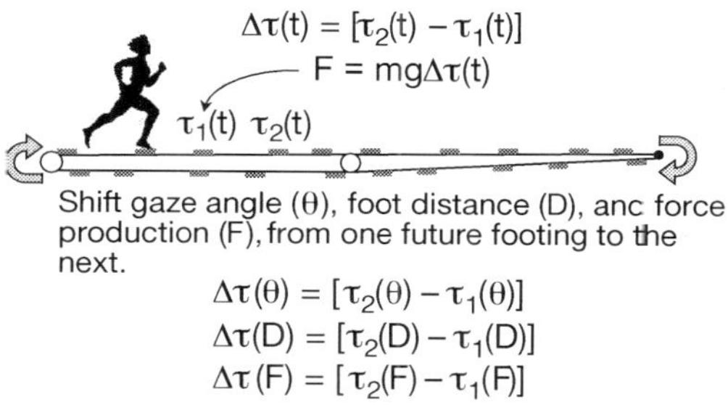

Figure 24.10 Experimental arrangement for investigating the optical basis for adapting running dynamics to the challenges of unevenly spaced footing.

(From Figure 2, Warren et al., Visual control of step length during running over irregular terrain. *Journal of Experimental Psychology: Human Perception and Performance, 12*, 259–266, 1986, APA, adapted with permission.)

that of the principle governing the closings of multiple different action gaps, the principle that renders them coherent (see Lee, 2009). General Tau Theory may not be general enough. Achieving greater generality is likely to follow from recognizing more fully that activity conducted in ordinary cluttered surroundings is very much a matter of what an agent's dimensions and realizable dynamics afford behaviorally. As highlighted by Fajen (2005, 2011, 2013), a theory of visually guided locomotion is incomplete in the absence of an account of how the agent's dimensions and the agent–environment dynamics are incorporated. Consider the following desiderata: (1) Information in the scale of eye heights that specifies dimensions of the environment relative to the dimensions of the body. (2) Self-calibration of the visual perceptual system to relations between dimensions of the body (e.g., eye height) and dimensions of attachments to the body (e.g., a hand-held raquet). (3) Registering the movements of things composing one's environment, and the speeds of those things in the coordinates of the environment, during the course of walking or running at this or that speed.

24.5 How is the Information that is Detected Related to the Energy that is Controlled?

By way of conclusion, let us return to the scenario of Figure 23.1 while keeping in mind the outfielder problem and the running over uneven terrain problem. The dragonfly preying upon a mosquito provides an important opportunity to elaborate on "seeing" as a state of affairs at the ecological scale.

At any point in the dragonfly's pursuit of a mosquito in flight, an intimate connection must hold between seeing direction to contact and seeing torque to contact, and likewise between seeing distance to contact and seeing work to contact (Turvey & Shaw, 1995). In pursuit of the insect, the optical information that is detected is related to the energy that is controlled. If it were to be otherwise—that is, if information about direction-to-contact and energy for torque-to-contact were independent and absent a common basis (i.e., arbitrary), then the dragonfly's success as a predator would likely be a matter of happenstance. The ecological perspective on the information–energy relation may be expressed as follows (Turvey & Shaw, 1995):

> When properly understood, information and energy are reciprocal aspects of nature. This reciprocity is neither required nor revealed by a physics that considers natural systems that exhibit "knowing about" as special systems. The reciprocity is brought to the forefront only when systems exhibiting "knowing about" are understood as more general in respect to the principles that underlie them than the material systems currently addressed by physics.
>
> (p. 161)

Notes

1 Z is in units of distance (e.g., cm), V is in units of distance and time (e.g., cm/s). Thus, Z/V is dimensionally cm × s/cm—that is, s.
2 To reiterate, if perception is not merely contingent but entailed, following necessarily from maximizing the global rate of entropy production (Lecture 20), then perception for all organisms is a phenomenon to be understood in terms of lawful regularities and symmetry principles defined at the ecological scale.
3 Here we elaborate on issues raised in Lectures 4 and 12. We do so in the manner of Kim and Turvey (1998) based on the deliberations of Rosen (1991; see also Rosen, 2000).
4 See Lecture 12, Section 2.
5 See Rosen (1991, p. 34).
6 Referred to as Tau-dot, Tau-gap and Tau-coupling. For details, see Lee (1998, 2009) and Pepping & Grealy (2007).
7 Data collection took place in a VENLab at Brown University, a 12m × 12m area in which participants were able to move about freely. Participants wore a head-mounted display. Synoptic images of a virtual environment were generated on a graphics workstation.

References

Adams, A. J. (2012). Physiological optics and vision science. *Optometry and Vision Science*, *89*, 953.

Bernstein, N. (1967). *The coordination and regulation of movements*. Oxford, UK: Pergamon Press.

Blancaflor, E. B., & Masson, P. H. (2003) Plant gravitropism. Unraveling the ups and downs of a complex process. *Plant Physiology*, *133*, 1677–1690.

Bootsma, R. (2009). The (current) future is here! *Perception*, *38*, 851.

Chapman S. (1968). Catching a baseball. *American Journal of Physics*, *36*, 868–870.

Darwin, C., & Darwin, F. (1880) *The power of movement in plants*. London: Murray.
Fajen, B. R. (2005). The scaling of information to action in visually guided braking. *Journal of Experimental Psychology: Human Perception and Performance, 31*, 1107–1123.
Fajen, B. R. (2011). Direct perception of action-scaled affordances: The shrinking gap problem. *Journal of Experimental Psychology: Human Perception and Performance*, 37, 1442–1457.
Fajen, B. R. (2013). Guiding locomotion in complex, dynamic environments. *Frontiers in Behavioral Neuroscience, 7*(85), 1–15.
Fink, P. W., Foo, P. S., & Warren, W. H. (2009). Catching fly balls in virtual reality: A critical test of the outfielder problem. *Journal of Vision*, 9(14), 1–8.
Gibson, J. J. (1958). Visually controlled locomotion and visual orientation in animals. *British Journal of Psychology*, 49, 182–194.
Gibson, J. J. (1966). *The senses considered as perceptual systems*. Boston, MA: Houghton Mifflin.
Gibson, J. J. (1986). *The ecological approach to visual perception*. Mahwah, NJ: Erlbaum (original work published 1979).
Goodman, N. (1965). *Fact, fiction and forecast*. Indianapolis, IN: Bobbs-Merrill.
Harrison, H., Turvey, M.T., & Frank, T. (2016). Affordance-based perception–action dynamics: A model of visually guided braking. *Psychological Review, 123*, 305–323.
Johansson, G. (1985). About visual event perception. In W. H. Warren & R. E. Shaw (Eds.), *Persistence and change: Proceedings of the first international conference on event perception* (pp. 29–54). Hillsdale, NJ: Erlbaum.
Kim, N.-G., & Turvey, M. T. (1998). Optical flow fields and Bernstein's "modeling of the future" In M. Latash (Ed.), *Progress in motor control, Vol I: Bernstein's traditions in movement studies* (pp. 221–266). Champaign, IL: Human Kinetics.
Koenderink, J. J. (1986). Optic flow. *Vision Research*, 26, 166–180.
Kugler, P. N., & Turvey, M. T. (1987). *Information, natural law and the self-assembly of rhythmic movement*. Hillsdale, NJ: Erlbaum.
Lee, D. N. (1974). Visual information during locomotion. In R. B. MacLeod & H. L. Pick Jr (Eds.), *Perception: Essays in honor of James J. Gibson* (pp. 250–267). Ithaca, NY: Cornell University Press.
Lee, D. N. (1978). The functions of vision. In H. L. Pick Jr & E. Saltzman (Eds.), *Modes of perceiving and processing information*, (pp. 159–170). Hillsdale, NJ: Erlbaum.
Lee, D. N. (1980). The optic flow field: The foundation of vision. *Philosophical Transactions of the Royal Society of London, Series B*, 290, 169–178.
Lee, D. N. (1998). Guiding movement by coupling taus. *Ecological Psychology, 10*, 221–250.
Lee, D. N. (2009). General tau theory: Evolution to date. *Perception*, 38, 837–851.
Lee, D. N., Weel, F. R., Hitchcock, T., Matejowsky, E., & Pettigrew, J. D. (1992). Common principle of guidance by echolocation and vision. *Journal of Comparative Physiology A: Neuroethology, Sensory, Neural, and Behavioral Physiology, 171*, 563–571.
Lee, D. N., Bootsma, R. J., Frost, B. J., Land, M., Regan, D., & Gray, R. (2009). Lee's 1976 paper. *Perception*, 38, 837–858.
Massa, G. D., & Gilroy, S. (2003). Touch modulates gravity sensing to regulate the growth of primary roots of *Arabidopsis thaliana*. *The Plant Journal*, 33, 435–445.
Michaels, C. F., & Oudejans, R. D. (1992). The optics and actions of catching fly balls: Zeroing out optical acceleration. *Ecological Psychology*, 4, 199–222.

Pepping, G-J., & Grealy, M. A. (Eds.). (2007). *Closing the gap: The scientific writings of David N. Lee*. Mahwah, NJ: Erlbaum.

Reed, E. S. (1996). *Encountering the world: Toward an ecological psychology*. Oxford, UK: Oxford University Press.

Rosen, R. (1985). Organisms as causal systems which are not mechanisms: An essay into the nature of complexity. In R. Rosen (Ed.), *Theoretical biology and complexity* (pp. 165–204). San Diego, CA: Academic Press.

Rosen, R. (1991). *Life itself*. New York: Columbia University Press.

Rosen, R. (2000). *Essays on life itself*. New York: Columbia University Press.

Runeson, S., & Frykholm, G. (1983). Kinematic specification of dynamics as an informational basis for person and action perception: Expectation, gender recognition, and deceptive intention. *Journal of Experimental Psychology: General, 112*, 585–615.

Shaw, R. E., & Kinsella-Shaw, J. (1988). Ecological mechanics: A physical geometry for intentional constraints. *Human Movement Science, 7*, 155–200.

Stoffregen, T. A., & Bardy, B. G. (2001). On specification and the senses. *Behavioral and Brain Sciences, 24*, 195–261.

Telewski, F. W. (2006). A unified hypothesis of mechanoperception in plants. *American Journal of Botany, 93*, 1466–1476.

Turvey, M. T. (2007). Action and perception at the level of synergies. *Human Movement Science, 26*, 657–697.

Turvey, M. T., & Shaw, R. E. (1995). Toward an ecological physics and a physical psychology. In R. Solso & D. Massaro (Eds.), *The science of the mind: 2001 and beyond* (pp. 144–169). Oxford, UK: Oxford University Press.

Turvey, M. T., Shaw, R. E., Reed, E. S., & Mace, W. M. (1981). Ecological laws of perceiving and acting: In reply to Fodor and Pylyshyn (1981). *Cognition, 9*, 237–304.

van de Langenberg, R., Kingma, I., & Beek, P. J. (2008). The perception of limb orientation depends on the center of mass. *Journal of Experimental Psychology: Human Perception and Performance, 34*, 624–639.

Warren, W. H. (1990). The perception-action coupling. In H. Bloch & B. I. Bertenthal (Eds.), *Sensory-motor organizations and development in infancy and early childhood* (pp. 23–38). Dordrecht, Netherlands: Kluwer.

Warren, W. H. (1998). Visually controlled locomotion: 40 years later. *Ecological Psychology, 10*, 177–219.

Warren, W. H. (2006). The dynamics of perception and action. *Psychological Review, 113*, 358–389.

Warren, W. H., Young, D.S., & Lee, D.N. (1986). Visual control of step length during running over irregular terrain. *Journal of Experimental Psychology: Human Perception and Performance, 12*, 259–266.

Lecture 25

The Mechanical Basis for "Getting About Among Things"

In varying degrees, all organisms encounter their surroundings mechanically. Such encounters induce tissue deformation at the segmental level, or whole body level, or both. This topic of getting about among things mechanically, and perceiving mechanically what to do or not to do with them, was broached in Lecture 8 in the course of addressing Berkeley's contribution to the "Space Enigmas," in Lecture 9 in the course of noting that the "outness problem" typically stated in respect to vision is commonplace in touch, and in Lecture 22 in the course of addressing the construction and maintenance of the mammalian body.

Specifically, in Lecture 8 we noted that for some members of Arachnida—particularly, the night-active wandering spider—the predominant perceptual means of getting about in their habitats is mechanical; in Lecture 9 we noted that a nonvisible distal surface contacted with a nonvisible hand-manipulated stick is felt at the end of the stick and *not at, or in, the hand*; and in Lecture 22 we noted that the microscopic fibroblasts construct and maintain the extracellular matrix on the basis of perceiving in any given region of the extracellular matrix the locomotion possibilities afforded by the region's stiffness and pliability. To the latter we might add dirt-living nematodes (a kind of worm). Mechanically they perceive (a) contacts with soil particles, (b) contacts with other members of Animalia, (c) forces arising from self-generated movement, and (d) bacteria that comprise a major food source.

In the present lecture, we expand our appreciation of this mechanical mode of perceiving surroundings of the body and attachments to the body under the designation *dynamic or effortful touching* (Gibson, 1966). For humans, it is perhaps the most basic form of touch in everyday activity, but hardly noticed as such[1] and only recently subject to sustained inquiry beginning with the investigations of Solomon and colleagues (e.g., Solomon, 1988; Solomon & Turvey, 1988; Solomon, Turvey & Burton, 1989). Its nature is expressed in Figure 25.1 in respect to the grasping and wielding[2] of an object occluded from view. The figure indicates what is perceptible about the object, the hand's relation to the object, and the object's relation to neighboring objects strictly on grounds of grasping the object, wielding the object, and contacting

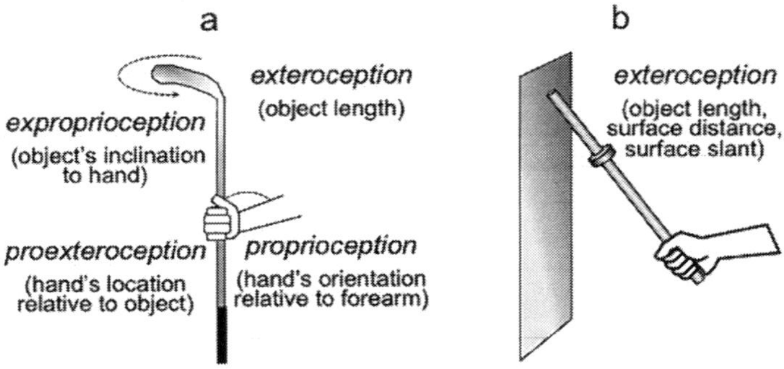

Figure 25.1 (a) Examples of the four kinds of dynamic (effortful) touching. (b) Three variants of extero-perception accompanying the striking of a nonvisible surface with a nonvisible rod. The mass and location of a metal ring attached to the rod affects the moments of the rod's mass distribution and, in consequence, the pattern of forces imposed upon the hand and arm during holding and striking (see text for details).

(From Figure 1, Carello & Turvey, 2015, *Scholarpedia*, adapted with permission, Elsevier.)

neighboring objects with it. The presumption guiding inquiry into dynamical (effortful) touch is that the functions of extero-perception, proprio-perception, proextero-perception and exproprio-perception are tied lawfully to the attendant deformations of the body's tissues (e.g., Carello & Turvey, 2016).

Dynamic (effortful) touch is part and parcel of the haptic perceptual system.[3] Its basis is the deformation of tissue, both temporary and prolonged. The haptic system, unlike the perceptual systems for hearing, tasting, smelling, and seeing includes the whole body, most of the body's parts, and the entirety of its surface. The body's segments are both exploratory subsystems in respect to perception and performatory subsystems in respect to action. That is to say, the body's apparatus for *feeling* is anatomically the same as its apparatus for *doing* (Gibson, 1966). It is an identity that will be addressed at the lecture's end in the terms of a 20th-century architectural concept—the concept of tensegrity.

25.1 A Core Ecological Hypothesis and Other Necessities

There are three necessities for getting this lecture underway. The first is recognition of the commonplace nature of dynamic (effortful) touch. Here is a sample of the multiplicity of words in the English language needed to capture its variant behavioral realizations in daily human activity: supporting, shaking, lifting, hefting, wielding, pushing, pulling, probing, pressing, chewing, prodding, groping, bending, stretching, striking, tugging, folding, twisting, squeezing, turning, rolling, vibrating.

The second necessity is familiarity with the primary forms of resistance to motion manifest in many of the preceding realizations, namely, the 0th, 1st, and 2nd moments of inertia. Consider a stick of uniform mass along its length. The 0th moment would be the rod held at its center (the center of mass), and held still. The 1st moment would be the rod held anywhere other than center, and held still. And the 2nd form would be the rod held anywhere, and moved freely. The three cases are, respectively, the mass, the static moment, and the moment of inertia. They are identified more formally in Figure 25.2.

The third necessity is appreciation of a core ecological hypothesis—namely, "*information about*" *is free of the peculiarities of perceptual systems* (Gibson, 1966). Information about x defined over the body's tissues (in the form of invariants of time-varying patterns of tissue deformation) *is the same as* information about x defined over the optic array (in the form of invariants of time-varying patterns of optic array transformations). In brief, despite the differences (in energy kind, anatomy, and physiology) the core hypothesis holds that seeing x and touching x entail detection of one and the same information kind.

Figure 25.3 shows experimental results consonant with the core hypothesis. It shows that perception of whether an inclined surface is stand-on-able[4] is the same for looking at the surface and touching the surface with a hand-held stick while blindfolded (Fitzpatrick, Carello, Schmidt & Corey, 1994). A related test of the core hypothesis entails the participant wearing a weighted vest that raises or lowers the height of the body's center of mass (Regia-Corte & Wagman, 2008). For both the higher and the lower body centers of mass, the limit of a stand-on-able slope perceived visually is found to be the same as the limit of a stand-on-able slope perceived by dynamic (effortful) touching absent vision. To be purposely redundant, whether the perception was by seeing or by touching, manipulation of body center of mass affected the perception of a stand-on-able slope *in the same way*.

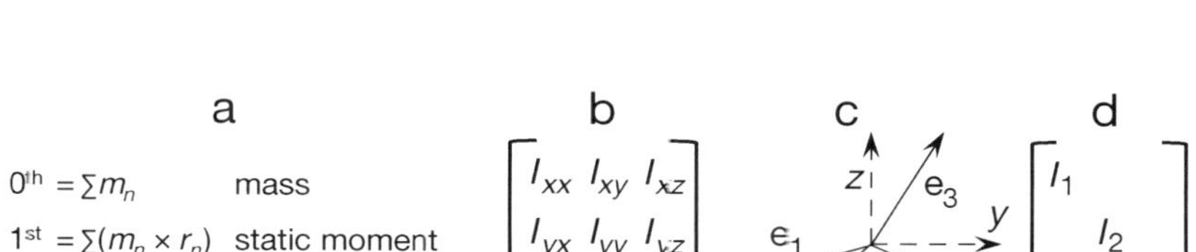

Figure 25.2 (a) The three kinds of inertial moments where m is a point mass and r is its distance from the point of rotation. (b) The moments of inertia (e.g., xx) and products of inertia (e.g., xy) comprising the inertia tensor. (c) The eigenvectors (e.g., e_3) of the inertia tensor. (d) The eigenvalues of the inertia tensor.

(From Figure 2, Carello & Turvey, 2015, *Scholarpedia*, adapted with permission, Elsevier.)

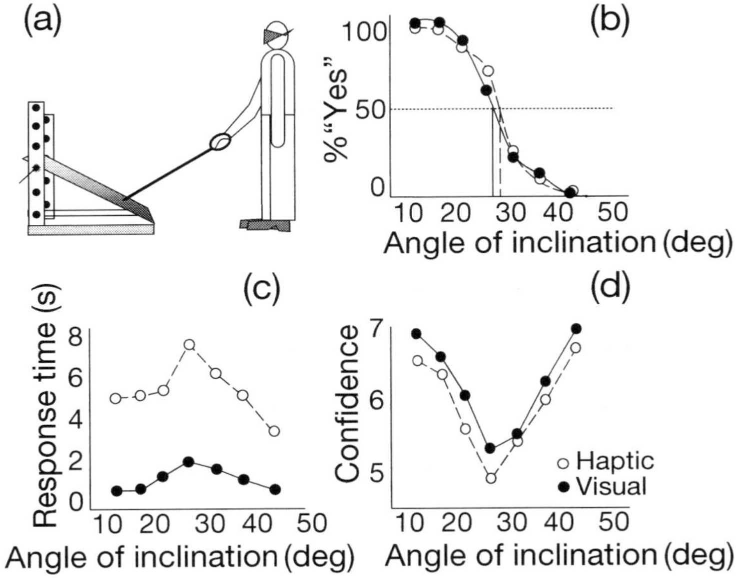

Figure 25.3 Perceiving whether a slanted surface supports upright stance. Perceiving was by looking or by dynamic (effortful) touching. (a) The latter was conducted with a 120 cm hand-held wooden dowel while wearing a blindfold. All participants performed both tasks. Slants were 12°, 17°, 22°, 27°, 33°, 39° and 45°. (b) The slope transition value between supportable and non-supportable was the same for looking and dynamic (effortful) touching. (c) Relative to perceiving by looking, dynamic (effortful) touching was slower and (d) less confident.

(From Figures 1–4, Fitzpatrick, Carello, Schmidt & Corey, 1994, adapted with permission, *Ecological Psychology*.)

An instance of the core hypothesis in a more classical setting is the sameness of the change in perception of size at a distance. The size of the separation between two blocks at a distance is the same for (a) freely looking back and forth at the blocks and (b) freely probing the gap between the blocks with a stick, with blocks and stick nonvisible (Garrett, Barac-Cikoja, Carello, & Turvey, 1996).

25.2 Variance and Invariance

A further telling feature of dynamic (effortful) touch is its dependence upon the variation of muscular forces and its independence from the magnitude of muscular forces. As Gibson (1966) observed:

> The mass of an object can be judged, in fact, by wielding it in any of a variety of ways, such as tossing and catching, or shaking it from side to side. One can only conclude that the judgment is based on information, not on the sensations. The stimulus information from wielding can only be an invariant of the changing flux of stimulation in the muscles and tendons, an exterospecific invariant in this play of forces. Whatever specifies the mass of the object presumably can be isolated from the change, and the wielding of the object has a function of separating off the permanent component from the changes.
>
> (p. 127)

In substantiation of this observation are experiments that examined perceiving the lengths of non-visible hand-held rods wielded freely about (a) the wrist (with elbow and shoulder firm), (b) the elbow (with wrist and shoulder firm), (c) the shoulder (with wrist and elbow firm) and (d) all three joints simultaneously (Pagano, Fitzpatrick & Turvey, 1993). Perceived length reported by adjusting a visible marker was the same for all four conditions, suggestive of *invariance detection over* torques and movements. Allied observations are that perceiving rod length is invariant over imposed levels of acceleration and over imposed levels of drag as engendered by wielding non-visible rods in water versus in air (Pagano & Cabe, 2003).

The partnership of change and non-change, variance and invariance, suggests, however, that a perceiver is mandated to modulate force during a bout of dynamic (effortful) touching. Such modulation and its benefits have been observed and may be allied with the observation that the structure of wielding differs for different object properties (e.g., Riley, Wagman, Santana, Carello & Turvey, 2002). An apparent challenge to the foregoing mandate is the fact that the length of a rod grasped in a hand can be perceived *without intended movement* (without the explicit and intended torque variations of wielding, hefting, etc.)—that is, by simply holding the rod still (e.g., Burton, Turvey & Solomon, 1990). That a capability is evident without intended movement does not mean that this capability occurs without movement. As depicted in Figure 25.4, the selective perception of the whole rod or the part rightward or leftward of the point of attachment can be achieved when standing still (so-called "quiet standing") on a force plate. Multifractal analysis (Lecture 9, Figure 9.8) reveals different spatiotemporal structure in the fluctuations of the body's center of pressure at the mm/ms scale between the perceiving of the whole and the perceiving of the part (Palatinus, Kelty-Stephen, Kinsella-Shaw, Carello, & Turvey, 2014). The implication of the foregoing is that selective perception by dynamic (effortful) touch entails differential force modulation, one kind for whole length report and one kind for part length report. The difference in the modulation of quiet standing is subtle and undetectable by the naked eye.

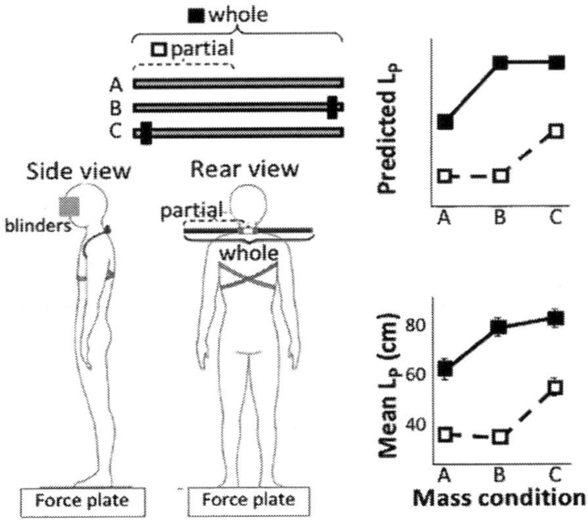

Figure 25.4 Judging shoulder-attached rods. (From Figures 1 and 3, Palatinus et al., Haptic intent in quiet standing affects multifractal scaling of postural fluctuations. *Journal of Experimental Psychology: Human Perception and Performance*, 40, 1808–1818, 2014, APA, adapted with permission.)

25.3 The Wandering Spider, the Web-Dwelling Spider, and Human Analogues

Functional similes in the dynamic (effortful) touching of spider and human provide significant insights into the informative-ness of mechanical contacts.

Wandering. We begin with the wandering spider and the twofold function of its legs: (i) propelling the body relative to the surfaces of support and (ii) embodying the four information kinds (propriospecific and exterospecific, expropriospecific and proexterospecific) in the exoskeleton deformation patterns induced by locomotion.

The eight-legged wandering spider employs all eight legs when walking in well-lit conditions, but only six when walking in darkness. It uses the first pair of legs much as an unsighted person uses a cane to probe adjacent and upcoming surfaces (Barth, 2002; Schmid, 1997). The walking legs, whether eight or six, are subject to patterns of ground reaction forces, and thereby patterns of strain in the exoskeleton, that are specific to the slope (Brüssel, 1987), mechanical resistance (surface viscosity) (Barnes & Barth, 1991) and, presumably, various other substrate properties of relevance to nocturnal navigation and place learning. The "blind" spider's ability to return to the location of a previously caught but not devoured prey, underscores the capability and significance of the legs' mechanoreceptors (Seyfarth & Barth,

1972; Seyfarth et al. 1982) and the importance of distinguishing information kinds in the manner laid out in Lecture 23 (see Figure 23.4). The exproprioceptive ability to orient to the direction and distance of the prey site (absent the prey, and absent landmarks) is severely impaired by inactivation of the legs' lyriform organs of mechanoreception (recall Lecture 8 and Figures 8.7, 8.8). In contrast, inactivation of lyriform organs does not impair the proprioceptive ability to coordinate the legs in the normal manner of walking.

The wandering spider's ability to get about mechanically has parallels in human dynamical (effortful) touch. Figure 25.5a depicts a minimal straight-path environment used to assess the ability of blindfolded human participants to orient to their surroundings strictly on the basis of mechanical contact (Harrison & Turvey, 2010). Figure 25.5b–d depicts the experimental task and the experimental manipulations.

Raised steps S_1, S_2, and S_3 indicated in Figure 25.5b constituted landmarks on the path. The mechanical contacts were those of walking, stepping, and probing with a soft-tipped cane. "Home" (*H*) was a mechanically indistinct location. The blindfolded participants learned to distinguish *H* in the course of exploring the minimal environment by means of the experimenter halting the participant and stating: "This location is home." More specifically, on each trial in the training phase the individual participant was indirectly guided to *H* from a distal location (either F_1, F_2, F_3 or F_4) before performing a simple homing task from one of four set distances (either D_1, D_2, D_3 and D_4). The locations and distances are identified in Figure 25.5b. On each trial in the test

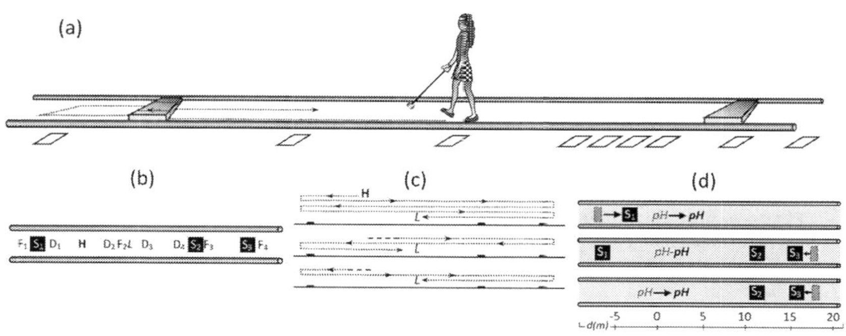

Figure 25.5 (a) The minimal mechanical environment for blindfolded human participants deployed in Harrison and Turvey (2010). The participant is shown standing at "home"—an unmarked place that was learned over the course of the experiment. The rectangular markers placed next to the environment allowed the experimenter to control the training and test phases by means of simple verbal instructions. (b–d) The experimental manipulations; details are spelled out in the text.

(From Figure 1, Harrison & Turvey, 2010, adapted with permission.)

phase, participants were led indirectly through hallways prior to entering the path at the test location *L* with the assigned task of walking to *H*. Travel routes prior to test are identified in Figure 25.5c: top is the Trial 1 route; middle is the Trials 2, 4 and 6 route, and bottom is the Trials 3 and 5 route. Figure 25.5d identifies (a) the perturbations of landmarks S_1 and S_3 at test (with gray squares showing landmark locations used during training) in Experiment 1 (top), Experiment 2 (middle) and Experiment 3 (bottom) and (b) the shift in perceived location of home (*pH*) as a function of non-perturbation (gray *pH*) and perturbation (black *pH*).

In a one-landmark (i.e., one-step) environment, *pH* in the experimental condition shifted in the same direction, with the same magnitude, as the shifted landmark. In an environment of two of the three landmarks located in the same direction from *H*, shifting the further landmark toward *H* resulted in a change in *pH* that preserved the original ratio of distances separating (a) *H*, (b) the nearer landmark, and (c) the further landmark. Both findings were invariant over the travel route to the test location and repetitions of testing. It seems that for both humans and wandering spiders, mechanical contact in the absence of vision can reveal the directions and spatial relations specifying places.

Web dwelling. The web-dwelling spider presents different kinds of challenges to dynamic (effortful) touching. The "information about" carried in the vibrations are often imposed, but they are also obtained by the spider setting the web into vibration. A minimal model system for studying this capability with "human spiders" is perceiving the distance of a non-visible object on a single taut strand (a minimal haptic web) either vibrated by the spider (the participant) or by the "intruder" (the experimenter) (Kinsella-Shaw & Turvey, 1992). The model system is depicted in Figure 25.6. As Figure 25.6 makes

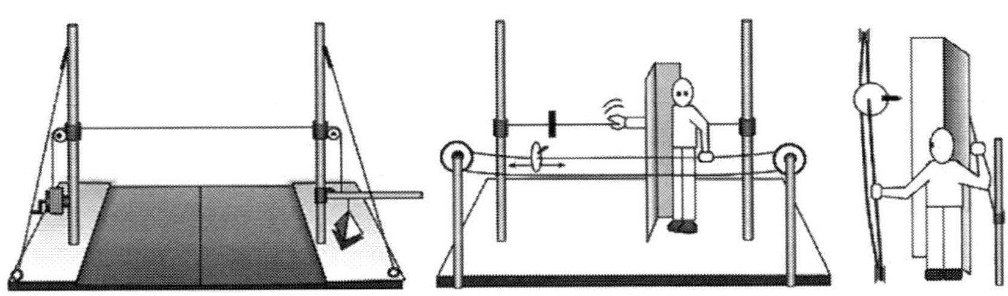

Figure 25.6 (*Left*) Minimal "haptic web" consisting of a strand of nylon under high tension. (*Middle*) Strand with an attached object is vibrated by the occluded right hand while the visible left hand positions a pointer to match its distance. (*Right*) View from behind the participant. See original text for details.

(From Figure 1, Kinsella-Shaw & Turvey, 1992, adapted with permission, Springer.)

evident, participants indicated where along the strand the object was attached by moving ("reeling in" or "reeling out") a report arrow to a position parallel to the object.

Vibrations were initiated manually by a sharp, single shake. The single strand's dynamics are those of the one-dimensional wave equation. In this equation, the elastic force is coupled to the strand's motions by the constant ratio of the strand's linear density μ to the strand's tension T (the horizontal component of force on the strand). The significance of T, and thereby μ/T, was demonstrated via manipulations of the hand's position on the strand. For vibrations induced by the participant (the "spider"), object distances of 30.5, 61, 91, 122 and 152 cm were perceived at mean values of 48.3, 66, 83.4, 101.6 and 141.6 cm without any practice in the task and at mean values of 33.7, 58.4, 89.4, 105.4, and 136.2 cm, respectively, with minimal practice in the task. For vibrations induced by the experimenter (the "intruder") perceived distances were similarly ordered well, but with less accuracy.

The upshot of the experiments conducted in this single-strand variant of a spider's web was that, by manually vibrating a solid medium, an ordinary person can perceive the distances of objects attached to that solid medium. Perceived distance was (a) linearly dependent on object distance with or without practice, (b) inversely related to strand tension, and (c) dependent on whether strand manipulations were vertical or horizontal. Of particular significance, perceived distance was manifest when the mechanical wave was other-initiated as well as self-initiated. In short, there are circumstances under which humans, like spiders and other members of the Kingdom Animalia, can perceive the distances of things on a tensed medium by means of vibrations in that tensed medium.

Non-neural reception. The preceding invites elaboration along lines suggested by Burton (1993). The web is a tensed medium but as such it is also receptor-like. In a very functional sense, it registers *and* transmits patterns of stimulation. The fact that non-neural things can serve a receptive function—such as a hand-held cane used by a person without vision (cf. Figures 25.3, 25.5)—suggests to Burton (1993, p. 107) that the phenomenon of perception may be more fundamental (and probably more ancient) than the phenomenon of specialized nervous systems. It is a conjecture that receives support from the perception–action abilities of the nerveless shelled amoebae discussed at length in Lecture 23. Although very far from being understood, a reasonable guess is that those abilities self-organize from the embedding of actin-myosin dynamics in the dynamics of plasmasol–plasmagel.[5]

The preceding can incline one to the argument that organisms without nervous systems relate to their surroundings in a categorically different way than organisms with nervous systems. It can also incline one to the somewhat more radical view that nervous systems are what they are because the self-organizing principles that beget the expertise of nerveless organisms are what they are.

25.4 Bishop George Berkeley, Sir Charles Bell, and Mr. Ian Waterman

The following three quotations span three centuries. They help one to acquire a visceral appreciation of dynamic (effortful) touch in particular and the perceptual system grounded in the body's tissues more generally.

> consider the case of an . . . unbodied spirit, which is supposed to see perfectly well, i.e., to have a clear perception of the proper and immediate objects of sight, but to have no sense of touch. Whether there be any such being in nature or no is beside my purpose to inquire; it suffices that the supposition contains no contradiction in it.
>
> (Berkeley, 1709/1948, Section 153)

> in standing, walking, and running, every effort of the voluntary power, which gives motion to the body, is directed by a sense of the condition of the muscles, and without this sense we could not regulate their actions.
>
> (Bell, 1826, p. 167)

> If the world was a cricket pitch I'd be happy. If it was a pebbled beach I might as well commit suicide.
>
> (Waterman in Cole, 1995, p. 129)

Although Bell's focus was the phylum Craniata (in the Kingdom Animalia), his observation of the significance of sensitivity to mechanical forces (self-generated or imposed) is now known to encompass all Six Kingdoms and perhaps all phyla.[6] Berkeley and Waterman are referring (albeit obliquely) to the loss of body perception identified by Bell. Whereas Berkeley *pondered* such a loss, Waterman *suffered* such a loss. An illness at the age of 19 rendered Mr. Waterman unable to feel his body and its motions with the exception of his head and neck. He suffered the sensory disorder of peripheral neuropathy. Mr. Waterman's achievements, trials, tribulations, and exhaustion in respect to getting about among things and perceiving what to do or not to do with them are described in a book entitled *Pride and a Daily Marathon* (Cole, 1995). He finds standing, walking, reaching, and manipulating objects extremely challenging and, on many an occasion, simply impossible. Perceiving that a surface affords walking upon, an opening affords passing through, a gap affords stepping over, etc., etc., are necessary requirements for getting about. They are, however, requirements that can be accomplished by Mr. Waterman only with considerable concentration and intellectual effort. Vision must substitute, however imperfectly, for the absence below the neck of the four functions identified in Figure 25.1a. Mr. Waterman's choice of food is dictated by the coordination challenges posed by the act of eating, notably, the use of the utensils and the arranging of the food to facilitate transport from plate to mouth. In the case of everyday walking in everyday architectural surroundings, Mr. Waterman must watch each leg in turn as it swings stiffly forward so that he can decide explicitly when and where that forward movement should be brought to a halt. A pebbled beach presents an even greater challenge: Vision cannot resolve the uncertainty of footing in sufficient degree for him to voluntarily prepare the musculature of lower limbs for contact with the terrain's unevenness prior to contact. (Hence, the contrast, in the earlier quotation, between a cricket pitch[7] and a pebbled beach.)

25.5 Haptic Perceptual Instruments: Smart, Determinate, Soft, and Scaled

An instance of dynamic (effortful) touching can be conceived of as the assembling of a measurement device, a perceptual instrument (e.g., Bingham, 1988; Runeson, 1977; Solomon, 1988; Solomon & Turvey, 1988). It can be said of such an instrument that it is smart, determinate, soft and scaled. *Smart* is in reference to the exploitation of special aspects of the situation (e.g., physical invariants) in achieving the perceptual task (Bingham, 1988; Runeson, 1977). *Determinate* is in reference to the uniqueness of the mapping of perception to the designated property. *Soft* is in reference to the facility of dynamic (effortful) touch to function as different kinds of measurement instruments.[8] Fundamentally, soft implies that the assembled system is specific to general dynamical principles as opposed to particular anatomical and neural components. *Scaled* expresses the close approximation of a perceived magnitude (e.g., angular direction, length) to the actual magnitude.

A prosaic but stunning human capability is that on provision of a given intent in the form of a task (e.g., "perceive object property π") a person can effectively assemble her- or himself into a smart instrument that serves just that purpose. The Palatinus et al. (2014) "quiet standing" study discussed earlier is a case in point. Here are two additional cases. Consider holding a uniformly dense rod occluded from view at intermediate positions 1/4, 1/2, and 3/4 along its length. For each position, the person can be given the intent of wielding the hand-held rod to determine *rod length if held at an end* (whole length intent). On a separate occasion the person can be given the intent of wielding to determine *length of the rod part forward of grasp* (partial length intent). For a variety of rods with mean actual length of 76 cm and a mean partial length of 37 cm, the respective mean perceptions for participants in Solomon and Turvey (1988) were 76 cm and 38 cm. This apparent ability to "fractionate" nonvisible hand-held objects on instruction gives emphasis to investigations of dynamic (effortful) touch in terms of "to intend perception of x requires attending to information about x." The additional empirical fact that rod fractions can be perceived when rods are simply held (no wielding) at different locations along their lengths underscores the theoretical challenge. The challenge is amplified if emphasis is given to 0th and 1st moments. The 0th (alias mass) is the same value for all hand positions. The 1st (alias static moment) is zero at the 1/2 position.

Experiments on perceiving the sweet spot of wielded occluded rackets and wielded wooden rods invite similar considerations (Carello, Thuot, Anderson & Turvey, 1999; Carello, Thuot, & Turvey, 2000). The "sweet spot" of an implement refers to the best location along its length (its center of percussion) to strike something. Perception given the "sweet spot intent" is distinguished from perception given the "length intent"[9] both in the measure of magnitude production and in dependence on mass moments. Perceived sweet spot follows closely the value of the ratio of the largest moment of inertia (I_1) to the static moment, both for tennis rackets of different lengths (from junior through stretch rackets) and for wooden rods with attached masses used to manipulate the moments. Figure 25.7 provides a useful summary of the so far identified abilities of dynamic (effortful) touch.[10]

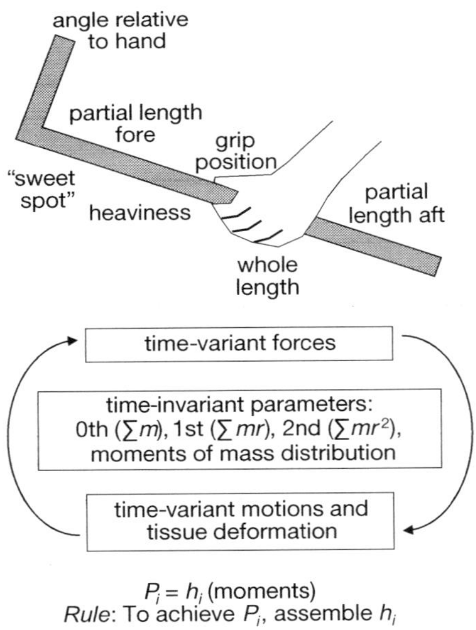

Figure 25.7 (*Top*) Properties of an L-shaped rod shown to be perceptible by wielding without benefit of vision. (*Bottom*) Schematic of the basis for perception of those properties by dynamic (effortful) touch: perception (P) as a function (h) of mass moments.

(From Figure 16, Turvey, 2007, adapted with permission, Elsevier.)

25.6 The Heaviness of Things (and Another So-Called Illusion that Isn't)

Common to everyday human behavior is changing the locations and orientations of things. Interactions with grasped objects (e.g., the pushing, turning, lifting, carrying, etc. of books, mugs, forks, cellphones, etc.) tend to involve translations and rotations. These interactions combine forces proportional to an object's resistance to translational acceleration (i.e., its mass or 0th moment) and torques scaled to an object's resistance to rotational acceleration (i.e., its tensor of inertia or 2nd moment). Research on the wielding of a nonvisible object suggests that the object's felt weight or heaviness depends on a quantity other than its mass. It depends on its 2nd moment as well as its 0th moment (e.g., Amazeen, 1997; Shockley, Carello & Turvey, 2004).

From the ecological perspective, this heaviness "illusion" (often referred to as the weight illusion) is a point of entry into what a hand-held object affords by way of neuromuscular control. It makes clear that one's perception of an object's heaviness does not refer to the object's weight (mass × gravity; see Amazeen & Turvey, 1996). Objects of the kind shown in Figure 25.8 can be referred to as tensor objects. They were introduced to study heaviness perception's dependence on any given object's inertial eigenvalues. Experiments have varied the mass M of the tensor objects and, independently, two scalar variables of their inertia ellipsoids, namely, symmetry $S = 2I_3/(I_1 + I_2)$ and volume $V = 4\pi/3(Det\ I_{ij})^{-1/2}$.[11] Together, S and V are physical characterizations of an object's resistance to rotational acceleration taken in reference to the movement system. Arguably, they are the right degrees of freedom. They bear,

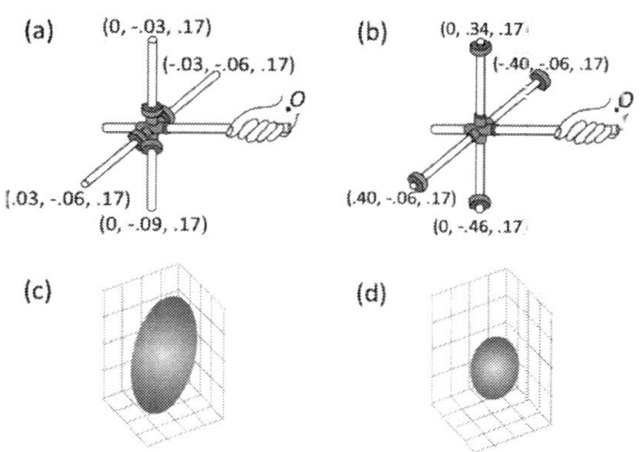

Figure 25.8 Two tensor objects (a and b) together with the coordinates of the hub and attached metal rings and their corresponding inertia ellipsoids (c and d). These objects were used in Experiment 1 of Shockley et al., 2004.

(From Figure 2, adapted with permission, Springer.)

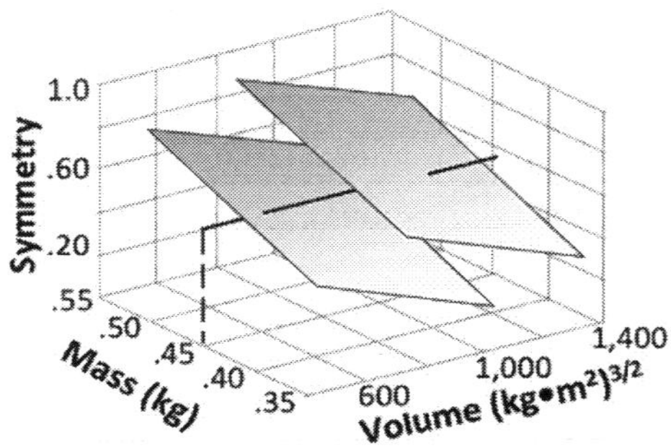

Figure 25.9 Heaviness/movableness space consisting of mass and the volume and symmetry of the inertia ellipsoid. Each point in a plane identifies a combination of the designated variables that yields the same heaviness/moveableness percept as the combination of variables corresponding to any other point in the plane. Parallel planes reflect different sets of metameric matches. The solid line intersecting more than one plane illustrates that a single mass (designated as .45 kg) may be perceived differently depending on the inertia tensor variables (a variant of the size–weight illusion). The lower plane represents heavier metamers (heaviness decreases with increases in both ellipsoid symmetry and ellipsoid volume).

(From Figure 1, Shockley et al., 2004, adapted with permission, Springer.)

respectively, on the patterning and level of muscular forces needed to move a hand-held object in a controlled fashion. Experiments with tensor objects reveal that the effects of *S*, *V* and mass are additive (e.g., Shockley et al., 2004). The understanding that mass matters to the perception of heaviness, but gravity does not, is affirmed by the demonstration that the (wrongly called) size-weight illusion is indifferent to the perception of weight (Plaisier & Smeets, 2012).

The observations of a change in perceived heaviness for a fixed mass have a complement in *weight metamers*: objects of different mass that have the same perceived heaviness (Turvey & Carello, 2011). As shown in Figure 25.9, combinations of mass, symmetry and volume yield metameric planes. Length perception by wielding a given object is different from heaviness perception (Amazeen, E., 1999). It can be expected, therefore, that metamers for heaviness are not metamers for length, an expectation that has been confirmed (Shockley et al., 2004, Experiment 5).

25.7 Is Dynamic (Effortful) Touch in General a Self-Similar (Fractal) Process?

The suggested power law behavior has important implications, most notably, that perception by dynamic touch is a self-similar or fractal process (Lecture

8)—that is, it depends on moments of the mass distribution at all object sizes or scales (e.g., consider very small objects with little resistance to being rotationally accelerated, such as sewing needles, and very large objects with great resistance, such as baseball or cricket bats), within largest and smallest scale sizes that have yet to be identified (Santana & Carello, 1999; Turvey, 1996; Turvey et al., 1998).

The importance of power laws for psychophysics was well respected by Stevens (1961, 1962), but the fullness of their implications would only become clear in subsequent years. A system whose functioning abides a power law, such as dynamic (effortful) touch in the perception of length, does not conform to the principle of superposition—that is, it does not parse into multiple non-interacting components and it is not understandable as the sum of separate components. To the contrary, the power law behavior indicates that the underlying processes are multiple and interdependent operating at many spatial and temporal scales that are distributed lognormally[12] (e.g., West & Deering, 1995). The perceiving of whole and partial lengths in quiet standing is a case in point.

25.8 Perceiving Limb Direction

One benefit of thinking about attachments to the body in terms of Figures 25.2 and 25.7 is that it transfers readily to thinking about the body itself. If the nonvisual perception of a hand-held object's orientation can be related to a measure of the object's mass distribution relative to the grasp, then perhaps the nonvisible perception of a limb's orientation can likewise be related to a measure of its mass distribution relative to its attachment to the body (Figure 25.10) (Pagano & Turvey, 1995; Pagano, Garrett, & Turvey, 1996; Turvey & Carello, 1995).

As inspection of Figure 25.10 (*top*) indicates, the arm's inertial quantities can be manipulated through a hand-held rod extending along the underside of the arm with a cross-bar to which masses can be added (reviewed in Turvey & Carello, 2011). From an inertia tensor perspective, masses evenly distributed on the left and right keep the inertia ellipsoid aligned with the long axis of the arm. Uneven distribution of those masses diverts the ellipsoid from the arm's axis. In such a case, an individual asked to point at a visible target with the occluded arm points with $\boldsymbol{e}_i$. Matching the positions of the left and right arms when splints are held in the two hands also result in matching the ellipsoids of the two limbs rather than matching the angles of the joints.

Subsequent experiments indicate, however, that these phenomena are tied to the arm's center of mass vector, *Vcm*, rather than the arm's eigenvector, Ve_i. The two cross-bars in Figure 25.10 (*bottom*) allow manipulations of added masses that disentangle *Vcm* and Ve_i. Such manipulations reveal *Vcm* to be the constraining invariant in the nonvisual (a) matching of joint angles (van de Langenberg, Kingma, & Beek, 2007), (b) pointing with a limb

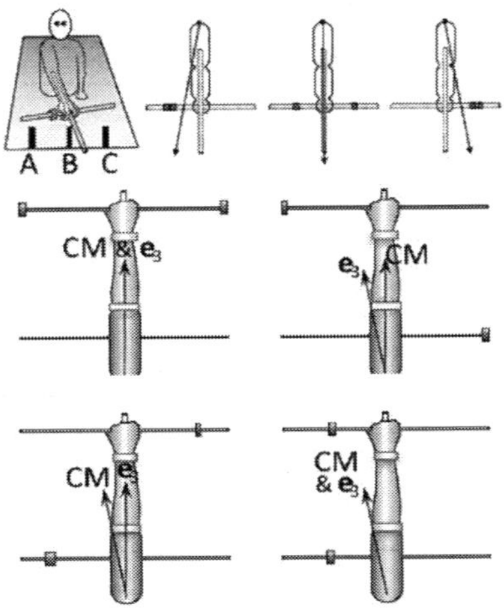

Figure 25.10 Contributions of inertia tensor eigenvectors (in particular e_3) and the center of mass (CM) vector to pointing with a nonvisible arm. (left) Positions of masses added to the hand-held cross-bar change felt direction of arm (e.g., felt to be pointing at B when leftward of B). (*Right*) Use of two cross-bars allows for the co-manipulation of $\mathbf{e}_3$ and CM. Participants point with CM vector, not $\mathbf{e}_3$

(From Figures 1 and 2, Pagano & Turvey, 1995, and Figure 3, van de Langenberg et al., *Journal of Experimental Psychology: Human Perception and Performance*, APA, adapted with permission.)

(van de Langenberg, Kingma, & Beek, 2008), and (c) inphase and antiphase rhythmic coordinations of left and right hand-held pendulums (Silva & Turvey, 2012).

25.9 Tensegrity Architecture: Equivalence of the Muscular-Connective Tissue-Skeletal System and the Optic Array

The common media for the perceptual systems of seeing, hearing, smelling and tasting, namely, air and water, share the features of being homogeneous (physical properties are place invariant) and isotropic (physical properties are direction invariant). They are suited to being structured reliably by events that tie the perceiver to the environment. The body interpreted as *tensegrity architecture*, a matter of continuous tension elements and intermittent compression elements at all of its scales, promises the requisite homogeneity and isotropy for the medium of haptic perception (Turvey & Fonseca, 2014).

Implicit in this lecture has been the assumption of this tension array as *information about* in the sense of specificity to (a) the layout of the body, (b) movements of the body, and (c) attachments to the body. It is the body's equivalent to optic array/optic flow. By hypothesis, it grounds the haptic perceptual system and, perforce, the phenomena of dynamic (effortful) touch. By hypothesis, it is, like the optic array, constituted as an indefinite nesting of functionally self-similar units subject to local and global transformations. If the arm is so characterized (see Figure 25.11) then we should expect that the act of wielding a hand-held rod about the wrist, elbow and shoulder (either singly or in combination) would deform this tensegrity structure in ways unique to the wielding activity, the inertial properties of the hand-held rod and, relatedly, the linear dimensions, of the hand-held rod. An experiment referred to previously (Pagano et al., 1993) can be revisited. A nonvisible rod held at one end and wielded freely is perceived to be of the same length whether wielded about the wrist, the elbow, or the shoulder, either singly or in combination. One reading of the preceding is that invariance of extero-perception across these conditions follows from a sameness of dynamics in the tensegrity architecture despite neuroanatomical differences from joint to joint and from scale to scale.

The force distributed within the multifractal tensegrity expressed in Figure 25.11 arises from multiple sources originating in the multifarious changing and persisting aspects of the mechanical relation of an organism and its environment. The primary question is how information about these sources is made available in the multifractal tensegrity. Taking the visual system and optic array as guide, we should ask: What would be the corresponding array for the haptic system? We intimated above that it would be in terms of deformation. This potential answer requires further detail on the optic array.

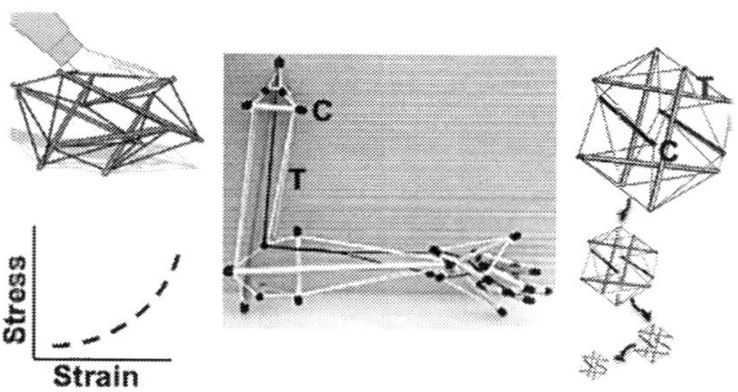

Figure 25.11 (*Upper left*) Deformation of an icosahedral tensegrity and (*lower left*) the underlying non-linear stress response to strain. The property of *pre-stress* is indicated by nonzero stress when applied strain is at and near zero. (*Middle*) A modeled tensegrity arm constituted by tension (T) and compression (C) elements. (*Right*) Biologically, instances of T and C would themselves be constituted by T and C elements at all scales.

Upper left: (from Figure 11b, Myers, 2004, reprinted with permission, Elsevier)
Lower left: (from Figure 17e, Fonseca & Turvey, 2014, adapted with permission, *Journal of Motor Behavior*).
Middle: (© T. Flemons 2008, reprinted with permission)

The conception of "optic array" (Gibson, 1966, 1979/1986) starts with the rejection of discrete points or spots of light, each with a locus indexed by coordinates, and each with a determinate intensity and frequency. (As implied above, it rejects the theory of local signs.) The nesting of optical solid angles replaces the point matrix, the relation of inclusion (optical solid angles within optical solid angles) replaces coordinates, and the relation of margin or contrast (e.g., differences of intensity and frequency in different directions) replaces individual magnitudes of point intensities. The optic array is an alternative description of the light distribution. It is a description that gives emphasis to relations (within an energy distribution) rather than energy. It is a description that expresses the structure in ambient light and, in consequence, provides a basis for identifying information about the conditions that give rise to it (see Gibson, 1966, 1979/1986; Lee, 1980).

Individual tensegrity icosahedra comprising the haptic array would be the functional equivalents of optic solid angles comprising the optic array with the exception of being defined independently of a point of observation. In the same manner that optical solid angles assume their forms in respect to the layout of surfaces, tensegrity icosahedra will assume their forms in respect to the layout of forces. Insofar as they have a form in isolation, their concerted responses to a layout of forces would be a change of form, a deformation. With an understanding of this deformed state of the body, locally and globally, comes the promise of an understanding of the hypothesized basis for *haptic information about*.

In sum, the haptic system as a multifractal architecture of compression-tension elements constitutes a medium that permits the propagation/distribution of mechanical forces generated by and imposed upon it. It is companion to air and water, which permit the flux of light, the transmission of vibrations, and the diffusion of volatile substances.

25.10 A Necessary Addendum: We Can Hear What a Struck Object Looks Like

A close affiliate of touching is hearing. For both, the conditions of stimulation are tied to mechanical events. In respect to hearing, the physical parameters of an object together with its spatial dimensions determine its natural modes of vibration and, thereby, the acoustic patterns it radiates when mechanically disturbed. The acoustical structure of a vibrating object is potentially information about the object's properties—both geometric (e.g., spatial dimensions) and material (e.g., steel) (Gaver, 1993a, 1993b). If the information contained in the radiating acoustic waveforms can be detected, then a listener can, in principle, hear what an object looks like. This expectation has been verified through experiments in which participants listened to suspended objects of commonplace geometric forms, set into vibration by a pendular hammer, whether responses were categorical (pointing at visible matches for

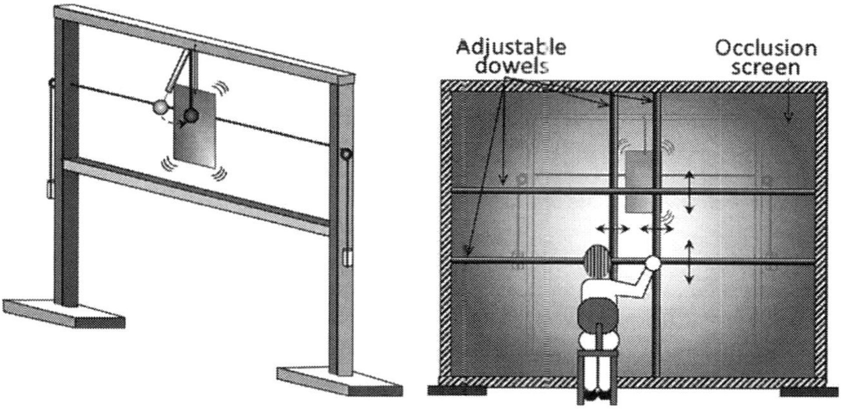

Figure 25.12 Hearing shape. (*Left*) The support apparatus with pendulum and suspended plate. (Right) A listener adjusts the positions of dowels to indicate the size of an object set into vibration on the other side of an occlusion screen.

(From Figure 1, Kunkler-Peck & Turvey, Hearing shape, *Journal of Experimental Psychology: Human Perception and Performance*, 26, 279–294, 2000, APA, adapted with permission)

occluded circles, triangles, squares) or metrical (Figure 25.12; Kunkler-Peck & Turvey, 2000).

Notes

1 Hoisington (1920) is an early exception.
2 Wield and wielding are intended to convey the activities one might conduct relative to a hand-held object and more generally to an object attached to the body. The intent is to encompass the common meanings of words such as shaking, twisting, swinging, turning, hefting, and so on.
3 The term "haptic" is said to be derivative of the Greek *haptesthai* (able to lay hold of—e.g., Revesz, 1950). The description of the haptic perceptual system given here follows Gibson's (1966, Chapters 6 and 7).
4 The *x* in the preceding sentence.
5 See Nakagaki & Guy (2008) for details on the analogous phenomena exhibited by the slime mold *Physarum*.
6 The shared basis of these forces is the stretching of the underlying cytoskeleton of individual cell membranes. In addition to Animalia, mechanoreceptors have been identified in Archea (e.g., Engelberth, Wanner, Groth, & Elmar, 1995; Kloda & Martinac, 2001), Bacteria (e.g., Hamill & Martinac, 2001), Fungi (e.g., Kumamoto 2008), Protoctista (e.g., Machemer, 2001), and Plantae (e.g., Visnovitz, Világi, Varró, & Kristóf, 2007).
7 The pitch in the game of cricket is renowned for being (near) perfectly flat.
8 Different meters (measuring instruments) can be assembled over the same neural-anatomical-muscular components and the same meter can be assembled over different neural-anatomical-muscular components.

9 The use of "length intent" in the preceding paragraphs is not ideal. "Length" is not an ecological predicate. A more apt phrasing of the participant's charge in the experiments just described is to perceive "distance reach-with-able." Likewise for "sweet spot": a more apt phrasing of the participant's charge is to perceive something akin to "region most efficaciously contact-with-able." Articulating the affordances in the domain of dynamic (effortful) touch is not a simple matter.

10 One does not have to wield a nonvisible rod to perceive its length. Rolling it back and forth on a firm surface with the palm of the hand yields reasonable length perception (Cabe, 2010).

11 The determinant (*Det* for short) in the equation for *V* is a general quantity calculable from the elements of a square matrix such as the inertia tensor.

12 The designation for a probability distribution in which the log of a random variable conforms to a bell-shaped curve.

References

Amazeen, E. L. (1997). The effects on perceived heaviness by dynamic touch: With and without vision. *Ecological Psychology*, 9, 245–263.

Amazeen, E. L. (1999). Perceptual independence of size and weight by dynamic touch. *Journal of Experimental Psychology: Human Perception and Performance*, *25*, 102–129.

Amazeen, E. L., & Turvey, M. T. (1996). Weight perception and the haptic size–weight illusion are functions of the inertia tensor. *Journal of Experimental Psychology: Human Perception and Performance*, *22*, 213–232.

Barnes W., & Barth, F. G. (1991). Sensory control of locomotor mode in semi-aquatic spiders. In D. M. Armstrong & B. M. H. Bush (Eds.), *Locomotor neural mechanisms in arthropods and vertebrates* (pp. 105–116). Manchester, UK: Manchester University Press.

Barth, F. G. (2002). *A spider's world: Senses and behavior*. Berlin, Germany: Springer.

Bell, C. (1826). On the nervous circle which connects the voluntary muscles with the brain. *Philosophical Transactions of the Royal Society of London*, *116*, 163–173.

Berkeley, G. (1948). Essay towards a new theory of vision. In A. A. Luce & T. E. Jessop (Eds.), *The works of George Berkeley, Bishop of Cloyne*. London: Nelson (original work published 1709).

Bingham, G. (1988). Task-specific devices and the perceptual bottleneck. *Human Movement Science*, *7*, 225–264.

Burton, G. (1993). Non-neural extensions of haptic sensitivity. *Ecological Psychology*, 5, 105–124.

Burton, G., Turvey, M. T, & Solomon, H. Y. (1990). Can shape be perceived by dynamic touch? *Perception & Psychophysics*, 48, 477–487.

Brüssel, A. (1987). *Belastungen und Dehnungen im Spinnenskelett unter natürlichen Verhaltensbedingungen*. (Unpublished doctoral dissertation). University of Frankfurt, Germany.

Cabe, P. A. (2010). Sufficiency of longitudinal moment of inertia for haptic cylinder length judgments. *Journal of Experimental Psychology: Human Perception and Performance*, 36, 373–394.

Carello, C., Thuot, S., Anderson, K. L., & Turvey, M. T. (1999). Perceiving the sweet spot. *Perception*, *28*, 307–320.

Carello, C., Thuot, S., & Turvey, M. T. (2000). Aging and the perception of a racket's sweet spot. *Human Movement Science*, *19*, 1–20.

Carello, C., & Turvey, M. T. (2016). Dynamic (effortful) touch. In A. Prescott, E. Ahisser, & E. Izhikevich (Eds.), *Scholarpedia of touch* (pp. 227–240). Paris: Atlantis Press.

Cole, J. (1995). *Pride and a daily marathon*. Cambridge, MA: MIT Press.

Engelberth. J., Wanner, G., Groth, B., & Elmar, W. (1995). Functional anatomy of the mechanoreceptor cells in tendrils of Bryonia dioica. *Planta*, 196, 539–550.

Fitzpatrick, P., Carello, C., Schmidt, R. C., & Corey, D. (1994). Haptic and visual perception of an affordance for upright posture. *Ecological Psychology*, 6, 265–287.

Garrett, S., Barac-Cikoja, D., Carello, C., & Turvey, M. T. (1996). A parallel between visual and haptic perception of size at a distance. *Ecological Psychology*, 8, 25–42.

Gaver, W. W. (1993a). What in the world do we hear? An ecological approach to auditory source perception. *Ecological Psychology*, 5, 1–29.

Gaver, W. W. (1993b). How do we hear in the world? Explorations in ecological acoustics. *Ecological Psychology*, 5, 285–313.

Gibson, J. J. (1966). *The senses considered as perceptual systems*. Boston, MA: Houghton Mifflin.

Gibson, J. J. (1986). *The ecological approach to visual perception*. Mahwah, NJ: Erlbaum (original work published 1979).

Hamill, O. P., & Martinac, B. (2001). Molecular basis of mechanotransduction in living cells, *Physiological Review*, 81, 685–740.

Harrison, S. J., & Turvey, M. T. (2010). Place learning by mechanical contact. *Journal of Experimental Biology*, 213, 1436–1442.

Hoisington, L. B. (1920). On the nonvisual perception of the length of lifted rods. *American Journal of Psychology*, 31, 114–146.

Kinsella-Shaw, J., & Turvey, M. T. (1992). Haptic perception of object distance on a single-strand vibratory web. *Perception & Psychophysics*, 52, 625–638.

Kloda, A., & Martinac, B. (2001). Mechanosensitive channels in Archaea. *Cell Biochemistry & Biophysics*, 34, 349–381.

Kumamoto, C. A. (2008). Molecular mechanisms of mechanosensing and their roles in fungal contact sensing. *Nature Reviews Microbiology*, 6, 667–673.

Kunkler-Peck, A., & Turvey, M. T. (2000). Hearing shape. *Journal of Experimental Psychology: Human Perception and Performance*, 26, 279–294.

Lee, D. N. (1980). The optic flow field: The foundation of vision. *Philosophical Transactions of the Royal Society of London, Series B*, 290, 169–178.

Machemer, H. (2001). The swimming cell and its world: Structures and mechanisms of orientation in Protoctista. *European Journal of Protistology*, 37, 3–14.

Myers, T. W. (2001). *Anatomy trains: Myofascial meridians for manual and movement therapists*. Edinburgh, UK: Churchill Livingstone.

Nakagaki, T., & Guy, R. D. (2008). Intelligent behaviors of amoeboid movement based on complex dynamics of soft matter. *Soft Matter*, 4, 57–67.

Pagano, C., & Cabe, P. A. (2003). Constancy in dynamic touch: Length perceived by dynamic touch is invariant over changes in media. *Ecological Psychology*, 15, 1–17.

Pagano, C., Fitzpatrick, P., & Turvey, M. T. (1993). Tensorial basis to the constancy of perceived object extent over variations of dynamic touch. *Perception & Psychophysics*, 54, 43–45.

Pagano, C., Garrett, S., & Turvey, M. T. (1996). Is limb proprioception a function of the limbs' inertial eigenvectors? *Ecological Psychology* 8, 43–69.

Pagano, C., & Turvey, M. T. (1995). The inertia tensor as a basis for the perception of limb orientation. *Journal of Experimental Psychology Human Perception and Performance*, *21*, 1070–1087.

Palatinus, Z., Kelty-Stephen, D., Kinsella-Shaw, J., Carello, C., & Turvey, M. T. (2014). Haptic intent in quiet standing affects multifractal scaling of postural fluctuations. *Journal of Experimental Psychology: Human Perception and Performance*, *40*, 1808–1818.

Plaisier, M. A., & Smeets, J. B. (2012). Mass is all that matters in size-weight illusion. *PLoS1*, *7*, e42518.

Regia-Corte, T., & Wagman, J. B. (2008). Perception of affordances for standing on an inclined surface depends on height of center of mass. *Experimental Brain Research*, *191*, 25–85.

Revesz, G. (1950). *The psychology and art of the blind*. London: Longmans Green.

Riley, M., Wagman, J., Santana, M-V., Carello, C., & Turvey, M. T. (2002). Perceptual behavior: Recurrence analysis of a haptic exploratory procedure. *Perception*, *31*, 481–510.

Runeson, S. (1977). On the possibility of "smart" perceptual mechanisms. *Scandinavian Journal of Psychology*, *18*, 172–179.

Santana, M. V., & Carello, C. (1999). Perceiving whole and partial extents of small objects by dynamic touch. *Ecological Psychology*, *11*, 283–307.

Schmid, A. (1997). A visually induced switch in mode of locomotion of a spider. *Zeitschrift für Naturforschung C*, *52*, 124–128.

Seyfarth, E-A., & Barth, F. G. (1972). Compound slit organs on the spider leg: Mechanoreceptors involved in kinesthetic orientation. *Journal of Comparative Physiology*, *78*, 176–191.

Seyfarth, E-A., Hergenröder, R., Ebbes, H., & Barth, F. G. (1982). Idiothetic orientation of a wandering spider: Compensation of detours and estimates of goal distance. *Behavioral Ecology and Sociobiology*, *11*, 139–148.

Shockley, K., Carello, C., & Turvey, M. T. (2004). Metamers in the haptic perception of heaviness and moveableness. *Perception & Psychophysics*, 66, 731–742.

Silva, P. L., & Turvey, M. T. (2012). The role of haptic information in shaping coordination dynamics: Inertial frame of reference hypothesis. *Human Movement Science*, *31*, 1014–1036.

Solomon, H. Y. (1988). Movement-produced invariants in haptic explorations: An example of a self-organizing, information-driven, intentional system. *Human Movement Science*, *7*, 201–224.

Solomon, H. Y., & Turvey, M. T. (1988). Haptically perceiving the distances reachable with hand-held objects. *Journal of Experimental Psychology: Human Perception and Performance*, *14*, 404–427.

Solomon, H. Y., Turvey, M. T., & Burton, G. (1989). Perceiving rod extents by wielding: Haptic diagonalization and decomposition of the inertia tensor. *Journal of Experimental Psychology: Human Perception and Performance*, *15*, 58–68.

Stevens, S. S. (1961). To honor Fechner and repeal his law. *Science*, *133*, 80–86.

Stevens, S. S. (1962). The surprising simplicity of sensory metrics. *American Psychologist*, *17*, 29–39.

Turvey, M. T. (1996). Dynamic touch. *American Psychologist*, *51*, 1134–1152.

Turvey, M. T. (2007). Action and perception at the level of synergies. *Human Movement Science*, *26*, 657–697.

Turvey, M. T., & Carello, C. (1995). Dynamic touch. In W. Epstein & S. Rogers (Eds.), *Handbook of perception and cognition, Vol. V. Perception of space and motion* (pp. 401–490). San Diego, CA: Academic Press

Turvey, M. T., Burton, G., Amazeen, E. L., Butwill, M., & Carello, C. (1998). Perceiving the width and height of a hand-held object by dynamic touch. *Journal of Experimental Psychology: Human Perception and Performance, 24*, 35–48.

Turvey, M. T., & Carello, C. (2011). Obtaining information by dynamic (effortful) touching. *Philosophical Transactions of the Royal Society B: Biological Sciences, 366*, 3123–3132.

Turvey, M. T., & Fonseca, S. T. (2014). The medium of haptic perception: A tensegrity hypothesis. *Journal of Motor Behavior, 46*, 143–189.

van de Langenberg, R., Kingma, I., & Beek, P. J. (2007). Perception of limb orientation in the vertical plane depends on center of mass rather than inertial eigenvectors. *Experimental Brain Research, 180*, 595–607.

van de Langenberg, R., Kingma, I., & Beek, P. J. (2008). The perception of limb orientation depends on the center of mass. *Journal of Experimental Psychology: Human Perception and Performance, 34*, 624–639.

Visnovitz, T., Világi, I., Varró, P., & Kristóf, Z. (2007). Mechanoreceptor cells on the tertiary pulvini of *Mimosa pudica L. Plant Signaling and Behavior, 2*, 462–466.

West, B. J., & Deering, B. (1995). *The lure of modern science: Fractal thinking*. Singapore: World Scientific.

Lecture 26
Strong Anticipation and Direct Perception

> "[T]he fundamental purpose of brains is to produce future."
>
> (Dennett, 1991, p. 177)

> "[O]ne of the deepest, most general functions of living systems is to coordinate with the future."
>
> (Jacob, 1982, p. 66)

Our concern in this final lecture is with the self-evident fact that, for all organisms in all phyla of all Six Kingdoms, the burden of getting about among things is carried by the ability to coordinate current control and coordination with *upcoming states of affairs*. Of the two quotations above, that of Jacob foreshadows our endeavor more so than that of Dennett.

As discussed in Lecture 20, all organisms in all Six Kingdoms exhibit agency and do so to greater or lesser degree. However minimal it might be, agency encompasses (a) variation of means to bring about an end (*flexibility*), (b) coordinating current control with preceding states of affairs (*retrospectivity*) and (c) coordinating current control with upcoming states of affairs (*prospectivity*) (Gibson, E., 1994). In everyday parlance, we refer to the retrospective dimension as memory and the prospective dimension as anticipation or expectation. Anticipation and what it entails is the primary focus of our final lecture. Here we seek to flesh out the means by which anticipation, in everyday parlance, applies to the future—that is, the not yet existent. Our efforts will be in the direction of what has come to be termed "strong anticipation" (Dubois, 2003; Stepp & Turvey, 2010, 2015, 2017), where the autonomy and control are grounded in laws at the ecological scale. Our efforts stand in contrast to efforts more commonly made under the guise of what can be termed "weak anticipation" where the autonomy and control are grounded in future-oriented mental representations. Here's one characterization of the latter perspective on anticipation:

> [T]he ability that characterizes and defines a true cognitive mind, as opposed to a merely adaptive system, is that of building representations

of the non-existent, of what is not currently (yet) true or perceivable, of what is desired . . . a real mental activity begins when the organism is able to endogenously (i.e. not as the concuence of current perceptual stimuli) produce an internal representation of the world in order to select and guide its conduct goal-directed: *the mind serves to coordinate with the future.*

(Pezzulo, 2008, p. 179)

Ideally, one should, at this final lecture, be fully appreciative that perception is not concerned with a distinct "present." William James (1890/1983), to whom we have often turned in this course of lectures, showed his appreciation of the preceding in the following terms:

> In short, the practically cognized present is no knife-edge, but a saddle-back, with a certain breadth of its own on which we sit perched, and from which we look in two directions into time. The unit of composition of our perception of time is a *duration*, with a bow and a stern, as it were—a rearward- and a forward-looking end. . . . We do not first feel one end and then feel the other after it, and from the perception of the succession infer an interval of time between, but we seem to feel the interval of time as a whole, with its two ends embedded in it.
>
> (p. 608)

Shaw, Flascher, and Mace (1996) took the appreciation a step further, identifying *event* as perception's concern:

> Events are not un-extended instantaneous points in a space-time but occupy a "window" which extends beyond the "here and now" continuously, both backward and forward to the "there and then." Events, therefore, are sources of retrospective, perspective and prospective information because the "current" state of an event is spatiotemporally extended from the past through the present to the future.
>
> (p. 356)

Our goal in this final lecture is to understand the coordination of the functional capabilities referred to colloquially as anticipation and perception. We will attempt to do so through conceptualizations of strong anticipation and direct perception (e.g., Stepp & Turvey, 2010). An alias for the former is *anticipating synchronization* (Stepp & Turvey, 2015; Voss, 2000; Voss & Stepp, 2016). Ideally, it should become evident in this lecture that the commonalities of the two conceptualizations suggest that a theory of one is likely to imply the theory of the other. Getting there, however, requires confronting the four fallacies that historically constitute what can be referred to as the "muddle of anticipation." We have met them in various guises and approximate forms in prior lectures. They are the fallacies of (a) subjective

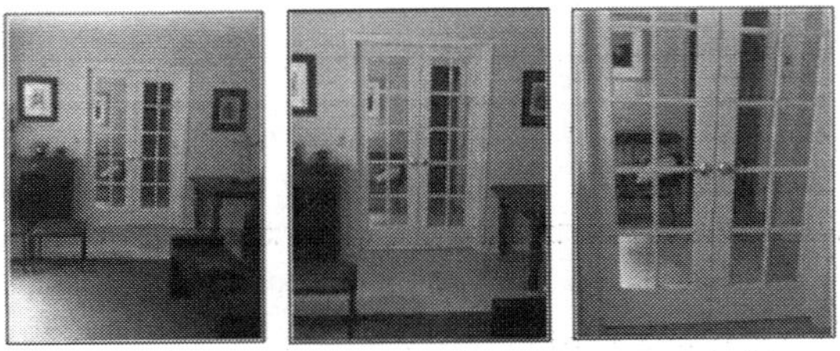

Figure 26.1 Transiting from one vista to another interpreted as assigning pattern to perception, sequence to expectation/anticipation, memory to past.

time, (b) sensation-based perception, (c) perception assigned to the present and (4) anticipation assigned to the future (as communicated in Figure 26.1). In the lecture, the aforementioned fallacies are in the background more so than in the foreground.

26.1 Significance of the Occluding Edge: Anticipation is Not a Special Faculty

It is commonplace for terrestrial and marine animals to encounter the "occluding, covering, or hiding of one thing by another" (Kaplan, 1969, p. 194). At any given location, some surfaces are visible and some are temporarily hidden from view. The sequence in Figure 26.1 illustrates Gibson's (1966b) way of expressing the unhiding or disoccluding of surfaces accompanying forward locomotion in a hallway. The doorway exemplifies the ecological fact of occluding edges. At its edges, more of the partially occluded room beyond comes into view with one's forward progression.

Figure 26.2 schematizes the general phenomenon in terms of one simple rectangular surface moving in a plane parallel to another. The *occluding surface* (the one in front) is that surface for which the (lettered) optical solid angles projected to the point of observation are unchanging. The *occluded surface* (the one in back) is that surface for which the (numbered) optical solid angles projected to the point of observation increase. Kaplan's (1969) key experimental observation is that both the contour separating two surfaces, and the surface to which the contour "belongs" (the direction of depth), are *specified by the accretion/deletion of optical solid angles.*[1] Gibson (1979/1986) summarized the broad implications of Kaplan's experimental findings as follows:

> The surface that was being covered was seen to persist after being concealed, and the surface that was being uncovered was seen to pre-exist before being revealed. The hidden surface could not be described as remembered in one case, or expected in the other. A better description would be that it was perceived retrospectively and prospectively. It is certainly reasonable to describe perception as extending into the past and the future, but note that to do so violates the accepted doctrine that perception is *confined* to the present.
>
> (Gibson, 1979/1986, p. 190, emphasis his)

To appreciate the usefulness of the occluding edge, consider why it is that anticipation, or perception of the future, is commonly thought to be a special faculty. In conventional perceptual terminology, a future event has not yet had a chance to be a "stimulus"—for example, to emit or reflect light to, and induce excitation in, the eye and visual cortex. Therefore, visual perception of the future is infeasible if light to the eye is the basis for visual perception. Experiments with the occluding edge comport, therefore, with the experiments with the light box that we encountered in Lecture 11: Both reveal that light as such is *not* the basis for visual perception. *The basis, rather, is light structured in a way that is informative about the source of its structure*. Not only does the fact of the occluding edge show that light to the eye is not the basis for visual perception, it also shows that structured light can carry information about something from which *no* light is reflected to the observer at that point in time. The information that an observer does have access to can be about something hidden or forthcoming. If such is the case then there is, in principle, no theoretical issue with information at a point of observation being about something that is not yet in view.

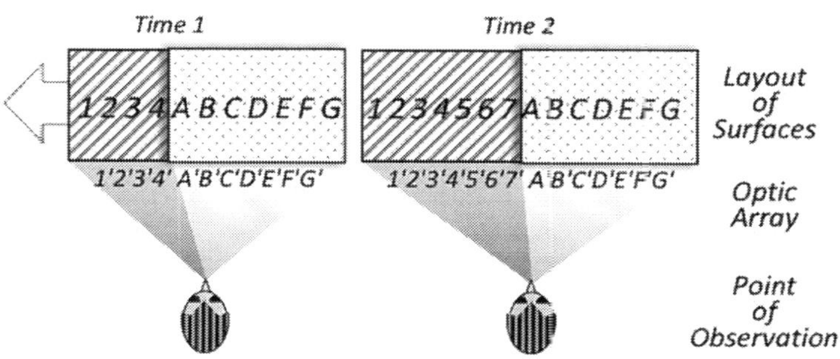

Figure 26.2 As the rear (darker) surface moves to the left, more of it is uncovered (depicted as an increase in numerals). The visibility of the occluding (lighter) surface does not change. Optical accretion at an edge specifies surface layout (cf. Kaplan, 1969).

26.2 The Current Future

An ecological approach to anticipation, then, will be one that takes advantage of causal laws of the form "what leads to what" (Gibson, 1966b; Tolman, 1932). Such a theory would not need to rely on prediction for access to the future, since the future would be specified, in a strong sense, by the present (Stepp & Turvey, 2015). The concept of *the current future* (Bootsma in Lee, Bootsma, Frost et al., 2009) defines the inquiry initiated by Lee (1974, 1976) in terms of the time to-contact concept commonly expressed as *tau* or τ (recall Lecture 24) and its extensions, namely, *tau-dot*,[2] *tau-gap* and *tau-coupling* (see Lee, 1998, 2009; Lee, Bootsma, Frost et al., 2009; and Pepping & Grealy, 2007, for summaries). The inquiry has been in respect to information about "what leads to what." In terms of the current future, it is that which will happen if things do not change (Bootsma in Lee, Bootsma, Frost et al., 2009). Moving radially toward or away from a hit baseball so as to keep the vertical acceleration of the ball's optical projection at zero brings an outfielder to the right place at the right time to effect a catch (Fink, Foo, & Warren, 2009). Moving so as to keep the rate of optical expansion of an approached branch at zero brings a bird into soft contact (minimal momentum exchange) with its landing site (Lee et al., 1992). The solution to the generic problem of visually controlled collisions (e.g., catching a ball, steering a car, a bird landing gently on a branch) is the equating of prospective control with the future that is optically specified in the current agent–environment relation. A change in that relation is a change in the current future.

Prospective control in any case of purposeful movement is realized in General Tau Theory (Lee, 2009) as the closing of so-called action gaps—the separations between the current states and end states of movement degrees of freedom needed to achieve the action. For a cat playing catch with a human, it must, at a minimum, guide its gaze. It does so by controlling the action gaps between head and shoulders, eyes and head, and gaze and (thrown) object (Lee, 1998). Figure 24.10 illustrates the kinds of action gaps comprising the case of running over a surface with uneven footing. In each case—that of gaze, step distance, and propulsive force—the metric of control is in terms of $\tau(t)$. A fundamental question is that of the principle governing the closings of these action gaps: How are they so organized as to realize a coherent action (see Lee, 2009, p. 858)? In broader terms, how are the multiple and temporally overlapping $\tau(t)$s of the action gaps of the current future coordinated? The argument to be developed is a possible answer to this question.

26.3 Strong Anticipation versus Weak Anticipation

For Dubois (2003), anticipation is *weak* if it arises from a model of the system via internal simulations and *strong* if it arises from the system itself, that is, by means of lawful regularities embedded in the system's ordinary mode of functioning. (For the outfielder problem, the system is ball-and-outfielder.) The strategic importance of this latter notion is that it invites a shift of focus from theorizing about a representation–anticipation relation to theorizing about a coupling–anticipation relation. The latter is consonant with the general ecological perspective. Rather than ask how the future is produced from an internal model, one asks about a lawful coupling (between organism and environment) that results in coordination with the future (Stepp & Turvey, 2010, 2015; Stepp, 2012; see also Zhao & Warren, 2015). Axiomatically, the ecological approach mandates a non-mediational theory of anticipation. *It must be so for the theory of direct perception to be self-consistent.* The mandate is that, for a given intent (e.g., "catch that ball"), there must be information about in the sense of specificity to the action that makes the intent implementable.

As previewed in Lecture 24, strong anticipation (or strong prospective control) is with respect to spatial layouts and events that do exist, necessarily. Weak anticipation, one might suggest, is with respect to spatial layouts and events that do not exist, but could (e.g., "I'm anticipating on the basis of my estimations of the ball's flight parameters at the current time t_i that if I *were to move* in direction z, at velocity v, I *ought to be* under the ball at time t_0"). For optically based strong anticipation, existing surface layouts and occurring events generate optical information about surfaces and events that are hidden at some points of observation during locomotion and unhidden at others.[3]

26.4 Anticipating through Coupling/Synchronizing: A General Framework

At base, "to anticipate" is for an aspect (or state) of one system S_i to maintain a negative phase relation to some other system S_j, in part or in whole, or for one aspect (or state) of S_i to maintain a negative phase relation with another aspect (or state) of S_i. The issue fundamentally is how it can be the case that a current state can be in respect to a future state. Addressing this issue is a matter of coming to terms with phenomena ranging from the prospective control of voluntary action to the automatic anticipatory regulation of the body's many steady states.

The most significant benefit of anticipation as dynamical rather than inferential is the promise of an understanding of anticipatory behavior that applies to all phyla (cf. Stepp & Turvey, 2010)—that is, an understanding of anticipation at the level of general principle. Given such, one would expect that each and every organism is necessarily anticipatory, whether the scope of their behavior be wide or narrow. Anticipation is another way of synchronizing. It is well appreciated as a phenomenon that occurs opportunistically (Pikovsky, Rosenblum, & Kurths, 2001).

Consider the following case. The slime mold is an entity that emerges from the tendency of multiple single-cell microscopic organisms under conditions of diminished nutrition to collect together as a single macroscopic entity with limb-like components. These pseudopods constitute a means of foraging, of travelling to a new food supply. If slime mold is subjected to a functional equivalent of the day-night cycle, it is active in the "day" and quiescent at "night." If this "day–night" cycle terminates, the slime mold continues in its absence for a complete cycle or more (Saigusa et al., 2008). We can view the day–night (light–dark) cycle as a master system that enslaves the slime mold. And we can view the slime mold behavior as an instance of anticipating by synchronizing.

It is of note that the aforementioned behavior is of a kind achievable by what can be termed *delay coupling* (e.g., Voss, 2000; Ciszak, Marino, Toral, & Balle, 2004).

$$\begin{aligned} \dot{x} &= f(x) \\ \dot{y} &= g(y) + k(x - y_\tau) \end{aligned} \tag{26.1}$$

In (26.1), f and g are intrinsic dynamics of two multidimensional systems x (a changing perceivable environmental feature) and y (a perception-action system), respectively, where k is coupling strength and y_τ is $y(t - \tau)$ that is, a past state of y delayed by τ (Stepp, 2009, 2012). Anticipating synchronization is expected when f and g are similar. In the cited research, f and g were assumed to be oscillatory, with characteristic periods close enough to engender, at a minimum, intermittent frequency locking.

A more general formulation of the delayed coupling function allows more complicated feedback structures (Stepp & Turvey, 2015). Equation 26.2 is intended to replace the simple $k(x - y_\tau)$ coupling function from Equation 26.1 with a coupling function K that admits arbitrary combinations of past and future feedback. It takes the form:

$$\int_0^\infty \int_0^\infty K(s,u)\big(x(t+u) - y(t-s)\big)\,ds\,du \tag{26.2}$$

where u and s are time shifts into future and past, respectively. K allows different coupling for different shifts. For example, choosing $K(s, u) = k\delta(s - \tau)\delta(u)$ (where δ is the Dirac delta function) recovers the coupling function in Equation 26.1.

A driving task can be used to investigate coupling to future values. The task is depicted in Figure 26.3. In this task, road width, under a perspective transform, falls off as 2π arctan $1/d$ after distance d. Accordingly, the function for coupling strength assumes the form:

$$K(s,u) = \frac{2}{\pi} \arctan\left(\frac{1}{u}\right)\delta(s - \tau) \tag{26.3}$$

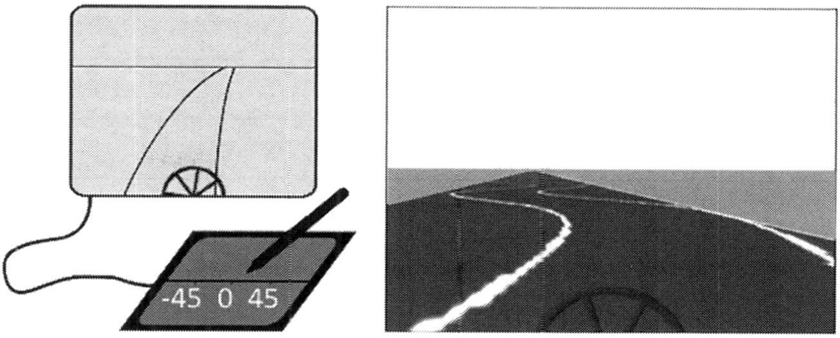

Figure 26.3 (left) Simple driving simulator displayed on a computer screen, with a participant-controlled steering wheel. The angle of the steering wheel corresponds to the position of the stylus on the tablet. (*Right*) Screenshot from the driving simulator, showing the road laid out ahead of the driver, and a small steering wheel that indicated current turning rate.

(From Figures 6 and 7, Stepp & Turvey, Anticipation in manual tracking with multiple delays. *Journal of Experimental Psychology: Human Perception and Performance*, 43, 914–925, 2017, APA, adapted with permission.)

The latter provides for the full coupling function:

$$h(x,y,t) = \int_{0}^{\infty} \frac{2}{\pi} \arctan\left(\frac{1}{u}\right)\left(x(t+u) - y(t-\tau)\right) du \tag{26.4}$$

Equation (26.4) instantiates a coupling to upcoming values that is fast and infinitely diminishing together with a self-feedback for a single delay. While the integral for $K(s, u)$ diverges, practical and physical limitations constrain it in practice. In respect to the foregoing, a distinction can be made between what may be called "weak anticipation" and "strong anticipation." Weak anticipation is a matter of (sophisticated) guessing. Strong anticipation is a matter of (lawful) perceiving.[4] The driving task in question is shown in Figure 26.3. It involved three primary functions corresponding to eye (E), hand (H), and road (R) expressed as the time-series, $E(t)$ and $H(t)$ and the space-series $R(z)$. The "driver" was charged with coordinating E, H, and R in a specific way.[5] An experiment conducted in respect to the foregoing aspects points to strong anticipation as the mode of coordination (Stepp & Turvey, 2017).

To reinforce understanding of strong anticipation, one may consider Figure 26.4. States over time are represented as circles. Transitions from one state to the next are represented as arrows. A coupling function, $k(x - y_\tau)$, couples the current state of $x(x_0)$ with a past state of y ($\tau = -2$). This particular coupling creates negative feedback aimed at minimizing the difference between x_0 and

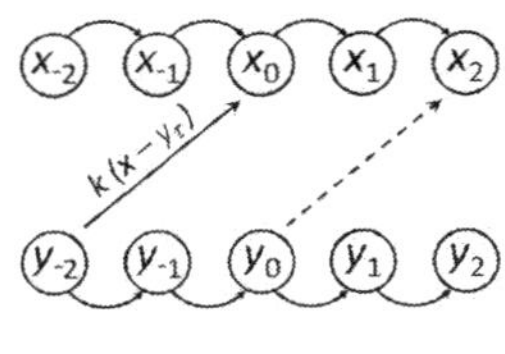

Figure 26.4 Delay coupling between two dynamical systems x and y. States over time are represented discretely as circles, with arrows as transitions between states, where x_0 and y_0 denote the states of each system at the current time. The coupling function sets up a negative feedback that minimizes the difference between x_0 and a past state of y, for instance y_{-2}. To the extent that this difference is minimized, the difference between y_0 and x_2 is also minimized.

y_{-2}. To the extent that this latter difference is minimized, the difference between y_0 and x_2 (dashed arrow) also tends to be minimized.[6]

26.5 Are Strong Anticipation and Direct Perception One and the Same?

As multiply underscored in the present and prior lectures, affordances are possibilities for action. They are in respect to forthcoming realizable states of affairs. Put bluntly, they deal in the future. A thing is graspable before it has been grasped. One might say, "I perceive that object to be graspable." In a strong sense this is equivalent to "I anticipate that I am able to grasp that object." The implication of this observation is the possibility that a theory of affordances, a theory of possibilities for action, is already a theory of perception of up-coming events, of perceiving the practical future. Intuitively, we can appreciate that Strong Anticipation and Direct Perception share many of the same qualities. Immediate examples are that each rejects a predicting model, each promotes lawful relations, and each mandates that organism and environment be taken together as a single system. The foregoing are enough to suggest that, at a minimum, Strong Anticipation is a generalization of Direct Perception. At a maximum the foregoing may suggest that the two conceptions are one and the same. Proof awaits an appropriate formalism for ecological realism.

26.6 By Way of Conclusion

> Explanations of perception based on sensory inputs fail because they all come down to this: In order to perceive the world, one must already have ideas about it. Knowledge of the world is explained by assuming that knowledge of the world exists. Whether the ideas are learned or innate makes no difference; the fallacy lies in the circular reasoning.

But if, on the other hand, perception of the environment is not based on a sequence of snapshots but on invariant–extraction from a flux, one does not need to have ideas about the environment in order to perceive it.

(Gibson, 1979/1986, p. 304)

Notes

1 Gibson's assertion (1966a, p. 313) that "information for length of a line . . . is not length of a line" can be generalized to "information about *x* is not *x*" (e.g., Turvey & Fonseca, 2014). Figure 26.3 is an expression of "information about a contour is not a contour."
2 The derivative of *tau*: it is typically written as $\dot{\tau}(t)$ or $\dot{\tau}$.
3 It is likewise the case for surfaces and events that are coming into and going out of existence. Simple everyday examples are the emergence of new environmental structure with the rupturing of a surface and erasure of environmental texture with the dissipation of a surface (Gibson, J., 1979/1986).
4 Even events that are not generated by a deterministic dynamical system are reasonably predictable by anticipatory coupling of a simple relaxation system. In so-called anticipatory relaxation dynamics, no prior knowledge is required about the event to be predicted (Voss, 2016).
5 There are other time-series, e.g., virtual vehicle position (V), virtual vehicle turning rate (Θ), virtual vehicle heading direction (D), and derivatives of $R(z)$.
6 Stepp (personal communication, September, 2017).

References

Ciszak, M., Marino, F., Toral, R., & Balle, S. (2004). Dynamical mechanism of anticipating synchronizations in excitable systems. *Physical Review Letters*, 93, 114102.

Dennett, D. (1991). *Consciousness explained*. Boston, MA: Little Brown.

Dubois, D. M. (2003). Mathematical foundations of discrete and functional systems with strong and weak anticipations. In *Anticipatory behavior in adaptive learning systems* (pp. 110–132). Berlin, Germany: Springer.

Fink, P. W., Foo, P. S., & Warren, W. H. (2009). Catching fly balls in virtual reality: A critical test of the outfielder problem. *Journal of Vision*, 9(14), 1–8.

Gibson, E. J. (1994). Has psychology a future? *Psychological Science*, 5, 69–76.

Gibson, J. J. (1966a). *The senses considered as perceptual systems*. Boston, MA: Houghton Mifflin.

Gibson, J. J. (1966b). The problem of temporal order in stimulation and perception. *Journal of Psychology*, 62, 141–149.

Gibson, J. J. (1986). *The ecological approach to visual perception*. Mahwah, NJ: Erlbaum (original work published 1979).

Jacob, F. (1982). *The possible and the actual*. New York: Pantheon.

James, W. (1983). *The principles of psychology*. Cambridge, UK: Cambridge University Press (original work published 1890).

Kaplan, G. A. (1969). Kinetic disruption of optical texture: The perception of depth at an edge. *Perception & Psychophysics*, 6, 193–198.

Lee, D. N. (1974). Visual information during locomotion. In R. B. MacLeod & H. L. Pick Jr (Eds.), *Perception: Essays in honor of James J. Gibson* (pp. 250–267). Ithaca, NY: Cornell University Press.

Lee, D. N. (1976). A theory of visual control of braking based on information about time-to-collision. *Perception, 5*, 437–459.

Lee, D. N. (1998). Guiding movement by coupling taus. *Ecological Psychology, 10*, 221–250.

Lee, D. N. (2009). General tau theory: Evolution to date. *Perception, 38*, 837–851.

Lee, D. N., Bootsma, R. J., Frost, B. J., Land, M., Regan, D., & Gray, R. (2009). Lee's 1976 paper. *Perception, 38*, 837–858.

Lee, D. N., Weel, F. R., Hitchcock, T., Matejowsky, E., & Pettigrew, J. D. (1992). Common principle of guidance by echolocation and vision. *Journal of Comparative Physiology A: Neuroethology, Sensory, Neural, and Behavioral Physiology, 171*, 563–571.

Pepping, G-J., & Grealy, M. A. (Eds.). (2007). *Closing the gap: The scientific writings of David N. Lee*. Mahwah, NJ: Erlbaum.

Pezzulo, G. (2008). Coordinating with the future: The anticipatory nature of representation. *Minds and Machines, 18*, 179–225.

Pikovsky, A., Rosenblum, M., & Kurths, J. (2001). *Synchronization: A universal concept in nonlinear sciences*. Cambridge, UK: Cambridge University Press.

Saigusa, T., Tero, A., Nakagaki, T., & Kuramoto, Y. (2008). Amoebae anticipate periodic events. *Physical Review Letters, 100*, 018101.

Shaw, R. E., Flascher, O. M., & Mace, W. M. (1996). Dimensions of event perception. In W. Prinz & B. Bridgeman (Eds.), *Handbook of perception and action, Vol. 1* (pp. 345–395). London: Academic Press.

Stepp, N. (2009). Anticipation in feedback-delayed manual tracking of a chaotic oscillator. *Experimental Brain Research, 198*, 521–525.

Stepp, N. (2012). *Emergence of anticipation at multiple time scales*. Unpublished doctoral dissertation, University of Connecticut, Storrs, CT, USA.

Stepp, N., & Turvey, M. T. (2010). On strong anticipation. *Cognitive Systems Research, 11*, 148–164.

Stepp, N., & Turvey, M. T. (2015). The muddle of anticipation. *Ecological Psychology, 27*, 103–126.

Stepp, N., & Turvey, M. T. (2017). Anticipation in manual tracking with multiple delays. *Journal of Experimental Psychology: Human Perception and Performance, 43*, 914–925.

Tolman, E. C. (1932). *Purposive behavior in animals and men*. New York: Appleton-Century-Crofts.

Turvey, M. T., & Fonseca, S. T. (2014). The medium of haptic perception: A tensegrity hypothesis. *Journal of Motor Behavior*, 46, 143–189.

Voss, H. U. (2000). Anticipating chaotic synchronization. *Physics Review E, 61*, 5115–5119.

Voss, H. U., (2016). Signal prediction by anticipatory relaxation dynamics. *Physical Review E*, 93, 030201(R).

Voss, H. U., & Stepp, N. (2016). A negative group delay model for feedback-delayed manual tracking performance. *Journal of computational neuroscience, 41*, 295–304.

Zhao, H., & Warren, W. (2015). On-line and model-based approaches to the visual control of action. *Vision Research*, 110, 190–202.

Index

Locators in *italics* refer to figures and those in **bold** to tables, though these are not indexed separately when concurrent with the related text.

Made in the USA
Las Vegas, NV
19 September 2026

52019214-b868-43a0-8aa7-4bb8eb000ca2R02